Medicolegal Update in

Obstetrics & Gynecology

A Journey Towards Safer Health Care

Medicolegal Update in
Obstetrics & Gynecology
A Journey Towards Safer Health Care

Editor

Virendar Pal Singh
MD LLB CC (Medical Laws) PGD Medicolegal Systems
CC (Healthcare Quality Management)
Professor
Department of Forensic Medicine
Dayanand Medical College and Hospital
Ludhiana, Punjab, India

Co-Editor

Harpreet Kaur
MD (Obstetrics and Gynecology)
Specialist (Obstetrics and Gynecology)
Professor and Unit Head
Guru Gobind Singh Medical College and Hospital
Faridkot, Punjab, India

Forewords

Niranjan Chavan
SM Kantikar

JAYPEE

JAYPEE BROTHERS MEDICAL PUBLISHERS
The Health Sciences Publisher
New Delhi | London

Jaypee Brothers Medical Publishers (P) Ltd

Headquarters
Jaypee Brothers Medical Publishers (P) Ltd
EMCA House, 23/23-B
Ansari Road, Daryaganj
New Delhi 110 002, India
Landline: +91-11-23272143, +91-11-23272703
+91-11-23282021, +91-11-23245672
Email: jaypee@jaypeebrothers.com

Corporate Office
Jaypee Brothers Medical Publishers (P) Ltd
4838/24, Ansari Road, Daryaganj
New Delhi 110 002, India
Phone: +91-11-43574357
Fax: +91-11-43574314
Email: jaypee@jaypeebrothers.com

Overseas Office
JP Medical Ltd.
83, Victoria Street, London
SW1H 0HW (UK)
Phone: +44 20 3170 8910
Fax: +44 (0)20 3008 6180
Email: info@jpmedpub.com

Website: www.jaypeebrothers.com
Website: www.jaypeedigital.com

Inquiries for bulk sales may be solicited at: jaypee@jaypeebrothers.com

Medicolegal Update in Obstetrics & Gynecology: A Journey Towards Safer Health Care

First Edition: **2025**

ISBN: 978-93-6616-085-6

Printed in India

Dedicated to

All those who strongly feel that medicolegal awareness is a must for all involved in patient care and to all the medical practitioners who want to practice their professional skills conscientiously and fearlessly and are ambitious to promote quality in health care.

Contributors

Amrita Ghosh
MBBS MD (Biochemistry) MSc (Medical Biochemistry)
Assistant Professor
Department of Biochemistry
Midnapore Medical College and Hospital
Midnapore, West Bengal, India

Anjali Suneel Mundkur
MBBS MS DNB MRCOG FRM
Associate Professor
Department of Reproductive Medicine and Surgery
Kasturba Medical College
Manipal, Karnataka, India

Antima Rathore MS MRCOG
Specialist in IVF and Reproductive Medicine
CREATE Fertility, Leeds, UK
Bourn-Hall Clinic, Cambridge
West Yorkshire, UK

Anupama Bhute-Anand
MBBS DGO DNB PhD FICOG FICMCH DIPMAS FMAS Masters in Reproductive Medicine
Chief Consultant and Associate Professor
Department of Obstetrics and Gynecology
Datta Meghe Medical College and Nelson Hospital
Nagpur, Maharashtra, India

Ashima Taneja MD (Obs & Gyne)
Professor and Head
Department of Obstetrics and Gynecology
Dayanand Medical College and Hospital
Ludhiana, Punjab, India

BL Chaudhary
MBBS MD (FMT) MBA (HR) LLB
Professor
Maulana Azad Medical College and Medical Superintendent
Acharya Shree Bhikshu Hospital
New Delhi, India

Charulata Chatterjee PhD
Senior Embryologist
MHRT Hospital and Research Center
Hyderabad, Telangana, India

Deepti Gupta MD (Obs & Gyne)
Associate Professor
Department of Obstetrics and Gynecology
Netaji Subhash Chandra Bose Medical College
Jabalpur, Madhya Pradesh, India

Divyanee Gulati MD (Obs & Gyne) FMAS (ICOG)
Senior Resident
Kukreja Nursing Home
Ganaur, Haryana, India

Gautam Biswas MD (Forensic Medicine & Toxicology)
Professor and Head
Department of Forensic Medicine and Toxicology
Dayanand Medical College and Hospital
Ludhiana, Punjab, India

Jagadeesh Narayanareddy
MBBS MD DNB LLB PGDMLE ACME
Professor and Head
Department of Forensic Medicine and Toxicology
Vydehi Institute of Medical Sciences and Research Centre
Bengaluru, Karnataka, India

Jyoti Sharma MD (Obs & Gyne)
Assistant Professor
Department of Obstetrics and Gynecology
Netaji Subhash Chandra Bose Medical College
Jabalpur, Madhya Pradesh, India

Kavita Mandrelle
MD FICOG FMAS Fellowship Reproductive Medicine ACME CIMP
Professor and Head
Department of Obstetrics and Gynecology
Christian Medical College and Hospital
Ludhiana, Punjab, India

Kunjan Modi
MBBS MD (Forensic Medicine) MBA LLB
Associate Professor
Department of Forensic Medicine
Banas Medical College and Research Institute
Banaskantha, Gujarat, India

MadhurimaArora
MD (Obstetrics and Gynecology)
Consultant
Department of Obstetrics and Gynecology
Madhu Nursing Home
Patiala, Punjab, India

Mahesh C Jariwala MD (Obs & Gyne)
IVF Specialist
Ahmedabad, Gujarat, India

Manpreet Kaur DGO MD (Obs & Gyne)
Obstetrician and Gynecologist
Patiala, Punjab, India

Monika Singh MBBS MS (Obs & Gyne)
Assistant Professor
Department of Obstetrics and Gynecology
Noida International Institute of Medical Sciences
Greater Noida, Uttar Pradesh, India

Muskan Soni MD (Obs & Gyne)
Assistant Professor
Department of Obstetrics and Gynecology
DMC & Hospital
Ludhiana, Punjab, India

Nivedita Vaja MD (Obs & Gyne)
Consultant Gynecologist
Ahmedabad, Gujarat, India

Panchampreet Kaur DGO DNB MNAMS FICMCH
Assistant Professor
Department of Obstetrics and Gynecology
Vardhman Mahavir Medical College and
Safdarjung Hospital
New Dehi, India

Pawneet Kaur MBBS MD (Obs & Gyne)
Associate Consultant
Department of Obstetrics and Gynecology
Dayanand Medical College and Hospital
Ludhiana, Punjab, India

Pinky Mishra
MBBS DGO DNB (Obs & Gynae)
Fellow Gynae-Oncology (AGOI)
Assistant Professor
Department of Obstetrics and Gynecology
Government Institute of Medical Sciences
Greater Noida, Uttar Pradesh, India

Pooja Sinha MD (Obs & Gyne)
Associate Professor
Department of Obstetrics and Gynecology
Pandit Bhagwat Dayal Sharma Postgraduate
Institute of Medical Sciences
Rohtak, Haryana, India

Pradyuman Vaja MD (Obs & Gyne)
Consultant and Head
Department of Obstetrics and Gynecology
ESIC Model Hospital
Ahmedabad, Gujarat, India

Prashanth Prabhu J MD (Anesthesiology)
Professor
Department of Anesthesiology
Sapthagiri Institute of Medical Science
and Research Centre
Sapthagiri NPS University
Bengaluru, Karnataka, India

Prateek Rastogi
MD (Forensic Medicine & Toxicology)
Professor
Department of Forensic Medicine
and Toxicology
Kasturba Medical College
Manipal Academy of Higher Education
Manipal, Karnataka, India

PV Varughese MD (Pediatrics)
Professor and Head
Department of Neonatology
Christian Medical College and Hospital
Ludhiana, Punjab, India

Ranabir Pal
MD PhD MBBS (Hon) DCH MBA
CMCL-Faimer Fellow MNAMS MNASc
Professor
Department of Community Medicine
MGM Medical College and LSK Hospital
Kishanganj, Bihar, India

Ritu Sharma
MBBS MD (Obs & Gyne) ACME Fellow Dip CR
Professor and Head
Department of Obstetrics and Gynecology
Government Institute of Medical Sciences
Greater Noida, Uttar Pradesh, India

Rohit Umakant Erande BCom LLB LLM
Advocate
Pune, Maharashtra, India

Ronakben Modi MBBS MD (Obs & Gyne)
Consultant (Obstetrics and Gynecology)
Harsh Maternity Home
Patan, Gujarat, India

Roya Rozati MD (Obs & Gyne)
Professor and Head
Department of Obstetrics and Gynecology
Shadan Institute of Medical Sciences
Medical and Research Director
Medical Health and Research Institute
Hyderabad, Telangana, India
National Advisor, IFS Telangana Chapter

RS Sharma
Professor
Department of Biotechnology
Sharda School of Engineering and Technology
Greater Noida, Uttar Pradesh, India

Sahir Bhatti MD (Physiology)
Demonstrator
Department of Physiology
Christian Medical College and Hospital
Ludhiana, Punjab, India

Sangeeta Pahwa MBBS MS (Obs & Gyne)
Professional and Head
Government Medical College
Amritsar, Punjab, India

Sarika Gautam MD (Obs & Gyne)
Associate Professor
Department of Obstetrics and Gynecology
Pandit Bhagwat Dayal Sharma Postgraduate
Institute of Medical Sciences
Rohtak, Haryana, India

Shashwat K Jani MS (Obs & Gyne) FICOG FIAOG
Consultant and Associate Professor
Department of Obstetrics and Gynecology
Sardar Vallabhbhai Patel Institute of Medical
Sciences and Research
Smt NHL Municipal Medical College
Ahmedabad, Gujarat, India

Sujjanna AL Manuel MD DNB MRCOG
Specialty Registrar
Department of Obstetrics and Gynecology
City Hospital Nottingham University Hospital
NHS Trust, Nottingham, UK

Sunil K Juneja DNB MNAMS FICOG
Professor
Department of Obstetrics and Gynecology
Dayanand Medical College and Hospital
Ludhiana, Punjab, India

T Srikala Prasad MD DGO MCh (Urology)
Professor and Head
Department of Urology
Government Kilpauk Medical College
Chennai, Tamil Nadu, India

Utsav Parekh MBBS MD DNB MNAMS
Assistant Professor
Forensic Medicine and Toxicology
All India Institute of Medical Sciences
Rajkot, Gujarat, India

Varun Modgil
MD (Forensic Medicine & Toxicology)
Assistant Professor
Department of Forensic Medicine
and Toxicology
Dayanand Medical College and Hospital
Ludhiana, Punjab, India

Virendar Pal Singh
MD LLB CC (Medical Laws) PGD Medicolegal Systems
CC (Healthcare Quality Management)
Professor
Department of Forensic Medicine
Dayanand Medical College and Hospital
Ludhiana, Punjab, India

Foreword

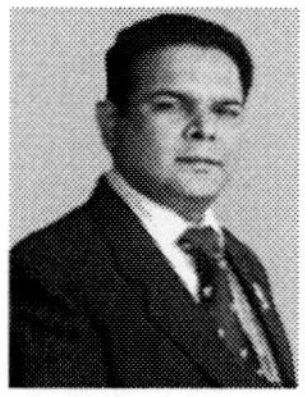

It is an honor to review this comprehensive and authoritative book on the medicolegal challenges faced by Obstetricians and Gynecologists in their routine clinical practice. With the increasing number of malpractice litigations against healthcare professionals and institutions, understanding medicolegal principles has become essential for ensuring safe and effective medical practice.

Medicolegal Update in Obstetrics & Gynecology: A Journey Towards Safer Health Care by Professor Dr Virendar Pal Singh and Dr Harpreet Kaur serves as a valuable resource, offering practical guidelines supported by relevant Indian Court Judgments. The book features chapters written by experts with proficiency in both clinical practice and medicolegal matters, providing a well-rounded perspective.

Dr Virendar Pal Singh has drawn upon his extensive academic and research expertise to compile and edit this work, ensuring a strong problem-solving focus. Dr Harpreet Kaur, a skilled Obstetrician and Gynecologist with significant clinical experience, has made meaningful contributions to this treatise. Together, they have created a dependable and insightful guide to assist practitioners in navigating the legal complexities of health care.

This book is an indispensable reference for obstetricians and gynecologists, equipping them with the knowledge and confidence to address medicolegal issues and safeguard their practice.

Warm regards,

Niranjan Chavan
MD FICOG FCPS DGO DFP MICOG DICOG
Diploma in Endoscopy (USA)
Professor and Unit Chief
Department of Obstetrics and Gynecology
Lokmanya Tilak Medical College and General Hospital
Mumbai, Maharashtra, India
Organizing Secretary
AICOG 2025 (Mumbai)
Treasurer, FOGSI
Past President, MOGS
Secretary, AFG

Foreword

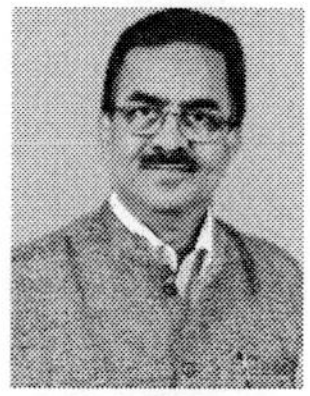

This book, *Medicolegal Update in Obstetrics & Gynecology: A Journey Towards Safer Health Care,* by Professor Dr Virendar Pal Singh and Dr Harpreet Kaur addresses the critical need for up-to-date legal knowledge and ethical guidelines in the practice of obstetrics and gynecology. By bringing together the latest legal precedents, regulatory changes and ethical considerations, this book serves as a comprehensive guide to help practitioners make informed, compassionate, and legally sound decisions.

Dr Virendar Pal Singh is a distinguished Expert in both medical and legal fields, offers a wealth of knowledge and practical insights of various Acts like MTP, PCPNDT, POSCO, and Domestic Violence, etc. Dr Harpreet Kaur is a Specialist in Obstetrics and Gynecology and her vast clinical experience. Both the Editors have contributed to make this treatise an authentic source of medicolegal knowledge relevant for the practitioners of obstetrics and gynecology.

The nexus of medicine and law is complex. I am sure that this book will serve as an indispensable day-to-day guide to provide the highest standard of care and a reference for medical documentation, informed consent, landmark judgments, and ethical issues in IVF.

Best Wishes

SM Kantikar

MD (Path) PhD Law (NLSIU)

Former Member

National Consumer Disputes

Redressal Commission

New Delhi, India

www.kantikarmedilaw.com

Preface

In today's era of consumerism, the perspective of society towards physicians has changed from life-savor to service provider. The privilege of being a physician has bestowed more liabilities than immunity. Providing the best possible care and acting in the best interest of the patient is not just enough. Physicians must regain the faith of their patients, without whom they could never transform from a disciple to a master of the noble medical profession.

A physician, ignorant towards the medical laws, is no excuse in a Court of Law. Medical Laws have emerged as a vast specialization that regulates the day-to-day practice of clinicians. Quality health care is incomplete without confirming to the legal expectations.

For a busy medical practitioner who finds legal expectations to be perplexing, *Medicolegal Update in Obstetrics & Gynecology: A Journey Towards Safer Health Care* is a humble presentation of the medicolegal knowledge in a lucid and easily understandable language.

The book has thoroughly discussed essential medicolegal issues related to the specialty of Obstetrics and Gynecology. This book has provided evidence-based guiding principles to tackle the actual medicolegal issues.

This authoritative treatise is written by distinguished experts who are authorities in their fields of specialization. We are confident that medical practitioners will find this book useful to prevent as well as solve the medicolegal conflicts.

We express our gratitude to all the authors and to the publisher for their cooperation. I am also grateful to all our readers for placing their reliance on us and for sharing our optimism. Feedback and suggestions from the esteemed readers is welcome and will be a boon to further improve the quality of this treatise.

Virendar Pal Singh
Harpreet Kaur

Contents

Section 8 Miscellaneous Topics

SECTION 1

Medical Laws

CHAPTER 1

Landmark Judgments Related to Obstetrics and Gynecology

Varun Modgil, Virendar Pal Singh

Landmark judgments related to medical professionals and the guiding principles laid by the courts are extremely helpful to understand the legal perspective related to reasonable care by the medical practitioners, and that how the court decided whether there is medical negligence or deficiency in service on the part of treating doctors. The landmark judgments related to Obstetrics and Gynecology have been discussed hereinunder so that the relevant medicolegal guidelines can be understood and implemented by Obstetricians and Gynecologists in their day-to-day clinical practice.

CASE 1: STATE OF HARYANA vs. SANTRA[1] [Supreme Court Case]

(Medical Negligence in Failed Sterilization)

Facts of the Case

- Smt. Santra filed a suit for recovery of ₹ 2 lakhs as damages for medical negligence, which was decreed for a sum of ₹ 54,000 with interest at the rate of 12% PA from the date of institution of the suit till payment of the decretal amount. Two appeals were filed against this decree in the court of District Judge, Gurugram, which were disposed of by Addl. District Judge, Gurugram, by a common judgment dated 10.5.1999. Both the appeals— one filed by the State of Haryana and the other by Smt. Santra were dismissed. The appeal filed by the State of Haryana was summarily dismissed by the Punjab & Haryana High Court on 3.8.1999. It is in these circumstances that the special leave petition was filed before the Hon'ble Supreme Court.
- The petitioner became pregnant despite having a sterilization operation under a state-run program to promote sterilization. On examination, it was revealed that her operation was "incomplete" as her left fallopian tube had not been operated upon. She was advised that termination of pregnancy could pose risk to her life.
- A suit for recovery of damages alleging negligence on the part of the doctor was decreed in her favor. Subsequently, appeals filed by each of the parties against the order of the trial court were dismissed.
- The State Govt. then appealed to the High Court of Punjab and Haryana which did not succeed.
- In this special leave petition filed by the State Govt, the issue before the Supreme Court was whether the doctor and the State could be held liable if the sterilization operation fails on account of the doctor's negligence.

Patient's Allegation

- The "sterilization scheme" was launched by the Haryana Government and taking advantage of that scheme, Smt. Santra approached the Chief Medical Officer, Gurugram, for her sterilization in 1988.

- Smt. Santra was assured that a full, complete and successful sterilization operation had been performed upon her and she would not conceive a child in future. But despite the operation, she conceived. When she contacted the CMO and other doctors of the General Hospital, Gurugram, she was informed that she was not pregnant. Two months later when the pregnancy became apparent, she again approached those doctors who then told her that her sterilization operation was not successful.
- She requested for an abortion, but was advised against it, as it could pose risk to her life. Later, she gave birth to a female child.
- Smt. Santra already had seven children, and the birth of a new child put her to unnecessary burden of rearing up the child as also to all the expenses involved in the maintenance of that child, including the expenses towards her clothes and education.

Doctor's Defense

- Sterilization operation performed upon Smt. Santra on 4.2.1988 was done carefully and successfully, and there was no negligence on the part of the doctor who performed that operation.
- Smt. Santra had herself put her thumb impression on a paper containing a recital that, in case the operation was not successful, she would not claim any damages. It was pleaded that she was stopped from raising the plea of negligence or from claiming damages for an unsuccessful sterilization operation from the State. It was further pleaded by the State that it was not liable even vicariously for any lapse on the part of the doctor who performed that operation.

Judgment by the Court (Summary)

i. The trial court and also the lower appellate court, both recorded concurrent findings of the fact that the sterilization operation performed upon Smt. Santra was not "complete" as in that operation only the right Fallopian tube was operated upon, while the left tube was untouched. The courts were of the opinion that this exhibited negligence on the part of the Medical Officer who performed the operation. Smt. Santra, in spite of the unsuccessful operation, was informed that the sterilization operation was successful and that she would not conceive any child in future.
ii. The plea of estoppel raised by the defendants was also rejected.
iii. It is an admitted fact that plaintiff Santra was operated on for the right tube and not for the left tube. Dr Sushil Kumar Goel, while appearing as DW2 has categorically stated so. If Santra, plaintiff, was not operated on the left side, in that event the doctor should not have issued certificate of sterilization to her. The doctors who operated plaintiff Santra should have advised her to come for second time for her operation of left side.
iv. The plaintiff has placed family sterilization case card Ex. P2 on the file. The defendant State has admitted in its written statement that she was successfully operated on 4.02.1988 in General Hospital, Gurugram. When admittedly Santra, plaintiff, was not operated, as discussed above, for her left tube in that event issuance of certificate of her sterilization amounts gross negligence.
v. If Smt. Santra, in these circumstances, had offered herself for complete sterilization, both the Fallopian tubes

should have been operated upon. The doctor who performed the operation acted in a most negligent manner as the possibility of conception by Smt. Santra was not completely ruled out as her left Fallopian tube was not touched. Smt. Santra did conceive and gave birth to an unwanted child.

vi. Very often, in a claim for compensation arising out of medical negligence, a plea is taken that it is a case of bona fide mistake which under certain circumstances may be excusable, but a mistake which would tantamount to negligence cannot be pardoned. In the former case, a court can accept that ordinary human fallibility precludes liability while in the latter the conduct of the defendant is considered to have gone beyond the bounds of what is expected of the reasonable skill of a competent doctor.

vii. The Doctor who performed the operation acted in a most negligent manner as the possibility of conception by Smt. Santra was not completely ruled out, as her left Fallopian Tube was not touched. Smt. Santra did conceive and gave birth to an unwanted child. The amount of ₹54,000 which has been decreed by the courts below represents the amount of expenses which Smt. Santra would have to incur at the rate of ₹3000 per annum in bringing up the child up to the age of puberty.

viii. In State of MP vs. Asharam[2] the High Court allowed the damages on account of medical negligence in the performance of a family planning operation on account of which a daughter was born after 15 months of the date of the operation. No other decision of any High Court has come to Supreme Court's notice where damages were awarded on account of a failed sterilization operation.

ix. India is a developing country where the majority of the people live below the poverty line. On account of the ever-increasing population, the country is almost at the saturation point so far as its resources are concerned. The principles on the basis of which damages have not been allowed on account of failed sterilization operation in other countries either on account of public policy or on account of pleasure in having a child being offset against the claim for damages cannot be strictly applied to Indian conditions so far as poor families are concerned. The public policy here professed by the Government is to control the population and that is why various programs have been launched to implement the State-sponsored family planning programs and policies. Damages for the birth of an unwanted child may not be of any value for those who are already living in affluent conditions but those who live below the poverty line or who belong to the labor class, who earn their livelihood on a daily basis by taking up the job of an ordinary labor, cannot be denied the claim for damages on account of medical negligence.

x. The contention as to the vicarious liability of the State for the negligence of its officers in performing the sterilization operation cannot be accepted in view of the law settled by this Court in N Nagendra Rao & Co. vs. State of AP (1994)[3], Common Cause, A Regd Society vs. Union of India (1999)[4] and Achutrao Haribhau Khodwa vs. State of Maharashtra (1996)[5]. The last case, which related to the fallout of a sterilization operation, deals, like the two previous cases, with the question of vicarious liability of the State on account of medical negligence of a doctor in a government hospital. The theory of sovereign immunity was rejected.

xi. Smt. Santra, as already stated above, was a poor lady who already had seven children. She was already under considerable monetary burden. The unwanted child (girl) born to her has created additional burden for her on account of the negligence of the doctor who performed the sterilization operation upon her and, therefore, she is clearly entitled to claim full damages from the State Government to enable her to bring up the child at least till she attains puberty."

xii. Hon'ble Supreme Court dismissed the appeal as there were no merits in the appeal.

CASE 2: STATE OF PUNJAB vs. SHIV RAM & ORS (2005)[6] [Supreme Court Case]

(Medical Negligence in Failed Sterilization)

Facts of the Case

- This case is based on failed sterilization surgery resulting in pregnancy. The defendant was working in Govt hospital and conducting tubectomies as part of the state-run public health program. The case of plaintiff was alleged negligence on the part of surgeon which led to pregnancy even after a sterilization operation which was also the result of impressive campaigning by the State population control program, thus a plea of vicarious liability was also invoked by the complainant.
- The plaintiffs, husband and wife (*respondents in the appeal before Supreme Court*) filed a suit against the State of Punjab (appellant *in the appeal before Supreme Court*) and a lady surgeon for recovery of damages to the tune of ₹3,00,000 on account of a female child having been born to them in spite of the wife-respondent no. 2 having undergone a tubectomy operation performed by the lady surgeon.

Patient's Allegation

- The plaintiffs already had a son and 2 daughters from the marriage of over 17 years. In response to a publicity campaign carried out by the Family Welfare Department of the appellant-State, the complainant underwent a sterilization operation on 1.08.1984. A certificate in this regard, duly signed by the lady surgeon who performed the said surgery, was issued to her.
- On 4.10.1991, she gave birth to a female child, attributing the birth of the child to carelessness and negligence of the lady surgeon.
- The plaintiff alleged that they considered abortion to be a sin and that is why after knowing of the conception, they did not opt for abortion.

Doctor's Defense

- It was submitted that there was no negligence or carelessness in the performance of the surgery. In authoritative medical textbooks, it is stated that pregnancy occurring after sterilization may be attributable to natural failure.
- The plaintiffs having learnt of the unwanted pregnancy, should have sought

medical termination of pregnancy within 20 weeks which is permissible and legal.

Judgment by Trial Court and First Appellate Court (Summary)

- The two courts have proceeded on the reasoning that on birth of a child to a woman who was allured into undergoing sterilization operation by the State in pursuance of its Family Planning Schemes, the State was liable to compensate for the consequences of the operation having failed.
- The suit was decreed for ₹50,000 with interest and costs.
- The first appellate court upheld the decree for compensation passed by the trial court. The second appeal preferred by the State has been summarily dismissed.

Judgment by Hon'ble Supreme Court (Summary)

i. The Supreme Court adjudged that no negligence could be found in this case as Bolam test[7] was not satisfied. This case was considered different from the view taken in the State of Haryana & Ors. vs. Smt. Santra[1] where complete sterilization was not performed. Explanation II appended to sub-section (2) of Section 3 of MTP Act 1971[8] which provides for termination of pregnancy on grounds of failure of any device or method used by any married woman or her husband. Further, it was made clear that sterilization failure owing to natural causes is not actionable.

ii. The methods of sterilization so far known to medical science, which are most popular and prevalent, are not 100% safe and secure. In spite of the operation having been successfully performed and without any negligence on the part of the surgeon, the sterilized woman can become pregnant due to natural causes. Once the woman misses the menstrual cycle, it is expected of the couple to visit the doctor and seek medical advice. A reference to the provisions of the Medical Termination of Pregnancy Act, 1971 is apposite. Section 3 thereof permits termination of pregnancy by a registered medical practitioner, notwithstanding anything contained in the Indian Penal Code, 1860 in certain circumstances and within a period of 20 weeks of the length of pregnancy. Explanation II appended to subsection (2) of Section 3 provides "Explanation II. Where any pregnancy occurs as a result of failure of any device or method used by any married woman or her husband for the purpose of limiting the number of children, the anguish caused by such unwanted pregnancy may be presumed to constitute a grave injury to the mental health of the pregnant woman." And that provides, under the law, a valid and legal ground for termination of pregnancy. If the woman has suffered an unwanted pregnancy, it can be terminated and this is legal and permissible under the Medical Termination of Pregnancy Act, 1971.

iii. The cause of action for claiming compensation in cases of failed sterilization operation arises on account of negligence of the surgeon and not on account of childbirth. Failure due to natural causes would not provide any ground for claim. It is for the woman who has conceived the child to go or not to go for medical termination of pregnancy.

iv. Having gathered the knowledge of conception in spite of having undergone sterilization operation, if the couple opts for bearing the child, it ceases to be an unwanted child. Compensation for maintenance and upbringing of such a child cannot be claimed.

v. For the foregoing reasons, we are of the opinion that the judgments and the decrees passed by the High Court and courts below cannot be sustained. The trial court has proceeded to pass a decree of damages in favor of the plaintiffs—respondents solely on the ground that in spite of the plaintiff-respondent No. 2 having undergone a sterilization operation, she became pregnant. No finding has been arrived at that will hold the operating surgeon or its employer-he State, liable for damages either in contract or in tort. The error committed by the trial court, though pointed out to the first appellate court and the High Court, has been overlooked. The appeal has, therefore, to be allowed and the judgment and decree under appeal have to be set aside.

CASE 3: ACHUTRAO HARIBHAU KHODWA vs. STATE OF MAHARASHTRA (1996)[9] [Supreme Court Case]

(Medical Negligence in Surgical Procedure; death due to complications of sterilization operation—a mop was left inside her body)

Facts of the Case

- Chandrikabai delivered a male child on 10.07.1963. Thereafter she got herself admitted to Civil Hospital Aurangabad for sterilization operation. After the operation, she developed a high fever and pain in her abdomen. Dr Divan, General Surgeon advised for an explorative surgery which was denied by the complainant, but as her condition deteriorated, later on, she agreed for the surgery. During the explorative surgery, a mop (towel) was found inside the abdomen of the patient which was left inside her body during sterilization procedure. There was collection of pus, which was drained out, but her condition did not improve and ultimately, she expired on 24.07.1963.
- A complaint was filed by husband of the deceased in a Civil Court, and a Civil Judge passed a decree for ₹36,000 as damages on account of death of Chandrikabai, after she had undergone a sterilization operation at Civil Hospital, Aurangabad.
- The State as well as the respondents 2 & 3 filed appeals to the High Court. Aurangabad Bench of Bombay High Court reversed the decree by Civil Court.
- Aggrieved by this judgment, an Appeal was filed before the Supreme Court by husband and children of the deceased.

Patient's Allegation

- The case of the appellants (patient party) before the trial court was that death of Chandrikabai was caused due to negligence of respondent no. 2 who had performed the sterilization operation irresponsible behavior of respondent no. 3.
- The appellants also alleged that the hospital lacked adequate medical aid and proper care and there was gross dereliction of duty on the part of the officers of Civil Hospital which directly resulted in the death of Chandrikabai.
- In support of their case, the appellants relied upon the evidence of Dr Divan. In addition thereto, the appellants also examined, on commission, Dr Ajinkya who was a Gynecologist and Obstetrician of Bombay. According to Dr Divan, after

the sterilization operation Chandrikabai had suffered from postoperative peritonitis. This was due to a mop which had remained inside the peritoneal cavity for a number of days and inflammatory condition had reached a stage from which recovery was very difficult. After removal of the mop Dr Divan said that he saw the condition of the intestine which continued to remain paralyzed. The treatment of peritonitis was started from 15th July 1963 and in his opinion, the death of the patient was due to the complications following the leaving of the mop inside the abdomen. The other expert witness Dr Ajinkya also came to the same conclusion, though his statement was recorded without his having the benefit of seeing the case papers.

Doctor's Defense

- Respondent doctors denied that there any negligence in the performance of the sterilization operation. Respondent no. 2 denied having left any mop inside the abdomen. In the alternative, pleaded that even if such a mop was left inside the body, the same could not have, either directly or remotely, caused the death. Respondent no. 3 also denied the recovery of the mop from the abdomen and generally supported the case of the other respondents.
- On behalf of the respondents, two experts, namely, Dr Marwa, Professor of Surgery, and Dr BV Purandare, a leading Obstetrician and Gynecologist of Mumbai were examined. But, the trial court did not rely upon the evidence of the experts examined by the respondents because it came to the conclusion that the original documents and case papers had been filed late, some relevant entries had also been tampered with and it was only the typed papers, which were copies of the tampered documents, which were supplied to the respondents' expert witnesses for their opinion.

Judgment by Hon'ble Court (Summary)

The SC accepted the plea of negligence and awarded penalty on following grounds:

i. *Res ipsa loquitur* doctrine was invoked by the Supreme Court, i.e., the thing or fact speaks for itself. Finding of pus in the subsequent operation confirms that the complication arose from leaving mop inside the peritoneal cavity and closing the operation. It is true that in a number of cases when foreign bodies are left inside the body of a human being either deliberately, as in the case of orthopedic operations, or accidentally no harm may befall the patient, but it also happens that complications can arise when the doctor acts without due care and caution and leaves a foreign body inside the patient after performing an operation and it suppurates. The formation of pus leaves no doubt that the mop left in the abdomen caused it, and it was the pus formation that caused all the subsequent difficulties. Established case law in but for the fact that a mop was left inside the body, the second operation on 19th July 1963 would not have taken place. It is the leaving of that mop inside the abdomen of Chandrikabai which led to the development of peritonitis leading to her death. She was admitted to the hospital on 10th July 1963 for a simple case of delivery followed by a sterilization operation. Bolam test[7], AS Mittal vs. State of UP[10] and Laxman Balkrishna Joshi (Dr) vs. Dr Trimbak

Bapu Godbole[11] was relied upon to objectify the criteria of negligence.

ii. The plea of vicarious liability of the state for the negligence of their employees was accepted and the non-sovereign role played by the State was recognized. Once death by negligence in the hospital is established, as in the case here, the State would be liable to pay the damages.

iii. The High Court clearly fell in error in reversing the judgment of the trial court and in dismissing the appellants' suit. The judgment of the High Court of Bombay under appeal is set aside and the judgment and decree of the trial court is restored. The appellants were also entitled to costs throughout.

CASE 4: SMT SAROJ CHANDHOKE vs. SIR GANGA RAM HOSPITAL[12] [NCDRC, New Delhi Case]

(Medical Negligence in Surgical Procedures)

Facts of the Case

- Complainant, a 43-year-old lady was suffering from bleeding for the last 2 to 3 months. She consulted the Opposite Party, Dr SK Bhandari, a senior doctor in Sir Ganga Ram Hospital and was diagnosed for dysfunctional uterine bleeding (DUB).
- As the DUB was not responding to medical therapy, she was advised for hysterectomy. Her consent was taken for removal of uterus through abdominal route. Total abdominal hysterectomy (TAH) was performed on 21.06.1993.

Patient's Allegation

- In a simple hysterectomy operation, the complainant suffered a lot, and she lost her kidney; her ovaries; she was required to undergo various further curative operations, because there was uncontrollable fecal discharge from vagina from 29.06.1993 onwards; and she suffered pain for months together after the operation. Her large intestines were exposed, and small intestines were infected with adhesions at various places.
- Further surgery was carried out for repair of the fistula and closure of fistula on 17.11.1993 and for closure of colostomy operation was performed on 21.02.1994. She remained in pitiable condition in the hospital. She was finally discharged on 14.03.1994.
- Her specific consent was taken for TAH under general anesthesia. She was not advised on the alternative routes of surgery, their comparative benefits. Complainant denied the contention of Dr Bhandari that the complainant and her husband left the decision to Dr Bhandari to choose the appropriate route. Hysterectomy was done without consent through vaginal route, and thereafter, via abdominal route, TAH.
- Complaint is filed contending that due to alleged deficiency in service by the expert doctors, the complainant, her husband and three young daughters suffered and experienced immense trauma and hardship. For this deficiency, she has claimed compensation of ₹25,50,000.

Doctor's Defense

- The most common reason for hysterectomy in this age group is dysfunctional uterine bleeding (DUB), which does not respond to hormone therapy and for which there is no organic pathology.
- D&C is only done in such cases to determine the cause of bleeding and not as a curative procedure and if the bleeding is continued, hysterectomy may have to be considered as the best option.

- Patients could possibly have undergone vaginal hysterectomy, but since she has had two previous cesarean sections, she should also have been prepared for abdominal hysterectomy, if indicated either as a result of her re-examination in the operation theater. Patient is normally re-examined again before undertaking hysterectomy when patient is sedated (EUA) or as a result of D&C. Re-examination is to check if there are any contraindications to vaginal hysterectomy.

Main Issues

- Whether a doctor who is an expert gynecologist was justified in carrying out operation of hysterectomy via vaginal route even though specific consent was obtained for total abdominal hysterectomy (TAH)?
- Whether the Doctor was justified in removing healthy ovaries while performing the operation for hysterectomy, that too, without the consent of the complainant?
- Whether the vein can avulse to such an extent that kidney is required to be removed?
- As there is no explanation as to how the vein had avulsed to such an extent that it could not be traced and clamped, whether the principle of *res ispa loquitor* (facts speak for themselves) could be applied?

Judgment by NCDRC, New Delhi (Summary)

i. In a simple hysterectomy operation, the complainant lost her ovaries and left kidney. She was required to undergo other operations for control of fecal discharge from vagina as a result of development of rectovaginal fistula as a consequence of surgery. She was required to stay in the hospital for a complete cure for months.
ii. Informed consent was obtained only for TAH. There was no necessity to try to operate via vaginal route. No consent was obtained for removal of ovaries in advance planned surgery. During left ovarian removal, there was avulsion of the left renal vein which is connected with left ovarian vein and not to uterine vessel. As a result, nephrectomy had to be done.
iii. In the present case, the question is not whether TAH is preferable to VH. The patient was prepared for TAH and had given written consent for TAH, and no consent was obtained, or no information was given to the patient that her ovaries would be removed. In such sets of circumstances, it cannot be said that because a surgeon is an expert in the field he/she can carry out the surgery of his choice. If he/she does so, he/she does it at his/her risk in case of mishap.
iv. Before performing surgery, properly informed written consent is a must. No doubt, while operating, to control adverse situation, or to save the life of the patient or for benefit of the patient, other procedure could be followed, or other part of the body could be operated but it was not the case here.
v. As held in Spring Meadows Hospital[13] it is to be seen that superiority of the Doctor is not abused in any manner. Further, if during the operation any mishap occurs because of error of judgment, it would be deficiency in service or negligence, if that would not have been committed by a reasonably competent professional man professing the standard and type of

skill that a surgeon held out as having. The Opposite Party No 2 is an expert gynecologist who has performed many such operations as contended by her and Opposite Party No. 1 is a well-known big Hospital. In such a case, it is difficult to accept that for no fault there was avulsion of vein to such an extent that the left kidney was required to be removed. Inference could be that there was some error, which resulted in a cut of a vein.

vi. Further, it was the duty of the Doctor to advise the patient that D&C should be performed reasonably well in advance of performing the operation for hysterectomy.

vii. For finding out deficiency in service, motive is not the relevant ingredient. Act may be bona fide. But, if it is performed negligently or if any error is committed which the ordinary skilled person would not commit, then it is deficiency in service.

viii. Original Petition filed by Smt. Saroj Chandoke is allowed. Both the Opposite Parties 1 & 2 are jointly and severally held liable to pay a sum of ₹5 lakhs to the complainant. There shall be no order as to costs.

CASE 5: DR (MRS) INDU SHARMA vs. INDRAPRASTHA APOLLO HOSPITAL (2015)[16] [NCDRC, New Delhi Case]

(Medical Negligence in Antenatal Check-up and Fetal Monitoring)

This is the 3rd case since Prasant S Dhananka[14] and Kunal Saha[15] where compensation of more than 1 crore was awarded.

Facts of the Case

- The complainant, Dr Indu Sharma, BAMS, during her first pregnancy, was under observation and follow-up of Dr Sohni Verma, at Indraprastha Apollo Hospital, New Delhi. Previously, she took treatment from Dr Sohni Verma, for infertility, thereafter, spontaneously; she conceived, after 4½ years.
- On 10.6.1999, after midnight, due to rupture of membranes, she got admitted in the Apollo Hospital for her delivery. No senior doctor was available at that time, so the resident doctor examined her. In the morning, Dr Sohini Verma examined her and advised her medicines, started IV fluid with 1 ampoule of syntocinon for speeding up the process of delivery. But, the patient noticed that the dose was maximum, and the cardiotopographic tracings (CTG) machine showed that the heart rate of the child began to sink (80/min), during the midnight of 11/12.06.1999. It was alleged that no one attended the patient, immediately.
- Thereafter, the patient was shifted to operation theater at 2:00 AM for emergency cesarean (LSCS), and at 3:36 AM a female baby was delivered by LSCS, weighing 3.7 kg.
- The baby did not cry immediately after birth, and it took almost five minutes. The baby was kept in a ventilator in NICU. The OP assured that all the reports were normal. The condition of baby deteriorated further, till 29.6.1999. The baby was unable to suck milk. Meanwhile, the patient was discharged on 16.6.1999, while the baby was discharged from Apollo Hospital, on 30.6.1999.

Patient's Allegation

- The complainant alleged that the doctor failed to perform LSCS within 12–18 hours after rupture of membrane. It was abnormally delayed for about 27 hours.

- The doctor advised excessive dose of Syntocinon, which caused fetal distress and cerebral anoxia-palsy.
- None attended the patient, immediately. Therefore, it was alleged that, baby suffered birth asphyxia and seizures.
- The hospital assured the patient party that all the reports were normal.
- The doctors/hospital made number of corrections/interpolations on the case sheets. The neonatal record was also tampered. The hospital purposely concealed cardiotocogram (CTG) tracings, which was the vital document in this case.
- The doctor failed to take proper care during delivery, which resulted in the birth of an asphyxiated baby.
- The hospital did not issue entire medical record, CTG graphs, etc.

Doctor's Defense

The complainant has not produced any medical expert evidence and has not produced any witnesses from Holy Family Hospital and AIIMS where the baby was treated after discharge from OP-1.

Judgment by NCDRC, New Delhi (Summary)

i. The nursing notes clearly establish hypertonic contractions suggestive of fetal distress, which OP-3 failed to take proper decision for emergency C-section. It was an act of omission, thus negligence considering the precious pregnancy.

ii. NCDR concluded that the patient with precious pregnancy unnecessarily suffered during prolonged labor; there was administration of excessive Syntocinon which caused birth asphyxia to the baby Nishtha, who further suffered cerebral palsy and 95% disability. She survived in such pathetic condition for 12 years.

iii. The statement of OP that, the patient was informed about emergency LSCS which was rejected by the patient or by her husband, but there is no evidence as such. The progress sheet clearly showed some insertion made by OP/staff to show that patient was informed. Thus, the entry was also tampered one.

iv. A delayed decision of emergency C-section delivery was made by OP-3. Fetal scalp pH should be checked if augmented labor is prolonged and higher dosages are given. However, the same was not done by OP-3; it was the act of omission.

v. The baby was born with very low Apgar scores, was not breathing. Resuscitation maneuvers were initiated right after birth, by mask ventilation and further intubation. The umbilical cord showed blood pH 7.12; indicated baby had acidosis during delivery, i.e., she was deprived of oxygen for a significant period of time. She began having seizures, which is also an indication that she experienced an oxygen depriving insult. In fact, hypoxic ischemic encephalopathy (HIE) is the most common cause of seizures in the newborn period. HIE is caused by oxygen deprivation/ asphyxia. The CT scan/head imaging of the baby showed edema which is also sign of asphyxia.

vi. NCDRC partly allowed this complaint, and the opposite parties were held responsible for medical negligence in this case, therefore affixing total compensation of ₹ One Crore; out of which, Indraprastha Apollo Hospital, will pay ₹80 lacs and, Dr (Mrs) Sohini Verma will pay ₹20 lacs to the patient/ complainant within 90 days from the date of receipt of this order.[16]

CASE 6: SMT VINITHA ASHOK vs. LAKSHMI HOSPITAL & ORS 2017[17] [Supreme Court Case]

(Medical Negligence in Medical Termination of Pregnancy)

This is an unfortunate case of a woman losing her uterus, a vital organ of regeneration consequent upon an ectopic pregnancy in the cervical canal.

Facts of the Case

The appellant gave birth to a male baby on 6.06.1989 after cesarean section. On 3.02.1990, having suspected that she was pregnant again, she and her husband went to Lakshmi Hospital for consultation. The appellant was examined by Dr Santha Warriar, Respondent No 2. On examination, respondent No. 2 informed the appellant that she was pregnant, and it was decided to terminate the pregnancy for which 10.02.1990 was fixed. On 9.02.1990, laminaria tent was inserted when the appellant went to the Hospital. Dr Santha Warriar, respondent No. 2, took the appellant to the labor room. At about 10 o' clock Dr Somalatha, respondent No. 3, informed the appellant's husband that the appellant was bleeding profusely and therefore, they have decided to conduct an operation. At about 4 o'clock the operation was over, and the appellant's relatives were informed that she was better but under sedation. Dr Santha Warriar informed the appellant's husband that it was a case of cervical pregnancy, and her uterus had been removed. The appellant was discharged from the Hospital on 22.02.1990.

Complaint's Allegations

- Doctor had not acted with due care and caution required of medical professionals in diagnosing the problem and in the performance of their duties.
- Lack of necessary facilities and infrastructure at the Hospital.
- Dilatation & Curettage (D&C) procedure was unnecessarily done on her which led to other problems resulting in loss of uterus at a very young age.
- Doctor being negligent for not doing ultrasound test prior to MTP.
- It was a normal pregnancy and not a cervical pregnancy, bleeding might have been caused as a result of instrumentation.

Doctor's Defense

- The appellant was having a cervical pregnancy extending to the lower segment of her uterus which is very complicated and rare and cannot be diagnosed by clinical or vaginal examination particularly in the early weeks of pregnancy; that hysterectomy is a recommended and established procedure for tackling excessive bleeding in the case of cervical pregnancy.
- There was no general practice anywhere in Kerala to do ultrasound in MTP case. The doctor adhered to acceptable guidelines. Authoritative medical textual contexts adduced by respondents were as follows:
    - *Te Linde's Operative Gynecology, 6th Edition by Richard F Mattingly*, it was observed that the treatment of cervical pregnancy is surgical and the condition usually requires an abdominal hysterectomy.
    - *Cervical Pregnancy by Macro Antonio Peloci, Vol IV*, it was noticed that most obstetricians would never see a cervical pregnancy and that those who did would wish that they had not. This statement is nearly as true now as it was then.

- *In Clinical Obstetrics by Mudaliar and Menon,* the authors state that perhaps in certain instances to diagnose ectopic pregnancy and incomplete abortion, a transabdominal sonography may afford a quick diagnosis.
- A different type called transvaginal sonography is only a recent development, which gives better results in Gynecology. It is stated by the respondents that this facility was not available anywhere nearby at the time of alleged negligence.

- *Factors affecting medical complications of a cervical pregnancy:*
  - *Hemorrhage:* In about 50% of the cases reviewed by Resnick, blood-tinged vaginal discharge or irregular bleeding was present 2–4 weeks after the patient missed her first period. Such bleeding often becomes progressively more severe and can result in more or less brisk hemorrhage once the ovum begins to separate from the cervical wall or ruptures through it. Unless the gestation is very early, spontaneous or induced abortion tends to bring on violent hemorrhage. Attempts at removing the placenta, which is usually accreta only augments the hemorrhage potential. Average blood loss is put at 6.4 units. Cervical pregnancies may also involve signs of intraperitoneal bleeding if the gestation has ruptured through the cervical wall. However, since the diagnosis is not generally suspected, the origin of the hemorrhage may not be clear until laparotomy.
  - *Location:* Paalman and Mc Elin suggested that instances of torrential bleeding are probably associated with the cervicoisthmic variety of placentation, which entails greater involvement.
  - *Availability of advanced medical facilities:* Dr Rajan in his article, Endovaginal Sonography in Infertility, Gynecology and Obstetrics, acknowledges the usefulness of Transvaginal Sonography until the introduction of this method the diagnosis precision was questionable.

Operative findings:

- While doing MTP, the patient started bleeding profusely and signs of internal bleeding were present. So, an exploratory laparotomy was done. There was plenty of blood in the peritoneal cavity. The bleeding was from the lateral end of the lower uterine segment. The lower segment was opened and the uterine cavity evacuated. The products were actually in the cervical canal perforating the lower segment. Since the bleeding was not controlled even after evacuation and suturing the lower segment, total hysterectomy was done. Both tubes and ovaries were retained. A small rent in the bladder was repaired by Dr CBC Abdomen closed in layers after perfect hemostasis. 3 units of blood transfused at the time of surgery. Urine drained by Foley's catheter continuously. The urine is clear. Output satisfactory.
- Dr Somalatha P Shenoy, respondent No 3 stated that when the uterus was open, she saw the amniotic sac with a small fetus and Dr Santha Warriar, respondent No. 2, evacuated this product and the site of implantation was noticed at the upper cervical canal and at the isthmic area.

Expert Evidence:

- The next allegation regarding negligence on the part of the doctors is that laminaria tent for dilating cervix was used instead of dilapan and again on this aspect certain textbooks were referred to. In the evidence of Dr Rajan, RW 1, it was stated that he was using laminaria tent for dilatation of cervical canal. The use of laminaria tent in dilatation of cervix is one of the accepted standard procedures and it cannot be stated that the use of that procedure by respondent No. 2 in respect of appellant constituted a negligent act.

- Placing reliance on the article of Dr GI Dhall on the subject of Suction Evacuation and Dilatation & Curettage in First Trimester MTP, it was contended that suction evacuation is a method of choice in dealing with termination of first trimester pregnancy and this method has replaced Dilatation & Curettage method. The author does not say that dilatation and curettage methods for purposes of terminating the first trimester pregnancy is a prohibited one.

Judgment (Summary)

The Hon'ble Supreme Court also disposed of the appeal and regarded the dismissal by NCDRC as correct as the appellant failed to prove the alleged negligence of the doctors.

i. Reliance was placed on *Achutrao Haribhau Khodwa* case as follows: The skill of medical practitioners differs from doctor to doctor. The very nature of the profession is such that there may be more than one course of treatment which may be advisable for treating a patient. Courts would indeed be slow in attributing negligence to the part of a doctor if he has performed his duties to the best of his ability and with due care and caution. Medical opinion may differ with regard to the course of action to be taken by a doctor treating a patient, but as long as a doctor acts in a manner which is acceptable to the medical profession and the court finds that he has attended on the patient with due care, skill, and diligence and if the patient still does not survive or suffers a permanent ailment, it would be difficult to hold the doctor to be guilty of negligence.[9]
ii. It was alleged that on the removal of the uterus and the products of conception were not sent to the outside Pathological Department to confirm the diagnosis. The court said it would not have helped the case of the appellant in any manner because that would not have established in any manner negligence on the part of the respondents in the course of the surgical procedure adopted in case of the appellant. If there was a suspicion of cancer, there would have been some manifestation of the same and, in such a circumstance histopathological examination would have been done to rule out the possibility of cancer. However, there was no complaint of any kind of cancer nor was there any such visible proof of the same.
iii. Operative findings and the expert evidence were relied upon to arrive at the decision in this case.

CASE 7: DR MOHANBHAI S PATEL vs. THAKKAR BALDEVBHAI KESHAVLAL & ORS[18] [NCDRC, New Delhi Case]

The first Appeal was filed by Dr Mohanbhai S Patel, OP No.1 before the Gujarat SCDRC and Appellant herein being aggrieved by the order of Gujarat SCDRC which had partly allowed the complaint of medical negligence filed by Thakkar Baldevbhai Keshavlal, Original Complainant No.1 (Respondent

No.1 herein) and others (his minor children) before the Gujarat SCDRC.

Facts of the Case

- Thakkar Baldevbhai Keshavlal (Respondent/Complainant) took his wife Gitaben on 06.05.1997 for medical check-up as she was having irregular menstruation and pain abdomen. She was examined by Dr Mohanbhai S Patel (Appellant) at Navjeevan Maternity Home, who advised an X-ray and sonography and on the basis of that report, informed that Patient was 3 months pregnant, and that D&C procedure was required to be conducted.
- D&C procedure was conducted on 06.05.1997 and patient was prescribed some medicines. After the operation was over at about 4.00 PM, patients continued to complain of severe pain. The appellant informed the patient party that this was normal following such an operation and there was no reason for worry.
- Respondent/complainant and patient remained in the maternity home till about 8.30 PM after which appellant advised that she may be taken back to their village.
- On 07.05.1997 at about 3.00 AM, patient again felt severe pain and took painkillers. However, since the pain continued, a local doctor (Dr Bhagwandas Patel) was called, who after examining the Patient told Respondent/Complainant that the uterus of the patient had been punctured and, referred the patient to Appellant. A referral letter was also given by Dr. Bhagwandas Patel for Appellant.
- The appellant prescribed some medicines, but the patient's condition continued to deteriorate. The respondent/complainant was informed that another operation was necessary, which would last for 10 min and Respondent/Complainant was also asked to arrange for blood and medicines. The operation, however, lasted for 2 hours. The patient's condition remained serious, and she expired on 09.05.1997 at about 2.00 PM.
- 15 days after her death, Respondent/Complainant approached the appellant with the request to furnish him necessary case papers. The appellant refused to give him the papers.

Complainant's Allegations

- The complainant attributed death of his wife to medical negligence by the Appellant while performing the D&C operation, during which the uterus was punctured, terminating the pregnancy without consent and thereafter in not taking proper care to check the severe pain and bleeding before discharging her on 06.05.1997 and later after the laparotomy on 07.05.1997.
- Respondent/Complainant filed a complaint before the SCDRC against appellant and others on grounds of medical negligence and deficiency in service and requested that appellant be directed to pay compensation.

Doctor's Defense Before SCDRC

- Patient was admitted to the Maternity Home with complaints of irregular menstruation and pain in the uterus, on examination it was found that she was 3 months pregnant with threatened abortion.
- Appellant denied that he had conducted a D&C procedure. Since there was a threat of abortion, patient was given the option to either undergo conservative treatment or to abort the pregnancy. The patient opted for termination of the pregnancy and was,

therefore, given medical treatment for the same, namely, Prostadin injection and cervi prime gel to facilitate the abortion.

- Since the patient herself volunteered for termination of pregnancy, no written consent from her was taken.
- Later, in the interest of her health, laparotomy operation was conducted with the help of OP No. 2 (Dr Shaileshbhai Patel) after obtaining written consent. The operation was successful, and the patient's condition was improving till the third day when her health deteriorated.
- Appellant further contended that he had advised the Respondent/Complainant and other relatives to get a postmortem done of the patient, so that the real cause of death could be ascertained but they refused to get the postmortem done.
- There was no medical negligence on the part of the Appellant who being a qualified doctor and using his best professional judgment and in consultation with other expert doctors tried his best to treat and save the patient.
- It was contended that patient's death occurred because against medical advice, she left the hospital without permission, which aggravated her condition.

Judgment by SCDRC (Summary)

i. The SCDRC allowed the complaint and found only Dr Mohanbhai S Patel (the Appellant) guilty of medical negligence and deficiency in service.

ii. The SCDRC concluded that the termination of pregnancy was carried out without consent for the same and the patient and her relatives were also not kept informed about the progress of her condition. After the administration of prostadin injection and cervi prime gel, patient was not advised about the possible side effects and the possible complications. Further, the patient was left under the care of a woman called Gangaben who may not have had the necessary skills and competency to supervise the effects of the medication/ injection given.

iii. Although there was no evidence that any D&C was done and her pregnancy was terminated by giving Prostadin injection and cervi prime gel, this led to complications, including rupture of uterus and bleeding, to which Patient ultimately succumbed.

iv. OP no. 1 when used drugs or procedure to terminate the pregnancy ought to have known the inherent danger of using the drugs and taken enough safeguard to either prevent those complications or at least should have remedied them recognizing them as they came (in this case since starting of initial treatment; danger signals had already started appearing). The lack of recognizing and not treating them in time amounts to negligence, more so when OP No.1 is claimed to be senior, highly qualified and experienced gynecologist and obstetrician.

v. Complications occurring during the treatment cannot be said to be negligent, but not recognizing them in time and not treating them or treating them too late when patient had reached end stage where results were certainly to the detriment to the patient certainly amounts to negligence.

vi. The patient who has reposed to full trust and faith in the hands of treating doctor for his or her life and if that trust and faith is negative, it is not only negligence but also deficiency in service.

Being aggrieved by the order of the SCDRC, the present First Appeal was filed.

Doctor's Defense Before NCDRC

- The appellant contended that the SCDRC erred by not taking cognizance of the fact that:
    - when the patient was brought for treatment to Appellant, she was threatened with imminent abortion and wanted termination of the pregnancy, for which she was given necessary medicines/injection.
    - No D&C procedure was conducted.
    - Since the patient herself wanted the pregnancy to be terminated and further since her life was at risk because of the immediate threatened abortion, as per provisions of Section 3(2)(i) of the MTP Act, 1971, which provides that *a pregnancy may be terminated by a registered medical practitioner if the continuance of the pregnancy involves a risk to the life of the pregnancy woman or grave injury physical or mental health*, no consent was required.
    - The patient unauthorizedly left the Maternity Home on the night of 06.05.1997 and this fact is also written in the medical case history of the patient which was also filed in evidence before the State Commission.
- The allegation that uterus got punctured during D&C procedure did not arise since even the State Commission had concluded that no D&C operation was conducted.
- As a diligent medical professional, even though the patient had left unauthorizedly, when she came back the next day with complaints of severe abdominal pain he immediately examined her and conducted a laparotomy which was necessary. Two other doctors assisted him in the procedure.
- Appellant had also produced expert opinion of a Physician and an Anesthetist in support of his case but unfortunately their statement was disregarded by the SCDRC on the ground that they were not Specialists in Gynecology and, therefore, their statement did not amount to expert opinion.
- The SCDRC itself had observed that there was no medical negligence per se in the actual treatment of the Appellant and he was being penalized on the ground that patient and her relatives consent was not taken prior to termination of the pregnancy and proper follow-up and treatment was not given to check the bleeding. However, these facts are not borne out by the case history of the Patient on record. The finding of the State Commission was, therefore, against the settled principles of the law with regard to medical negligence.

Complainant/Respondent's Submission before NCDRC

- Counsel for the Respondent/Complainant reiterated that there was no evidence to support appellants contention that the patient, who was three months pregnant at the time of visiting the Appellant, wanted the termination of the pregnancy.
- She had come with complaints of pain in the uterus and although a provisional diagnosis of threatened abortion was made, after due examination the medical history does not indicate that there was imminent threat of abortion. Further, after the clinical tests nowhere was it mentioned that the abortion was inevitable. In fact, as per the clinical notes, it was confirmed that the patient was

14 weeks pregnant, and the advice given was Os tightening and complete bed rest.

- Thereafter in the same case sheet, it was recorded patient refuses for conservative treatment and wants to undergo termination. Patient never wanted to terminate the pregnancy, and she was administered medicines/injections to terminate the same without her knowledge or consent.
- Appellant's contention that as per the provisions of the MTP Act, 1971 no consent was required is not correct. Except when life of the patient is at extreme risk, the doctor is statutorily bound under the provisions of the above Act to obtain the written consent of the pregnant woman. Further, with respect to termination of pregnancy, which exceeds 12 weeks, the opinion of 2 RMPs is necessary to opine that continuance of pregnancy involves a risk to the life of the pregnant woman.
- In the instance case, as per the medical records of the patient, it has nowhere been indicated that life of the patient was at risk. Therefore, merely recording in medical case history that the patient wanted medical termination of pregnancy does not amount to consent nor does it give the medical practitioner the right to have terminated the pregnancy.
- It is incorrect that the patient left the maternity home unauthorizedly and without medical permission. In fact, after taking his fees from the Respondent/ Complainant, Appellant himself discharged the patient even though she continued to complain of severe abdominal pain at that time.
- When the patient was brought back on 07.05.1997 and the laparotomy was conducted on her. Patient's relatives were never informed about the seriousness of her condition by the Appellant, who kept assuring that the patient was recovering satisfactorily. Had the Respondent/ Complainant known that her condition was serious, he would have taken her to Ahmedabad where better medical facilities were available.

Judgment by NCDRC

National Commission concurred with the State Commission decision and reasoned as below:

i. It is an admitted fact that no written consent of the patient was taken by the Appellant before terminating the pregnancy. Appellants explanation for the same, namely, that the patient herself had volunteered for termination of pregnancy and that under the Medical Termination of Pregnancy Act, 1971 if the patient's life is at risk, the doctor can terminate the pregnancy without seeking consent, are not supported by the evidence on record. There is, for example, no clinical indication that the patient's life was at a risk. In fact, as recorded in the medical history of the patient, the appellant himself had recorded after the X-ray and the ultrasound that the patient required bed rest and conservative treatment.

ii. If abortion was indeed imminent or threatened, a recording of this effect should have been made in the final diagnosis, i.e., after X-ray and ultrasound tests. In any case, even if the patient herself had volunteered for termination of the pregnancy, under the Medical Termination of Pregnancy Act, 1971, her written consent was necessary. Merely recording the same by a doctor in her medical records is not adequate in such cases. This is also confirmed by a ruling of the Hon'ble Supreme Court of India in Samira Kohli v/s Dr Prabha Manchanda,[19] wherein the Hon'ble Apex Court has categorically ruled that unless it is necessary to save the life or preserve the health of a patient, valid consent is a must.

iii. It is well established as per medical literature that the drugs prostadin injection and cervi prime gel can have serious side effects and complications and a patient need to be cautioned about the same and the witness on record has observed a rent in the uterus further testifies the fact.

CASE 8: DR (Smt.) PRABHA AGARWAL vs. KAMAKHYA SINGH & ANR[19] [NCDRC, New Delhi Case]

Facts of the Case

- On 10.12.2001, complainant Kamakhya Singh had taken his wife Lalti Devi to the clinic of the appellants. She was suffering from abdominal pain. The appellants gave certain medicines to her and advised her to take a rest in the nursing home. After taking the medicine, her pain increased. At the relevant time, Lalti Devi was pregnant.
- Appellant No. 1 Dr (Smt) Prabha Agarwal advised termination of pregnancy by D&C operation. An amount of ₹10,000 was demanded for conducting the operation. However, Kamakhya Singh could manage payment of only ₹5000 and sought time to pay the remaining amount. Lalti Devi was operated at about 1:00 AM in the night of 10th and 11th Dec 2001. When she gained consciousness the next morning, she felt acute pain in the abdomen.
- On the next date, the appellants asked the complainant whether the remaining amount was arranged and deposited. He could not arrange for the money and, therefore, further treatment was refused.
- On 12.12.2001, complainant Kamakhya Singh, took his wife to Bose Clinic. He was advised to take her to higher medical center. So, he took her to Patna Medical College Hospital (PMCH), Patna. She was admitted in the said hospital on 13.12.2001.
- At the PMCH, it was noticed that there was a history of abortion on 10.12.2001, complaints of vomiting and she had not passed stools for 3 days. Further investigation revealed that there was poor prognosis due to perforation over the anterior surface of the uterus as well as in the SJ. The risk of the operation was explained to the patient and, thereafter, she was operated. She died on 15.12.2001 at 6:26 AM.

Complainant's Allegations

- Due to negligent surgical procedure done by the appellants, his wife lost her life.
- Appellant no. 1 Dr Prabha Agarwal had no adequate knowledge of conducting the MTP.
- He claimed compensation of ₹5,75,000 by filing a complaint before the State Commission.

Doctor's Defense

- The appellants denied the allegations and submitted that there was nothing in their records to show that deceased Lalti Devi was ever admitted in their nursing home. They denied having provided any treatment to the deceased Lalti Devi.
- The appellants submitted that Dr (Smt) Prabha Agarwal is a qualified Gynecologist

and is practicing since 18 years. They contended that false complaint was filed against them in order to malign their high reputation.

Sequence of Events in State Commission

i. The complainant filed photocopies of prescription and *chithas* issued by the clinic of the appellants. He also placed on record discharge card dated 12.12.2001 issued by Bose Clinic and death certificate issued by the PMCH.
ii. The appellants produced the indoor patient register and claimed that deceased Lalti Devi was not admitted in their hospital for any medical treatment.
iii. The State Commission came to the conclusion that the sequence of events and the record was sufficient to infer gross medical negligence on part of the appellants. Hence the complaint was partly allowed vide the impugned order.

Issues Before the National Commission

i. Whether it is duly proved by complainant Kamakhya Singh that his wife was subjected to Medical Termination of Pregnancy at the clinic of the appellants on or about 10.12.2001?
ii. Whether it is duly proved that the appellants committed gross negligence while conducting the D&C procedure and as a result of such negligence, the wife of complainant Kamakhya Singh lost her life?
iii. Whether the impugned order of the State Commission is legal, proper, and correct?

Judgment by NCDRC (Summary)

i. This is a case in which principle of *res ipsa loquitor* is squarely applicable having regard to the attending circumstances, conduct of the appellants and the fact that within a short span after the Medical Termination of Pregnancy the young woman lost her life. Hence, the National Commission upheld the order passed by the State Commission holding the doctors guilty of negligence.
ii. The National Commission took into consideration that the State Commission had compared handwriting on the prescription and the *chitthas*. It was noted by the State Commission that both the *chitthas* were in the handwriting of the same person. One of the *chitthas* shows that medicines prescribed were for the treatment of septicemia and intravaginal infection.
iii. The complainant had no previous enmity with appellants. He is a rustic, poor and illiterate person. He had no reason to falsely implicate the appellants as the treating doctors.
iv. The State Commission noticed that the register was apparently tampered with by re-stitching some of the pages. It also noticed that there was some re-writing in respect of the entries pertaining to the relevant period. The appellants attempted to manipulate the indoor registers record which was produced before the State Commission.
v. Complainant produced the prescription and the chitthas issued by the appellants, hence the onus shifted on them to show that wife of complainant Kamakhya Singh was not at all treated in their clinic.
vi. Bed-head ticket of PMCH shows that deceased Lalti Devi was subjected to operation on 10.12.2001. It was found that she had not passed flatus and stool for three days. It was also found that there were three perforations in the SI and one perforation over the anterior surface of uterus.

vii. Going by the sequence of events, the fact that the appellants prescribed medicines like Cifran, etc. indicated that they were aware about the complications which had occurred as a result of the medical termination of pregnancy.

CASE 9: SAMIRA KOHLI vs. DR PRABHA MANCHANDA & ANR (2008)[20] [Supreme Court Case]

(Medical Negligence in Context of Consent)

- Appeal was filed to Hon'ble Supreme Court against the order dated 19.11.2003 passed by the NCDRC, New Delhi rejecting the appellant's complaint under the Consumer Protection Act, 1986 alleging negligence on part of the surgeon.
- In this appeal, the issue before the Supreme Court was whether "informed consent" of a patient is required for a surgical procedure which involves removal of reproductive organs and if so, what should be the nature of such consent.
- Further, it examined if and under what circumstances consent given for a particular procedure be treated as consent for an additional surgical procedure.

Facts of the Case

- On 9.05.1995, the appellant, an unmarried woman, aged 44 years, visited the clinic of the first respondent with complaint of prolonged menstrual bleeding for 9 days. The respondent examined and advised her to undergo an ultrasound test on the same day. After examining the report, the respondent had a discussion with the appellant and advised her to come on the next day (10.05.1995) for a laparoscopy test under GA to make an affirmative diagnosis.
- On 10.05.1995, the appellant went to the respondent's clinic with her mother. On admission, the appellant's signatures were taken on:
  i. Admission and discharge card
  ii. Consent form for hospital admission and medical treatment
  iii. Consent form for surgery.
- The admission card showed that admission was "for diagnostic and operative laparoscopy on 10.05.1995". The consent form for surgery filled by Dr Lata Rangan (respondent's assistant) described the procedure to be undergone by the appellant as "Diagnostic and Operative Laparoscopy. Laparotomy may be needed."
- Thereafter, the appellant was put under general anesthesia and subjected to a laparoscopic examination. When the appellant was still unconscious, Dr Lata Rangan who was assisting the respondent, came out of the OT and took consent from appellant's mother waiting outside, for performing hysterectomy under GA. Thereafter, the respondent performed an abdominal hysterectomy and bilateral salpingo-oopherectomy (removal of ovaries and fallopian tubes). The appellant left the respondent's clinic on 15.05.1995 without settling the bill.

Patient's Allegation

- On 19.01.1996, the appellant filed a complaint before the NCDRC claiming compensation of ₹25 lakhs from the respondent. The appellant alleged that the respondent was negligent in treating her; that the radical surgery by which her uterus, ovaries and fallopian tubes were removed without her consent, when she was under general anesthesia for a laparoscopic test, was unlawful, unauthorized and unwarranted; that on account of the removal of her reproductive organs, she had suffered premature menopause necessitating a prolonged medical treatment and a hormone replacement therapy (HRT) course, apart from making her vulnerable to health problems by way of side-effects.

- The compensation claimed was for the loss of reproductive organs and consequential loss of opportunity to become a mother, for diminished matrimonial prospects, for physical injury resulting in the loss of vital body organs and irreversible permanent damage, for pain, suffering emotional stress and trauma, and for decline in the health and increasing vulnerability to health hazards.

Doctor's Defense

- The appellant voluntarily visited the respondent's clinic for treatment and consented for diagnostic procedures and operative surgery.
- The hysterectomy and other surgical procedures were done with adequate care and caution; and
- The surgical removal of uterus, ovaries, etc. was necessitated as the appellant was found to be suffering from endometriosis (Grade IV), and if they had not been removed, there was likelihood of the lesion extending to the intestines and bladder and damaging them.

After hearing the arguments, the National Commission dismissed the complaint by order dated 19.11.2003.

Issues for Consideration before the Hon'ble Supreme Court:

i. Whether informed consent of a patient is necessary for surgical procedure involving removal of reproductive organs? If so, what is the nature of such consent?

ii. Whether consent given for diagnostic surgery can be construed as consent for performing additional or further surgical procedure—as conservative treatment or as radical treatment—without the specific consent for such additional or further surgery?

iii. Whether there was consent by the appellant, for the abdominal hysterectomy and bilateral salpingo-oopherectomy performed by the respondent?

iv. Whether the respondent had falsely invented a case that the appellant was suffering from endometriosis to explain the unauthorized and unwarranted removal of uterus and ovaries, and whether such radical surgery was either to cover-up negligence in conducting diagnostic laparoscopy or to claim a higher fee?

v. Even if the appellant was suffering from endometriosis, the respondent ought to have resorted to conservative treatment/surgery instead of performing radical surgery?

vi. Whether the respondent is guilty of the tortious act of negligence/battery amounting to deficiency in service, and consequently liable to pay damages to the appellant?

Judgment by the Supreme Court (Summary)

i. Consent in the context of a doctor-patient relationship, means the grant of permission by the patient for an act to be carried out by the doctor, such as a diagnostic, surgical, or therapeutic procedure. Consent can be implied in some circumstances from the action of the patient. For example, when a patient enters a dentist's clinic and sits in the dental chair, his consent is implied for examination, diagnosis and consultation. Except where consent can be clearly and obviously implied, there should be express consent. There is, however, a significant difference in the nature of express consent of the patient, known as "real consent" in UK and as "informed consent" in America. In UK, the elements of consent are defined with reference to the patient and a consent is considered to be valid and "real" when (*i*) the patient gives it voluntarily without any coercion; (*ii*) the patient has the capacity and competence to give consent; and (*iii*) the patient has the minimum of adequate level of information about the nature of the procedure to which he is consenting to. On the other hand, the concept of "informed consent" developed by American courts, while retaining the basic requirements of consent, shifts the emphasis on the doctor's duty to disclose the necessary information to the patient to secure his consent.

ii. In *Canterbury vs. Spence*[21], the United States Court of Appeals, District of Columbia Circuit, emphasized the element of doctor's duty in "informed consent" thus: (F 2d pp. 782–783, paras 11–12)
   a. "... It is well established that the physician must seek and secure his patient's consent before commencing an operation or other course of treatment. It is also clear that the consent, to be efficacious, must be free from imposition upon the patient. It is the settled rule that therapy not authorized by the patient may amount to a tort—a common law battery—by the physician. *And it is evident that it is normally impossible to obtain consent worthy of the name unless the physician first elucidates the options and the perils for the patient's edification*. Thus, the physician has long borne a duty, on pain of liability for unauthorized treatment, to make adequate disclosure to the patient."

iii. The basic principle in regard to patient's consent may be traced to the following classic statement by Cardozo, J *Schloendorff vs. Society of New York Hospital*[22]

iv. "... Every human being of adult years and sound mind has a right to determine what shall be done with his own body; and a surgeon who performs an operation without his patient's consent commits an assault, for which he is liable in damages." This principle has been accepted by an English court also in the House of Lords while dealing with a case of sterilization of a mental patient[23] reiterated the fundamental principle that every person's body is inviolate and performance of a medical operation on a person without his or her consent is unlawful.

v. The next question is whether in an action for negligence/battery for performance of an unauthorized surgical procedure, the doctor can put forth as defense the consent given for a particular operative procedure, as consent for any additional or further operative procedures performed in the interests of the patient. In *Murray vs. McMurchy*[24], the Supreme Court of British Columbia, Canada, was considering a claim for battery by a patient who underwent a cesarean section. During the course of cesarean section, the doctor found fibroid tumors in the patient's uterus. Being of the view that such tumors would be a danger in case of future pregnancy, he performed a sterilization operation. The Court upheld the claim for damages for battery. It held that sterilization could not be justified under the principle of necessity, as there was no immediate threat or danger to the patient's health or life, and it would not have been unreasonable to postpone the operation to secure the patient's consent. The fact that the doctor found it convenient to perform the sterilization operation without consent as the patient was already under general anesthesia, was held to be not a valid defense.

vi. The doctor is required to communicate all inherent and potential hazards of the proposed treatment, the alternatives to that treatment. This stringent standard of disclosure was subjected to only two exceptions: (1) In cases of emergency, e.g., the patient was unconscious, and (2) If the information would be harmful to the patient, e.g., where it might cause psychological damage.

vii. A doctor has to seek and secure the consent of the patient before commencing a "treatment". The consent so obtained should be real and valid, which means that: the patient should have the capacity and competence to consent; his consent should be voluntary; and based on adequate information concerning the nature of the treatment procedure, so that he knows what he is consenting to.

viii. The admission card makes it clear that the appellant was admitted only for diagnostic and operative laparoscopy. It does not refer to laparotomy. The consent form shows that the appellant gave consent only for diagnostic operative laparoscopy, and laparotomy if needed. Laparotomy is a surgical procedure to open up the abdomen or an abdominal operation.

ix. Laparotomy by itself is not hysterectomy or salpingo-oopherectomy. Laparotomy does not refer to surgical removal of any vital or reproductive organs.

x. The respondent next contended that the consent given by the appellant's mother for performing hysterectomy should be considered as valid consent for performing hysterectomy and salpingo-oopherectomy. The appellant was neither a minor, nor mentally challenged, nor incapacitated. When a patient is a competent adult, there is no question of someone else giving consent on her behalf. There was no medical emergency during surgery. The appellant was only temporarily unconscious, undergoing only a diagnostic procedure by way of laparoscopy. The respondent ought to have waited till the appellant regained consciousness, discussed the result of the laparoscopic examination and then taken her consent for the removal of her uterus and ovaries. In the absence of an emergency and as the matter was still at the stage of diagnosis, the question of taking her mother's consent for radical surgery did not arise. Therefore, such consent by mother cannot be treated as valid or real consent.

xi. The Court denied the entire fee charged for the surgery and in addition, directed to pay ₹25,000 as compensation for the unauthorized AH-BSO surgery to the appellant.

CASE 10: DR STEPHEENA & ANR vs. LILLY JOSEPH[25] [NCDRC, New Delhi Case]

(Revision Petition filed to NCDRC, New Delhi)

- Two revision petitions were filed by the Opposite Party for dismissal of Complaint. Another revision petition was filed by the complainant, the patient Lily Joseph, for enhancement of compensation.
- The District Forum allowed the complaint and directed the OPs to pay a sum of ₹5,60,000 as compensation, together with costs of ₹5,000.
- The State Commission passed a common order and confirmed the negligence of OP/Petitioner. It modified the order of District Forum, and directed the OPs to pay ₹3,69,000, with interest @12% per annum and the liability of compensation on the first Petitioner was quantified at ₹1,00,000.

Facts of the Case

- The Complainant, Lily Joseph, a Laboratory Technician, went to Dr Stepheena (OP-1) working at Fathima Mission Hospital (OP-2) for complaints for physical uneasiness.
- She underwent abdominal hysterectomy, which was performed by OP-1, Dr Stepheena at OP-2 Hospital, Fathima Matha Mission Hospital on 02.04.2003.
- During the operation, she suffered an injury to the bladder which was noticed on 10th postoperative day when it was diagnosed as vesicovaginal fistula (VVF).
- Thereafter, she remained admitted in the hospital for 25 days for further treatment, the leaking of urine persisted, therefore, she approached OP-2 on 19.05.2003 for VVF repair.
- Thereafter, she underwent 2 major operations at Malabar Hospital, Kozhikode on 24.05.2003 and on 09.08.2003 but her condition did not improve.
- Hence, she took treatment at Kasturba Hospital at Manipal, Karnataka, where on 29.01.2003 she was operated again and was discharged.

Patient's Allegation

- The operating surgeon was grossly negligent in conducting the operation which resulted in injury to the bladder and subsequent complications due to which patient had to undergo multiple corrective surgeries and had to remain admitted in the hospital for extended periods of time.
- Due to negligence of the OPs, the patient was subjected to long treatment, she lost her profession, suffered mental agony.
- OP-2 acquired her MD degree from Italy; it is not recognized in India by MCI.

Doctor's Defense

- Patient was suffering from fibroid uterus with endometriosis, and during surgery, it was noticed that the uterus was having multiple intramural fibroids, ruptured (L) ovarian cyst, endometriotic patches over the anterior and posterior uterine wall, pouch of Douglas.
- There were dense bladder adhesions. During surgery while separating bladder adhesions from the anterior uterine wall; an accidental injury was occurred to the bladder.
- OP doctor took immediate steps, called the surgeon Dr VJ Sebastian, FRCS working in the hospital, who repaired the bladder injury and done the vault closure. Bladder leak was checked by pushing gentian violet into the bladder. Postoperatively,

patient was given antibiotics and catheter drainage continued. As per advice by the Urologist, bladder wash was given, and the catheter was changed.

- But, on the 10th postoperative day, i.e., on 12.04.2003, a frank leaking of urine through the vagina was noticed. The urologist diagnosed it as VVF and swab tests were done. The patient was put on Amikacin injection. The patient was discharged on 23.04.2003 with an advice for Urology and review after 2 weeks. Thus, the Counsel for OP finally concluded that the injury to bladder and VVF are accepted complications of hysterectomy.
- It is contended that OP-2 is a well-qualified and experienced gynecologist and the surgeon repaired the bladder injury completely. She was given postoperative antibiotics and bladder drainage to aid healing of the wound.
- The VVF was developed due to impaired healing of the repaired bladder injury. On detection of VVF, urologist intervention was done. Therefore, there was no negligence on the part of OPs.

Judgment by NCDRC (Summary)

On the basis of medical literature and textbooks on gynecology, it was concluded:

i. Firstly, prior to hysterectomy, the OP-1 should have treated the patient for endometriosis, primarily for 28 days with medicines, like injection Lupride or Danzole.

ii. Secondly, during operation, OP-1 noted multiple fibroids and dense adhesions between anterior uterine wall and the bladder. Therefore, in such a case, the OP-1 should have been more vigilant while separating and dissection of bladder adhesions. It was the duty of OP to immediately seek opinions or assistance from the Urologist Dr Santosh, who was working in the same hospital, during that period. But she took help from another surgeon who repaired the bladder injury. The records show that the OP took help from urologist on 10th postoperative day, when the patient developed VVF.

iii. Thirdly, in view of the court, the consent taken prior to hysterectomy was a '*Blanket Consent*' and not an '*Informed Consent*'. The consent does not show details about whether the patient was informed about, endometriosis or adhesions, which may cause possible injury to bladder during operation.

iv. Fourthly, the OP had not produced a histopathological report to support her diagnosis of multiple fibroids and endometriosis.

v. *Case law relied upon to ascertain Negligence:* The Hon'ble Supreme Court in the case of Dr Laxman Balkrishna Joshi vs. Dr Trimbak Babu Godbole and Anr.[11] and AS Mittal vs. State of UP.[10] laid down that, when a doctor is consulted by a patient, the doctor owes to his patient certain duties which are:

   a. duty of care in deciding whether to undertake the case,
   b. duty of care in deciding what treatment to give, and
   c. duty of care in the administration of that treatment.

   A breach of any of the above duties may give a cause of action for negligence and the patient may on that basis recover damages from his doctor.

vi. In the case on hand, OP-1 failed on all 4 counts (*as discussed above*), OP-1 cannot take advantage on the basis of known complication hence, it was an Act of omission, it is negligence.

Quantum of Damages

- The quantum of damages awarded is justified by evidence of economic loss and non-economic harm. Economic damages include past and future medical expenses, lost, past and future income, and other costs.
- The State Commission has made well-considered observations and awarded the proper compensation; therefore, it does not warrant our interference.

CONCLUSION

Knowledge of law related to medical practice is a must for every doctor involved in patient care. One of the most effective tools for ethical and safe practice of medicine. Ignorance of the law of the land (due to any reason whatsoever) is no excuse, and for safe clinical practice, it is a must that every doctor should spare some time from their busy schedule to learn the medicolegal aspects related to their day-to-day practice. There is no dearth of medicolegal information, the only thing required is the willingness to learn. To have a clear insight into the legals from medical practitioners, knowledge of medical laws is a must. Judgments related to medical professionals are the excellent source of guidelines for safe clinical practice as per the provisions of law.

REFERENCES

1. State of Haryana & Ors vs. Smt. Santra (2000) 5 SCC 182. [Accessed 06 April 2024]; Available from: https://indiankanoon.org/doc/53543700/.
2. MP vs. Asharam [1997 ACJ 1224 (MP)]. [Accessed 06 April 2024]; Available from: https://indiankanoon.org/doc/810994/
3. N. Nagendra Rao & Co. vs. State of AP (1994) 6 SCC 205. [Accessed 06 April 2024]; Available from: https://indiankanoon.org/doc/1929784/.
4. Common Cause, A Regd. Society vs. Union of India (1999) 6 SCC 667. [Accessed 06 April 2024]; Available from: https://indiankanoon.org/doc/1707158/.
5. Achutrao Haribhau Khodwa v. State of Maharashtra [(1996) 2 SCC 634. [Accessed 06 April 2024]; Available from: https://indiankanoon.org/doc/1917076/.
6. State of Punjab vs. Shiv Ram & Ors. (2005) 7 SCC 1. [Accessed 13 April 2024]; Available from: https://indiankanoon.org/doc/1599759/.
7. Bolam vs. Friern Hospital Management Committee (1957) 1 WLR 583.
8. The Medical Termination of Pregnancy Act, 1971. Act No. 34 Of 1971.
9. Achutrao Haribhau Khodwa vs. State of Maharashtra (1996) 2 SCC 634. [Accessed 13 April 2024]; Available from: https://indiankanoon.org/doc/1917076/.
10. AS Mittal vs. State of UP [(1989) 3 SCC 223 : 1989 SCC (Cri) 539 : AIR 1989 SC 1570.
11. Laxman Balkrishna Joshi (Dr) vs. Dr Trimbak Bapu Godbolee [AIR 1969 SC 128: (1969) 1 SCR 206: 71 Bom LR 236].
12. Smt Saroj Chandhoke vs. Sir Ganga Ram Hospital and Dr SK Bhandari. III (2007) CPJ189 (NC). Available from: http://indiankanoon.org/doc/235317/.
13. M/s Spring Meadows Hospital & Anr vs. Harjol Ahluwalia. 1998 (4) SCC 39. Available from: http://indiankanoon.org/doc/1715546/.
14. BN Agrawal, J, Harjit Singh Bedi, J, GS Singhvi, J. Nizam's Institute of Medical Sciences vs. Prasanth S. Dhananka & Ors., Civil Appeal No.4119 of 1999, with CA No. 3126 of 2000, Date of Judgment: 14.05.2009; [2009 (7) SCALE 407]. Available from: URL:http://judis.nic.in/supremecourt/imgs1.aspx?filename=34648.
15. Prasad vs. Dr. Kunal Saha & Ors., Civil Appeal No. 2867 of 2012, with Civil Appeal No. 692 of 2012, Advanced Medicare and Research Institute Ltd vs. Dr Kunal Saha & Ors, with Civil Appeal No.2866 of 2012 Dr Kunal Saha & Ors. vs. Dr. Sukumar Mukherjee & Ors., with Civil Appeal No.731 of 2012, Dr. Baidyanath Haldar vs. Dr. Kunal Saha &

Ors., and with Civil Appeal No.858 of 2012, Dr. Sukumar Mukherjee & Ors. vs. Dr. Kunal Saha & Ors., Date of Judgment: 24th Oct 2013; (2014) 1 SCC 384. [Online] [2015 May 12]. Available from: URL: http://judis.nic.in/supremecourt/imgs1.aspx?filename=40897.
16. Dr (Mrs) Indu Sharma vs. Indraprastha Apollo Hospital and Ors. 2015 April 27. Available from: https://indiankanoon.org/doc/64183895/.
17. Smt. Vinitha Ashok vs Lakshmi Hospital & Ors [2001 (8) SCC 731]. Available from: https://indiankanoon.org/doc/504385/.
18. Dr Mohanbhai S Patel vs Thakkar Baldevbhai Keshavlal & Ors. on 27th August, 2013 Available from: https://indiankanoon.org/doc/59413580/.
19. Dr. Prabha vs Kamakhya Singh, [2011, FA No. 117/07, NCRDC]. Available from: https://indiankanoon.org/doc/162323274/.
20. Samira Kohli vs Dr. Prabha Manchanda (2008) 2 SCC 1. Available from: https://indiankanoon.org/doc/438423/.
21. Canterbury vs. Spence [464 F 2d 772: 150 US App DC 263 (1972)]
22. Cardozo, J. Schloendorff vs. Society of New York Hospital [211 NY 125 : 105 NE 92 (1914)]: (NE p. 93, paras 5-6).
23. In re [(1990) 2 AC 1 : (1989) 2 WLR 1025: (1989) 2 All ER 545 sub nom F. v. West Berkshire HA].
24. Murray vs. McMurchy [(1949) 2DLR 442: (1949) 1 WWR 989].
25. Dr Stepheena & Anr. Vs. Lilly Joseph on 10 December, 2014. Available from: https://indiankanoon.org/doc/34794666/.

CHAPTER 2

Medicolegal Aspects of the Clinical Establishment Act

Rohit Umakant Erande

INTRODUCTION

The common saying, '*Health is Wealth*' is relevant to everyone's life. Good health is the most important part of our life, without which one cannot live life to the fullest. In India, the healthcare sector is widely unorganized. Various types of healthcare systems are being practiced in India, and quackery is one of the biggest challenges. Many patients are not even aware as to whether the treating doctor is really a qualified doctor or just a quack. The Government of India has an obligation to protect rights and privileges of its citizens. Hon'ble Apex Court has already held that *right to health and healthcare* is the part of Article 21 of the Constitution.[1] Article 47 of the Constitution casts a duty on the State to raise the level of nutrition and the standard of living and to improve public health. It further provides that, the State shall regard the raising of level of nutrition and standard of living of its people and improvement of public health as among its primary duties, and in particular, the State shall endeavor to bring about prohibition of the consumption except for medicinal purposes of intoxicating drinks and of drugs which are injurious to health. The Clinical Establishment Act (hereinafter may be referred to as CEA, for short and for the sake of brevity) has been passed on 19th August, 2010 in consonance with Article 47. The Act aims at:

i. Bringing the entire healthcare sector under one roof by using digital records.
ii. To end or to prevent the quackery.
iii. To improve the healthcare sector by prescribing minimum standard of facilities and services for all the clinical establishments.

WHAT IS A CLINICAL ESTABLISHMENT?

The scope of Definition is wide and includes almost all the doctors, clinics, etc. According to Section 2(c) of the Act, *clinical establishment* means:

i. A hospital, maternity home, nursing home, dispensary, clinic, sanatorium or an institution by whatever name called that offers services, facilities requiring diagnosis, treatment or care for illness, injury, deformity, abnormality or pregnancy in any recognized system of medicine established and administered or maintained by any person or body of persons, whether incorporated or not; or
ii. A place established as an independent entity or part of an establishment referred to in *sub-clause (i)*, in connection with the diagnosis or treatment of diseases where pathological, bacteriological, genetic, radiological, chemical, biological investigations or other diagnostic or investigative services with the aid of laboratory or other medical equipment, are usually carried on, established and

administered or maintained by any person or body of persons, whether incorporated or not, and shall include a clinical establishment owned, controlled or managed by (a) Government or a department of the Government; (b) a trust, whether public or private; (c) a corporation (including a society) registered under a Central, Provincial or State Act, whether or not owned by the Government; (d) a local authority; and (e) a single doctor.

To Whom the CEA is not Applicable?

- According to Section 2(c) of the Act, the clinical establishments owned, controlled or managed by the Armed Forces are not covered under this Act.
- Also, those categories of Clinical Establishment which are exempted by the state Government and Clinical Establishments located in the States/UTs mentioned in the schedule to the Act; unless these States/UTs repeal their existing Act and adopt Clinical Establishments Act.

Whether the CEA Applicable in the Entire Country?

- The CEA is not directly applicable in all the states of India. The subject "Health" comes in State list, and The CEA being a Central Legislation, will be applicable only in the States where a necessary resolution is passed by the respective State Legislative Assemblies. The Central could passed this Act, in view of Article 252 of the Constitution, only when the States like Himachal Pradesh, Arunachal Pradesh, Sikkim, and Mizoram passed resolution.
- As per the information available on the website of Ministry of Health and Family Welfare, Government of India, the Act has been implemented in four states, viz. Arunachal Pradesh, Himachal Pradesh, Mizoram, and Sikkim and all the Union Territories, except the NCT of Delhi. Later, the States of UP, Rajasthan, Uttarakhand, Bihar, Jharkhand, Haryana, and Assam have adopted the Act as per Article 252(1) of the Constitution.[2]
- Other states may adopt the CEA by passing a resolution in their state assemblies under clause (1) of Article 252 of the Constitution.

KEY FEATURES OF THE CLINICAL ESTABLISHMENT ACT

The Clinical Establishment Act runs into 56 sections and separate rules have also been framed under the Act, in 2012. This Act is very helpful in generating a reliable and comprehensive database for all types of clinical establishments in the country at district, state and national levels. It classifies various types of clinical establishments into categories and determines category wise basic minimum standards. The Act defines basic minimum standards for operation, using participatory and consultative approach to ensure uniformity across all establishments. Minimum standards indicate basic mandatory and certain desirable standards.

The key features of the Act are as follows:

- It establishes the National Council for Clinical Establishments at National level, State Council for Clinical Establishments at the state level, and District Registration Authority in each district. Implementation of the Act is by the respective state through the State Council and the District Registration Authority.
- There is a provision for *a two-step registration process*: (i) provisional

registration and (ii) permanent registration. Provisional registration is performed through a process of self-declaration without any inquiry or inspection. Permanent registration would be undertaken after categorization, classification and notification of category-wise minimum standards.
- The entire registration process and data of clinical establishments are placed in the public domain, which ensures transparency.
- Details of charges, and facilities available are to be prominently displayed at a conspicuous place at each establishment.
- There is a provision for cancellation of registration at any time, if conditions for registration are not complied with.
- The Clinical Establishments are required to provide emergency medical treatment, within the staff and facilities available (this provision has been attacked by the Medicos). The healthcare providers are required to maintain records and reporting as prescribed and provide information and statistics that may be asked for by the authority.

Registration Under the Act

The owner of the *clinical establishment* has the responsibility to register the establishment under Act. This Act has provided a separate registration for all the doctors, hospitals, clinics in addition to their earlier registration with the respective Medical Councils. *The Registration is Mandatory under the Act and without registration, a Clinical Establishment can't be run* (Section 11). Thus, for example, even if any clinic is having NABH accreditation, still registration under this Act shall be mandatory, once the Act is applicable in the State.

Requirements for Registration

The establishment has to fulfill certain conditions like minimum standards of facilities and services, minimum requirement of personnel, maintenance of records, etc. (Section 12). The Central Rules provide for other requirements for continuance and registration of the Establishment, that may be summarized as under (Rule no. 9):[3]

- It is mandatory for the Establishment *to display* at such conspicuous place, in English as well as in local language, *rates to be charged* for the services provided and facilities available in the Establishment.
- Such rates shall be fixed within such range as may be determined by the Central Government, in consultation with State Government.
- The Establishment has to comply with standard Treatment Guidelines, that may be framed from time to time by the respective Governments.
- The Establishment shall maintain and provide Electronic Medical/Health record of every patient.
- Every establishment has to maintain information and statistics in accordance with all other laws for the time being in force.

Provisional Certificate

The registration can be applied for online or in person. Those establishments which are already established, should apply for registration within a year from the date of commencement of this Act and those establishments which come into existence after this Act, those have to apply within 6 months of its establishment. Initially, a provisional certificate shall be granted by the Authority within 10 days from application, without conducting enquiry. The Provisional certificate shall be valid for a period of 12 months. The Authority shall cause to be published, within such time limit and in such manner, that may be prescribed, names of those establishments whose registration is expired.

Renewal of Provisional Certificate

The provisional registration shall not be renewed after a period of 2 years from the date of notification of minimum standards, in case of existing Clinical Establishments and the same shall not be renewed after a period of 6 months in case of Clinical Establishments which come into existence after date of notification of Minimum Standards.

Duplicate Certificate

If the Certificate is lost, destroyed, mutilated or damaged, then on Application and after paying such fees that may be prescribed, a Duplicate Certificate can be issued by the Authority.

Change in Ownership

This certificate shall be nontransferable. Thus, if there is any change in ownership or management, etc., such changes are to be notified to the Authority. Thus, for example, if a doctor buys a clinic already registered, such changes have to be notified. However, in case of change of location or category, a fresh certificate has to be applied for.

Permanent Certificate (Section 24)

Permanent registration is to be considered after notification of Minimum Standards. The establishment has to produce proof of fulfillment of the conditions. Once the objections, if any, are removed and the Authority is satisfied about the fulfillment of its conditions, the Permanent Certificate shall be granted and it is for 5 years. However, if the application for registration is not allowed, it can be applied afresh.

Cancellation of Certificate

The registration may be cancelled if the Authority finds that conditions are not fulfilled or the person entrusted with the management of the establishment has been convicted of offense under this Act.

Appeal against Refusal to Grant or Renew Certificate

If the certificate of registration or renewal of registration is refused or if the certificate is revoked by the Authority, then the aggrieved person has the right to file an appeal to the State Council within such time limit that may be prescribed. If the appeal is disallowed or it is not made in time prescribed, then the order of Authority shall become final and the Establishment cannot function.

Penalties for Doctors!

- The penalty for running the establishment without registration is ₹50,000 for 1st contravention, ₹2,00,000 for 2nd contravention and for subsequent contravention it may rise up to ₹5,00,000.
- Whoever knowingly works in an unregistered establishment, shall be fined up to ₹25,000.
- For any offense, for which no penalty has been prescribed, shall be fined ₹10,000, ₹50,000 and up to ₹5,00,000 for the 1st, 2nd and subsequent offenses respectively.
- However, holding of an inquiry by the Authority is the condition precedent before saddling such penalty and the authority shall take into consideration the category, size, type of establishment as well as local investigation.

- *Minor deficiencies:* Whoever contravenes any provision of the Act or the rules made thereunder, resulting in deficiencies that do not pose any immediate danger to the health and safety of any patient and can be rectified within a reasonable time, then it shall be punishable with fine not exceeding ₹10,000.

Recovery of Fines/Penalties

If any person fails to pay the fine saddled upon, then the Authority shall prepare the certificate and shall send it to the District Collector where such person resides or carries on the business, and such fine shall be recovered like arrears of land revenue. In simple words, it shall get preference over other dues.

Offenses Committed by Companies and Government Departments

- If the offence is committed by Company-establishment, then the person who was responsible at the time of commission of offence shall be held liable.
- In case of Government Department, the Head of the Department shall be held liable. However, there is saving clause for Department Departments. If such Head could prove that offence was committed without his knowledge or after due diligence, then such head will not be held liable. Such exception is not available to other Doctors.

Inspection of Registered Establishments

The Authority under this Act or any officer authorized by it have power to inspect the Establishments registered under this Act, its buildings, laboratories, equipment and the work done by the establishment. The Authority shall advise necessary changes/action to be made after such inspection and accordingly the Establishment shall in turn report the authority the implemented action. If the establishment does not take necessary action as advised, then after giving the opportunity of being heard, the Authority may issue necessary directions to the Establishment.

THE CEA RULES

In 2012, the CEA Rules were passed.[3] In 2018, amendment has been made, and thereby Minimum Standards for Medical Diagnostic Laboratories (or Pathological Labs) have been prescribed. The Rules also provide for Infrastructure, Safety Signage, Space Requirement, Human Resource, Instruments or Drugs, Legal Requirements under Bio-Medical Waste Management Rules, Record Maintenance, etc. The State Government has also been empowered to make various such rules regarding registration and other things. Various States and UTs in which the Act has been passed, have implanted the rules.[4]

Why Doctors are Opposing the CEA?

The Medical Fraternity, however, seems to be unhappy with the passing of this Act. The Medical Fraternity foresees this Act as a gateway to more dependency on Bureaucracy and accumulation of power in one hand, which shall lead to known complications. Further Medicos fear that so much of record keeping might consume their precious time or if they employ someone to do it, then it shall increase their expenses. The medical fraternity is opposing the Act mainly on grounds that it may create another License Raj. The Doctors are also apprehensive that this Act will increase operational cost and more paperwork, the amount of penalty is also very high. As any Act is "developed" by passage of time, this Act too shall be amended as the time passes. The maintenance of Record is going to be a great task for the Doctors. Nevertheless, in any medical negligence cases, record plays a very important role. It is said that *"Poor Records is a Poor Defence and No Record is No Defence".*

There are certain provisions which certainly would require reconsideration like Section 12(2). This Section provides that the establishment shall undertake to provide within the staff and facilities available, such medical examination and treatment as may be required to stabilize the emergency medical condition of any individual who comes to the establishment. This provision saddles too much responsibility on the establishment and whatever may be the condition of a patient, it should be stabilized first. Similarly, there is a provision that, the Head of the Government Department can be set free if he proves that breach of the provisions of the Act was beyond his knowledge or that he took all the diligence. Such relaxation is not available to other establishments. The author is of the opinion that such provision is discriminatory.

CONCLUSION

The Clinical Establishment Act has been passed to further improve the healthcare sector in India. To improve any healthcare system, mere enactment of the Act is not enough. Let's hope that the aims and objects of the Act are achieved, but without detriment to the doctors and the patients. During the current pandemic of coronavirus disease 2019 (COVID-19), we all have realized that there must be a robust healthcare system in the country. Few of the Doctors have given their lives while treating COVID patients. Although society is appreciating the services being provided by the healthcare professionals by calling doctors, paramedics and hospital staff as Corona Warriors, but at the same time, these professionals are facing problems like attacks, violence, and allegations of negligence. Many senior doctors have already started asking their next generation to stay away from this profession or they themselves are thinking of stopping the practice. There should be an effort to make the society aware that Healthcare System is for them, and they also have some responsibilities towards the healthcare providers.

REFERENCES

1. State of Punjab v/s. Ram Lubhaya Bagga & Ors., (1998) 4 SCC 117 and Navtej Singh Johar v/s. Union of India, (2018) 10 SCC 1 (Famous for LGBTQ equality judgement).
2. The Clinical Establishments Act, 2010 Available from: http://clinicalestablishments.gov.in/cms/Home.aspx.
3. Ministry of Health and Family Welfare, Department of Health and Family Welfare, Notification. New Delhi, 23 May 2012. [online] Available from http://clinicalestablishments.gov.in/WriteReadData/386.pdf. [Last accessed December, 2024].
4. Clinical Establishments Act, 2010. State and UTs (Rules and Notification). [online] Available from http://clinicalestablishments.gov.in/En/1077-state-and-uts-rules-and-notification.aspx. [Last accessed December, 2024].

CHAPTER 3

The Ethics of Medical Practice

Virendar Pal Singh, Gautam Biswas, Varun Modgil

"Justice consists not in being neutral between right and wrong, but in finding out the right and upholding it, wherever found, against the wrong."

—**Theodore Roosevelt**[1]

INTRODUCTION

Medicine is a profession that incorporates technological advancements in science and technology to alleviate the suffering. In the 21st century with advances in medical sciences, patient care has become more effective with better medications having fewer side effects. Surgery has moved towards less invasive modes of management, with lesser morbidity and faster recovery. The artificial intelligence (AI) controlled bionic arm is going to revolutionize the surgical specialty throwing a multitude of legal problems in the medical domain. With so much advancement in the field of *medicine*, the medical fraternity is becoming dependent on technology and further progress is mainly driven by technological demand. Market forces also tend to influence decision making by the doctors. Amidst all these developments, the medical practitioners often face ethical and legal challenges in their clinical practice. Keeping in mind the recent trends of medicolegal issues, the importance of ethical standards in the practice of medicine becomes even more relevant.

MEDICAL ETHICS

Medical ethics is a system of moral principles that apply values and judgments to the practice of medicine. It guides the medical practitioners in their behavior and decision making related to their relationship with patients, professional brethren and society at large. A physician is expected to be compassionate towards his patient, willing to take time to explain all the aspects of illness, mode of treatment, alternative forms of therapy and their individual benefits and expected outcomes with adverse effects (if any) so as to enable the patient to take an informed decision. The primary values of medicine insist that every physician has an obligation to keep the patient's interest above everything else. We have deviated from the earlier Paternalistic approach to the present concept of patient autonomy, as exemplified by the words of Judge Cardozo in Schloendroff vs. Society of New York Hospital[2] and the United Nations Universal Charter of Human Rights adopted by the General Assembly in 1948 which declares each human being to be born free and equal in dignity and human rights. The basic principles of medical ethics that guide the medical practitioners in clinical decision making are: (i) Autonomy; (ii) Beneficence; (iii) Non-maleficence; and (iv) Justice.[3]

Autonomy

Autonomy literally described as self-rule, is the principle that recognizes the rights of individuals to self-determination. In the medical profession, respecting the patient's autonomy requires the medical practitioners to give full information and get permission before doing anything to the patient, i.e., obtaining '*informed consent*' prior to treatment. Apart from ethical concerns, informed consent is also a legal obligation. Another implication of respecting the patient's autonomy is *'medical confidentiality'*. Medical practitioner impliedly promises his patients that he will keep confidential the information confided in him and hence the nature of doctor-patient relationship is fiduciary. Keeping promises is a way of respecting people's autonomy. Every effort should be made to ensure that confidentiality is maintained. However, in medical practice absolute confidentiality cannot exist. Often, it becomes necessary to share patient's information with other healthcare providers, so as to provide appropriate patient care as the medical care is being recognized more and more as a teamwork. In healthcare system, safeguarding confidentiality is far more challenging. With the advent of electronic health records, the risk of misuse of patient's confidential information has increased manifold. While discussing the patient's condition at the bedside where other patients are also present, confidentiality is not protected. There are occasions when law mandates disclosure of confidential information, like informing to the police about medicolegal cases, reporting certain notifiable diseases, disclosing professional secrets to the Court if asked to do so. While treating the patients suffering from mental illness, physician has a duty to disclose and warn others if the patient threatens to be violent or has self-harm tendency, in the latter case, divulging professional secrets to next of kin becomes necessary.

Respect for autonomy obligates the physicians not to deceive patients, and tell the truth about their diagnosed illness, unless they clearly wish not to be told about the illness. In the practice of medicine, sometimes there are situations where telling the absolute truth may not be the best option. Medical professionals often have to give bad news of poor prognosis or impending death to the patients. The Six-Step Protocol for Delivering Bad News in the context of oncologic practice (SPIKES) is well known for training the physician in an empathetic way to deliver the information related to terminal illness of the patient with limited survival.[4] They should weigh the benefit against the detriment before disclosing the truth as it may be more ethical to withhold the truth partially for the time being and disclose it in bits over time to avoid overwhelming the patient or relatives. If on a specialist psychiatric evaluation, there is a tangible risk of exacerbating existing medical condition due to the attendant stress response, the doctor may take into confidence the next of the kin, in whom disclosures regarding prognosis may be done. But the same should be documented to avoid any ambiguity. In medical practice, there are situations that challenge the principle of autonomy and create ethical dilemmas in decision making.

Beneficence

Beneficence refers to the actions that promote well-being of others. It is the moral obligation to do good for others and to help them in an active way. In medical practice, it means taking actions that are beneficial to the patient based on the patient's point of view as well.

Nonmaleficence

Nonmaleficence is a concept of *not causing harm* to others. This principle is well expressed in the Latin phrase, *'primum non nocere'* which means *'first do no harm.'*[5] It is not enough to just prevent intentional harm, but, one must be appropriately cautious not to cause harm. In the practice of medicine, however, almost all treatments carry some risk of injury. It is significant to know how likely it is that the proposed treatment will cause harm to the patient. This needs empirical information from reliable medical research about the probabilities of various harms and benefits possible with the proposed intervention. This concept also explains the need for practicing 'evidence-based medicine'. The obligation to provide net benefit over harm requires the medical professionals to be clear about the risks present and their probability, when they make assessments of benefit over harm. The medical practitioner, must therefore, consider the principles of beneficence and non- maleficence together and try to produce net benefit over harm. A single action may have combined implications of beneficence and nonmaleficence, which in medical ethics is referred to as *"double effect"*. A classic example of the double effect is administration of high dose of morphine to relieve pain in a patient suffering from advanced stage of malignancy. Such an act has combined effect of beneficence (relieving the pain) and maleficence (respiratory suppression leading to death of the patient).

Conflict Between Autonomy and Beneficence/Nonmaleficence

Sometimes the patient may disagree with the proposed management, which the physician believes to be the best for the patient, on the basis of medical literature. This usually occurs when a patient's interest clashes with patient's welfare leading to conflict between the principles of autonomy and beneficence. For example, a Jehovah patient may refuse blood transfusion due to religious or cultural views. Also, the patient may want unnecessary treatment which may cause medically unnecessary potential risks as in case of hypochondria or with body dysmorphic syndrome where the patient demands cosmetic surgery without indication. In such ethical dilemmas, usually the physician, just to nurture healthy physician-patient relationship, submits to the principle of autonomy and acts as per the patient's desires but the physician must do his best to balance the patient's welfare. In such cases if complication/undesired outcome occurs, the chances of allegation of medical malpractice is higher and it is far more challenging for the treating medical professional to defend his actions. He must get the written informed consent signed by the patient; documenting in detail the treatment to be followed and the probability of risks involved.

Equitable and Distributive Justice

Justice is the moral obligation to act on the basis of fairness. In simplistic sense, justice refers to equality. However, it does not mean treating all individuals the same. It is important to treat equals equally and to treat unequals unequally, in proportion to their morally relevant inequalities. Medical practitioner must recognize the competing moral concerns and take fair decisions. In the context of healthcare resources, justice requires providing sufficient healthcare to meet the needs of all who need it and if this is impossible, to provide healthcare resources in proportion to the extent of individual's need for healthcare. The concept of Triage is borne out of this principle. The medical resources are limited but the patient demand is unlimited. So, allocating or rationing medical resources in a proper way following the principles of justice is the best way forward. The same came under limelight in the wake of COVID-19 pandemic quite frequently where allocation of intensive care unit (ICU) beds on the basis of bonafide criteria was felt.

PATERNALISM vs. AUTONOMY: WHAT SERVES THE PATIENT BEST?

Paternalism

Paternalism comes from the Latin word, *"pater"* which means *to act like a father* or to *treat another person like a child*. Paternalism propounds that someone can better protect the interests of others, based on the value that *'father knows what is best for the children'*. Paternalism has a long history in the medical profession. From the days when the *Hippocratic* principles were developed, the physician has been recognized as a guardian who uses his specialized knowledge and experience to decide the patient's benefit. The primary theory behind the *Hippocratic Oath* is the principle of beneficence which clearly reflects in the original oath as the resolve to serve "for the benefit of the sick, according to the physician's ability and judgment". The relation between physician and the patient resembled that between a caring father and his child, hence the term *"paternalism"*. Such a father-child relationship stood firm and unchallenged for centuries. Until much of the 20th century, society acknowledged that the physicians were in the best position to make medical decisions on behalf of the patients.

Does Paternalism Really Serve the Purpose?

Medical ethics obligates the medical practitioner to do what is in the best interest of the patient. The real challenge is the interpretation: *"what is the best interest of the patient?"* In patient-physician interaction, there is asymmetric information, as the physician has access to technical knowledge and skill which the patient lacks, and the patient has access to personal preferences that are at times difficult to express. This bifocal vision may result in different perceptions and the physician's opinion may not coincide with the patient's view. The physician's efforts to do the best for the patient may advertently or inadvertently disregard the patient's wishes.

When the patient is not in a position to act willingly or autonomously, the paternalistic approach to prevent the patient from doing harm to himself, seems justified. For instance, emergency treatment to save the life of a dying patient at the critical time when there is no time to wait for patient's autonomy, termed as *weak paternalism*, might be morally justified. On the other hand, *strong paternalism*, which overrides the clearly voluntary action, is difficult to justify.

Paternalism is argued on the notion that, "It is the patient's life or health which is at stake, not the physician's so it must be the patient, not the physician, who must be allowed to decide whether the game is worth the candle."[6] John Stuart Mill, a British philosopher expressed that a competent person's freely made decision should never be overridden, even for that person's own good. He wrote: *"the only purpose for which power can be rightfully exercised over any member of a civilized community, against his will, is to prevent harm to others. His own good, either physical or moral, is not a sufficient warrant. He cannot rightfully be compelled to do or forbear because it will be better for him to do so, because it will make him happier, because in the opinion of others, to do so would be wise or even right."*[7]

Changing Ethos: Paternalism to Patient Autonomy

Paternalistic philosophy has a long history from the time of Hippocrates well into the 20th century until 1960s. After this long era of unchallenged and well-accepted paternalism, tremendous changes occurred that transformed predominantly paternalistic ideology: "*doctor knows the best*" to "*patient autonomy or self-determination*". In the present era, the medical paternalism has come under criticism through the concept of patient's authority to take decision on his medical needs. The concept of patient autonomy or self-determination has emerged as dominant ethos in the medical practice, worldwide.[8] The MCI Regulations, 2002,[9] as amended up to date, clearly stipulates the need to respect the patient's autonomy and doctor's obligation to adequately inform the patient for self-determination. The nature of the patient–doctor relationship has to be examined in the light of education and access to the knowledge of ordinary citizen in the present day. In the light of these facts and statutory provisions, the "Bolam Test" can no longer be applied to a doctor's advice to his or her patient, unless it complies with the statutory provisions. Much has changed nowadays. It is said that Bolam to Montgomery is the new journey and the UK Court in "Montgomery (Appellant) vs. Lanarkshire Health Board (Respondent) (Scotland)"[10] has almost diluted the effect of Bolam Test in view of the present-day advancement and availability of information to the patients and their attendants. While taking the medical decisions, it requires that medical benefits be weighed, not only against medical risks, but nonmedical values as well. For illustration, a medical decision that advises a couple to refrain from reproduction due to the genetic risks that they may face in having children, has not addressed the ethical issue from the couple's perspective. In such a situation patient autonomy empowers the couple, after receiving all the necessary medical information, to take the final decision to beget a child or not.

Supporters of paternalism may criticize that, "*offering full information and allowing patients to take crucial medical decisions may lead to unwise and irrational decisions even by technically competent patients*". However, this criticism does not offer any explanation, why a person is presumed as requiring protection from his so-called unwise decisions once they become medical patients, and yet are otherwise entitled to take decisions outside the medical setup (like choosing a life partner, selecting a career option, etc.). There are situations that challenge the principle of pure autonomy and make it complicated to follow on a consistent basis. For example, children, mentally incapacitated patients and patients who are otherwise incompetent to take decisions will be unable to exercise autonomy.

Should Physicians do Whatever Patients Say?[11,12]

The principle of patient autonomy providing moral right to the patients to control their own treatment, may be conceived as imparting obligation to the physicians to respect the medical decisions of their patients. Does that mean physicians have an obligation to do whatever patients say? Nonetheless, a physician should keep in mind that the obligation towards patient's decisions is not absolute as the same is to be weighed upon with other ethical values deserving commitment from the physician. Physicians are bound by their obligation to the medical profession, which may supersede the duty to respect a patient's choice. For example, a patient's wish to terminate life cannot be fulfilled as it violates the values of the medical profession. A more challenging situation may arise when a dying patient (or his family) asks for continuing treatment which is futile as per the physician's opinion. In continuing treatment that will do no good to the patient may be viewed as contrary to the values of the medical profession particularly in the backdrop of limited resources and does not obligate the physician to honor the patient's wishes. An obligation to practice patient autonomy cannot be taken as a simplistic directive to comply with all the expressed wishes of the patient, as the same may run into conflict with other moral values.

What Serves the Patient Best?[13,14]

Acting in the patient's best interest is one of the most fundamental convictions of the medical profession. But, "*what serves the patient best*?" is sometimes an ambiguous decision indeed. Although it is the patient who has to bear the consequences of medical decisions, absolute freedom of patient without necessary deliberations can be counterproductive in patient care. There are many factors that affect even the competent person's ability to make rational choices. Instead of evaluating the choices simultaneously people in reality evaluate them in succession and in this process, they often choose the first option that they consider to offer satisfactory outcome, even though that choice may not be the most rational outcome. These limitations have been called "bounded rationality". Decisions of a competent patient which are rational within the constraints of this "bounded rationality" may not appear rational to the physician without considering these constraints. The exercise of autonomy may fulfill the patient's desire but may not necessarily serve the patient best.

Having said all this, a primary concern remains here, i.e., *what serves the patient best?* One thing is clear that to serve the patient best, patient's involvement in decision making is inevitable, rather the most accepted concept in the current scenario. Generally accepted and much referred concept of "*shared decision making*" lays emphasis on "active participation from both patient and professional in decision making process, and agreement on decision". Both patient and physician discuss the preferences and facts into the decisional process to reach a shared decision. This decision might involve a compromise between the parties as they may not consider it to be the best decision, yet both accept it as treatment to be followed. Trying to find a compromise, which both parties are committed to agree on, will nurture the patient-physician relationship, then simply allowing the patient to make the decision on his own.

ETHICAL GUIDELINES FOR MEDICAL PRACTITIONERS

In India, ethical guidelines for medical practitioners were framed by Medical Council of India (MCI) in the year 2002, titled "Indian Medical Council (Professional Conduct, Etiquette and Ethics) Regulations, 2002. It was further amended in 2016 and 2020 when the detailed guidelines regarding monetary grants/gifts/aids and telemedicine practice guidelines were published respectively.

National Medical Commission Registered Medical Practitioner (Professional Conduct) Regulations, 2023[15]

In exercise of the powers conferred by section 27(1)(b), read with sections 10(b) (f), 16(2), 57(2) zd, zi, zl and zh of the National Medical

Commission Act, 2019 (No. 30 of 2019), the National Medical Commission made Regulations relating to Professional Conduct of Registered Medical Practitioners. These regulations titled as the "National Medical Commission Registered Medical Practitioner (Professional Conduct) Regulations, 2023" were notified on 2nd August, 2023. *The full version may be downloaded from: www.nmc.org.in.*

National Medical Commission Registered Medical Practitioners (Professional Conduct) (Amendment) Regulations, 2023[16]

- On 23rd August 2023, the National Medical Commission amended the said regulations and notified that
- the National Medical Commission Registered Medical Practitioner (Professional Conduct) Regulations, 2023, are hereby held in abeyance with immediate effect.
- National Medical Commission hereby adopts and makes effective with immediate effect the "Indian Medical Council (Professional Conduct, Etiquette and Ethics) Regulations, 2002", as if the same have been made by the Commission by virtue of the powers vested under the National Medical Commission Act, 2019 (Act No. 30 of 2019).
- Indian Medical Council (Professional Conduct, Etiquette and Ethics) Regulations, 2002, shall come into force with immediate effect.
- The National Medical Commission Registered Medical Practitioner (Professional Conduct) Regulations, 2023, shall not be operative and effective till further Gazette Notification on the subject by the National Medical Commission.

Salient features of National Medical Commission Registered Medical Practitioner (Professional Conduct) Regulations, 2023 are compared with theIndian Medical Council (Professional conduct, Etiquette and Ethics) Regulations, 2002 in **Table 1**.

INDIAN MEDICAL COUNCIL (PROFESSIONAL CONDUCT, ETIQUETTE AND ETHICS) REGULATIONS 2002

Chapter 1: Code of Medical Ethics

- A physician shall uphold the dignity and honor of his profession. Reward or financial gain will be a subordinate consideration.
- Only the doctors having qualification recognized by MCI and registered with MCI/State Medical Council(s) are allowed to practice modern system of medicine or surgery.
- A physician should affiliate with associations of allopathic medical professions.
- Physicians should attend CMEs for at least 30 hours every 5 years.

Maintenance of Medical Records

- Physicians shall maintain the medical records of their indoor patients for 3 years from the date of start of the treatment in a standard proforma. If any request is made for medical records by the patients/ authorized attendant or legal authorities, the same may be duly acknowledged and documents shall be issued within 72 hours.
- A physician shall maintain a register of Medical Certificates giving full details of certificates issued. When issuing a

TABLE 1: Quick comparison between Indian Medical Council (Professional Conduct, Etiquette and Ethics) Regulations, 2002 and National Medical Commission Registered Medical Practitioner (Professional Conduct) Regulations, 2023.

Features	*IMC PCEE 2002 [Indian Medical Council (Professional Conduct, Etiquette and Ethics) Regulations, 2002]*	*NMC RMP Professional Conduct Regulations, 2023 [National Medical Commission Registered Medical Practitioner (Professional Conduct) Regulations, 2023]*
Nomenclature	Indian Medical Council (Professional Conduct, Etiquette and Ethics) Regulations, 2002	National Medical Commission Registered Medical Practitioner (Professional Conduct) Regulations, 2023
Composition	8 chapters	5 chapters
Disciplinary action	No levels of disciplinary action as per breach of conduct	Levels of disciplinary action (as per breach of conduct) are graded at five levels
Issuance of medical records on demand	Within 72 hours	Within 5 days
Generic medicine	No detailed guidelines	Generic medicine and prescription guidelines
Declaration by RMP	Not updated	Declaration of Geneva 2017 included and updated
Professional development	Guidelines focus on CMEs	Included guidelines on CPDs (Continuous Professional Development Guidelines)
Punishment and disciplinary action	No provision of monetary penalty	Monetary penalty as per Section 30 of the NMC Act, 2019 can be given by SMC/EMRB

medical certificate enter the identification marks of the patient and keep a copy of the certificate.

- Try to computerize medical records for quick retrieval.

Display of Registration Numbers

- A physician shall display his registration numbers in his clinic and in all his prescriptions, certificates, money receipts given to his patients.
- Physicians shall display as suffix to their names only recognized medical degrees or such certificates/diplomas and memberships/honors which confer professional knowledge or recognize any exemplary qualification/achievements.

Use of Generic Names of Drugs

Every physician should, as far as possible, prescribe drugs with generic names and he shall ensure that there is a rational prescription and use of drugs.

Highest Quality Assurance in Patient Care

A physician shall not employ any attendant who is neither registered nor enlisted under the Medical Acts in force and shall not permit such persons to attend, treat or perform operations upon patients wherever professional discretion or skill is required.

Exposure of Unethical Conduct

A physician should expose incompetent or corrupt, dishonest or unethical conduct of members of the profession.

Payment of Professional Services

A physician should announce his fees before rendering service and not after the operation or treatment is under way. It is unethical to enter into a contract of "no cure no payment." Physician rendering service on behalf of the state shall refrain from anticipating or accepting any consideration.

Evasion of Legal Restrictions

The physician shall observe the laws of the country in regulating the medical profession and shall also not assist others to evade such laws. He should cooperate in observance and enforcement of sanitary laws and regulations in the interest of public health.

Chapter 2: Duties of Physicians to their Patients

Obligations to the Sick

- Though a physician is not bound to treat each and every person asking his services, he should be ever ready to respond to the calls of the sick and the injured.
- A physician should try to make his visits at the hour indicated to the patients.
- A physician advising a patient to seek the service of another physician is acceptable; however, in case of emergency a physician must treat the patient. No physician shall arbitrarily refuse treatment to a patient.
- When a patient is suffering from an ailment which is not within the range of experience of the treating physician, he may refuse treatment and refer the patient to another physician.

Secrecy

- Confidences entrusted by patients to him should never be revealed unless it is a legal requirement.
- Physician must determine whether his duty to society requires him to disclose confidential information to protect a healthy person against a communicable disease.

Prognosis

Physician should neither exaggerate nor minimize the gravity of a patient's condition. He should ensure that the patient or his family have such knowledge of the patient's condition as will serve the best interests of the patient and the family.

Never Neglect the Patient

- Physician should not neglect the patient, nor should he withdraw from the case without giving adequate notice to the patient and his family.
- Physicians shall not willfully commit an act of negligence that may deprive his patients from necessary medical care.

Engagement for an Obstetric Case

When a physician engaged to attend an obstetric case is absent and another is sent for and delivery accomplished, the acting physician is entitled to his professional fees, but should secure the patient's consent to resign on the arrival of the physician engaged.

Chapter 3: Duties of Physician in Consultation

Unnecessary Consultations should be Avoided

In case of serious illness and in doubtful or difficult conditions, physician should request consultation. Such consultation should be in the interest of the patient only. Consulting pathologists/radiologists or other diagnostic laboratory investigations should be done judiciously.

Statement to Patient after Consultation

All statements to the patient/representatives should take place in the presence of the consulting physicians, except as otherwise agreed. Differences of opinion should not be divulged unnecessarily but when there is irreconcilable difference of opinion the circumstances should be frankly and impartially explained to the patient/representative.

Treatment after Consultation

- Attending physician may make subsequent variations in the treatment if any unexpected change occurs. At the next consultation, reasons for such variation should be discussed/explained. The same privilege and obligations belong to the consultant who treats patient in emergency, during the absence of attending physician.
- The attending physician may prescribe medicine at any time for the patient, whereas the consultant may prescribe only in case of emergency or as an expert when called for.

Patients Referred to Specialists

When the attending physician refers the patient to a specialist, a case summary should be given to the specialist, who should communicate his opinion in writing to the attending physician.

Fees and Other Charges

- The physician shall display his fees and other charges on the board of his chamber and/or the hospitals he is visiting. The prescription should make clear if the physician himself dispensed any medicine.
- The physician shall write his name and designation in full along with registration number in his prescription letterhead (In Government hospital where the patient load is heavy, name of the prescribing doctor must be written below his/her signature).

Chapter 4: Responsibilities of Physicians to Each Other

Conduct in Consultation

No insincerity/rivalry should be indulged in during consultations. No statement/discussion should be carried on, which would impair the confidence reposed in physician in charge of the case.

Consultant not to Take Charge of the Case

- When a physician has been called for consultation, he should normally not take charge of the case, especially on the solicitation of the patient.
- The consultant shall not criticize the referring physician and shall discuss the diagnosis treatment plan with the referring physician.

Appointment of Substitute

- If a physician requests another physician to attend his patients during his temporary absence, professional courtesy requires the acceptance of such appointment only when he has the capacity to discharge the additional responsibility along with his other duties.
- The physician acting under such an appointment should give the utmost consideration to the interests and reputation of the absent physician and all such patients should be restored to the care of the latter upon his return.

Visiting Another Physician's Case

- When it becomes the duty of a physician occupying an official position to see and report upon an illness or injury, he should communicate to the physician in attendance so as to give him an option of being present.

- The physician occupying an official position should avoid remarks upon the diagnosis or the treatment that has been adopted.

Chapter 5: Duties of Physician to Public and Paramedical Profession

- Physicians should disseminate advice on public health issues. They should play their part in enforcing the laws of the community.
- Physicians, especially those engaged in public health work, should enlighten the public concerning quarantine regulations and measures for the prevention of epidemic and communicable diseases.
- The physician should notify the communicable disease under his care, in accordance with the laws, rules and regulations. When an epidemic occurs, a physician should not abandon his duty for fear of contracting the disease himself.

Chapter 6: Unethical Acts

Physician shall not aid or abet or commit any of the following unethical Acts:

Advertising

- Soliciting of patients directly or indirectly, by a physician, group of physicians or institutions or organizations is unethical. A physician shall not make use of him (or his name) as subject of any form of advertising or publicity through any mode either alone or in conjunction with others which tantamount to invite attention to him or to his professional position, skill, qualification, achievements, attainments, specialties, appointments, associations, affiliations or honors and/or of such character as would ordinarily result in his self-advertisement.
- A physician shall not give to any person, whether for compensation or otherwise, any approval, recommendation, endorsement, certificate, report or statement with respect of any drug, medicine, nostrum remedy, surgical, or therapeutic article, apparatus or appliance or any commercial product or article with respect to any property, quality or use thereof or any test, demonstration or trial thereof, for use in connection with his name, signature, or photograph in any form or manner of advertising through any mode nor shall he boast of cases, operations, cures or remedies or permit the publication of report thereof through any mode.

A physician is permitted to make a formal announcement in press regarding the following:

i. Starting practice.
ii. Change of type of practice.
iii. Changing address.
iv. Temporary absence from duty.
v. Resumption of another practice.
vi. Succeeding to another practice.
vii. Public declaration of charges.

- Printing of self-photograph, or any such material of publicity in the letter head or on sign board of the consulting room or any such clinical establishment shall be regarded as acts of self-advertisement and unethical conduct on the part of the physician. However, printing of sketches, diagrams, picture of human system shall not be treated as unethical.

Patent and Copyrights

A physician may patent surgical instruments, appliances and medicine or copyright applications, methods and procedures. However, it shall be unethical if the benefits of such patents or copyrights are not made available in situations where the interest of large population is involved.

Running an Open Shop (Dispensing of Drugs and Appliances by Physicians)

- A physician should not run an open shop for sale of medicine for dispensing prescriptions prescribed by doctors other than himself or for sale of medical or surgical appliances. It is not unethical for a physician to prescribe or supply drugs, remedies or appliances as long as there is no exploitation of the patient.
- Drugs prescribed by a physician or brought from the market for a patient should explicitly state the proprietary formulae as well as generic name of the drug.

Rebates and Commission

- A physician shall not give, solicit, or receive nor shall he offer to give solicit or receive, any gift, gratuity, commission or bonus in consideration of or return for the referring, recommending or procuring of any patient for medical, surgical or other treatment.
- A physician shall not directly or indirectly, participate in or be a party to the act of division, transference, assignment, subordination, rebating, splitting or refunding of any fee for medical, surgical or other treatment.

The above-mentioned provisions shall apply to the referring, recommending or procuring by a physician or any person, specimen or material for diagnostic purposes or other study/work. However, there is no prohibition on payment of salaries by a qualified physician to other duly qualified person rendering medical care under his supervision.

Secret Remedies

The prescribing or dispensing by a physician of secret remedial agents of which he does not know the composition, or the manufacture or promotion of their use is unethical and as such prohibited. All the drugs prescribed by a physician should always carry a proprietary formula and clear name.

Human Rights

The physician shall not aid or abet torture nor shall he be a party to either infliction of mental or physical trauma or concealment of torture inflicted by some other person or agency in clear violation of human rights.

Euthanasia

- Practicing euthanasia shall constitute unethical conduct. However, the question of withdrawing supporting devices to sustain cardiopulmonary function even after brain death, shall be decided by a team of doctors and not merely by the treating physician alone.
- A team of doctors shall declare withdrawal of support system. Such team shall consist of the doctor in- charge of the patient, Chief Medical Officer/Medical Officer in-charge of the hospital and a doctor nominated by the in-charge of the hospital from the hospital staff or in accordance with the provisions of the Transplantation of Human Organ Act, 1994.

Code of Conduct for Doctors and Professional Association of Doctors in their Relationship with Pharmaceutical and Allied Health Sector Industry

In dealing with pharmaceutical and allied health sector industry, a physician shall follow the stipulations given below:

a. *Gifts:* A physician shall not receive any gift from any pharmaceutical or allied healthcare industry and their sales people or representatives.
b. *Travel facilities:* A physician shall not accept any travel facility inside the country or outside, from any pharmaceutical or allied healthcare industry or their representatives for self and family members for vacation or for attending conferences, seminars, workshops, CMEs, etc. as a delegate.
c. *Hospitality:* A physician shall not accept individually any hospitality like hotel accommodation for self and family members under any pretext.
d. *Cash or monetary grants:* A physician shall not receive any cash or monetary grants from any pharmaceutical and allied healthcare industry for individual purpose in individual capacity under any pretext. Funding for medical research, study, etc. can only be received through approved institutions by modalities laid down by law/rules/guidelines adopted by such approved institutions, in a transparent manner. It shall always be fully disclosed.
e. *Medical research:* A physician may carry out or participate in research projects funded by pharmaceutical and allied healthcare industries. A physician is obliged to know that the fulfillment of the following items (i) to (vii) will be an imperative for undertaking any research assignment/project funded by industry—for being proper and ethical:

   A physician shall ensure that:
   i. Research proposal(s) has due permission from the competent concerned authorities.
   ii. Research project(s) has the clearance of national/state/institutional ethics committees/bodies.
   iii. It fulfills all the legal requirements prescribed for medical research.
   iv. Source and amount of funding is publicly disclosed at the beginning itself.
   v. Proper care and facilities are provided to human volunteers, if they are necessary for the research project(s).
   vi. Undue animal experimentations are not done and when these are necessary, they are done in a scientific and a humane way.
   vii. While accepting such an assignment a medical practitioner shall have the freedom to publish the results of research in the greater interest of the society by inserting such a clause in the MoU or any other document/agreement for any such assignment.
f. *Maintaining professional autonomy:* In dealing with pharmaceutical and allied healthcare industry, a medical practitioner shall always ensure that there shall be no compromise either with his/her own professional autonomy and/or with the autonomy and freedom of the medical institution.
g. *Affiliation:* A physician may work for pharmaceutical and allied healthcare industries in advisory capacities, as consultants, as researchers, as treating doctors or in any other professional capacity. In doing so, physician shall always ensure that:
   i. His professional integrity and freedom are maintained.
   ii. Patient's interests are not compromised in any way.
   iii. Such affiliations are within the law.
   iv. Such affiliations/employments are fully transparent and disclosed.
h. *Endorsement:* A physician shall not endorse any drug or product of the

industry publicly. Any study conducted on the efficacy or otherwise of such products shall be presented to and/or through scientific bodies or published in scientific journals in a proper way.

Chapter 7: Misconduct

The following acts of commission or omission on the part of a physician shall constitute professional misconduct rendering him/her liable for disciplinary action:

Violation of the Regulations

If a physician commits violation of any of these regulations:

- *Adultery or improper conduct:* Abuse of professional position by committing adultery or improper conduct with a patient or by maintaining an improper association with a patient will render a physician liable for disciplinary action.
- *Conviction by Court of law:* Conviction by a Court of Law for offences involving moral turpitude/criminal acts.
- *Sex determination tests:*
    - Sex determination test shall not be undertaken with intention to terminate a female fetus, unless there are other absolute indications for termination of pregnancy as specified in the MTP Act, 1971.
    - Any act of termination of pregnancy of normal female fetus amounting to female feticide is a professional misconduct by the physician leading to penal erasure besides rendering him liable to criminal proceedings as per the provisions of this Act.
- *Signing Professional Certificates, Reports and other Documents*
    - Physicians may be required to give certificates, notification, reports and other similar documents in their professional capacity for subsequent use in the courts or for administrative purposes, etc.
    - Any physician who is shown to have signed or given under his name and authority any such certificate, notification, report or similar document which is untrue, misleading or improper, is liable to have his name deleted from the Register.
- Physicians shall not contravene the provisions of the Drugs & Cosmetics Act and regulations made thereunder. Prescribing steroids/psychotropic drugs when there is no absolute medical indication or selling Schedule H & L drugs and poisons to the public except to his patient; in contravention of the above provisions shall constitute gross professional misconduct on the part of the physician.
- Performing or enabling unqualified person to perform an abortion or any illegal operation for which there is no medical, surgical or psychological indication.
- A physicians shall not issue certificates of efficiency in modern medicine to unqualified or nonmedical person.
- A physician should not contribute to the lay press articles and give interviews regarding diseases and treatments which may have the effect of advertising himself or soliciting practices; but is open to write to the lay press under his own name on matters of public health, hygienic living or to deliver public lectures, give talks on the radio/TV/internet chat for the same purpose and send announcement of the same to lay press.
- An institution run by a physician for a particular purpose such as a maternity home, nursing home, private hospital,

rehabilitation center or any type of training institution, etc. may be advertised in the lay press, but such advertisements should not contain anything more than the name of the institution, type of patients admitted, type of training and other facilities offered and the fees.

- It is improper for a physician to use an unusually large sign board and write on it anything other than his name, qualifications obtained from a University or a statutory body, titles and name of his specialty, registration number including the name of the State Medical Council under which registered. The same should be the contents of his prescription papers. It is improper to affix a signboard on a chemist's shop or in places where he does not reside or work.
- Physicians shall not disclose the secrets of a patient that have been learnt in the exercise of their profession except—(i) in a court of law under orders of the Presiding Judge; (ii) in circumstances where there is a serious and identified risk to a specific person and/or community; and (iii) notifiable diseases. In case of communicable/notifiable diseases, concerned public health authorities should be informed immediately.
- The physicians shall not refuse on religious grounds alone to give assistance in or conduct of sterility, birth control, circumcision and medical termination of pregnancy when there is medical indication, unless the medical practitioner feels himself/herself incompetent to do so.
- Before performing an operation, the physician should obtain in writing the consent from the husband or wife, parent or guardian in the case of minor, or the patient himself as the case may be. In an operation which may result in sterility the consent of both husband and wife is needed.
- Physicians shall not publish photographs or case reports of his/her patients without their permission, in any medical or other journal in a manner by which their identity could be made out. If the identity is not to be disclosed, consent is not needed.
- In the case of running of a nursing home by a physician and employing assistants to help him, the ultimate responsibility rests on the physician.
- Physician shall not use touts or agents for procuring patients.
- Physician shall not claim to be specialist unless he has a special qualification in that branch.
- In vitro fertilization or artificial insemination shall not be undertaken without informed consent of the female patient and her spouse as well as the donor. Such consent shall be obtained in writing only after the patient is provided, at her own level of comprehension, with sufficient information about the purpose, methods, risks, inconveniences, disappointments of the procedure and possible risks and hazards.

Chapter 8: Punishment and Disciplinary Action

The offences and misconduct given above do not constitute a complete list of the infamous acts which calls for disciplinary action. MCI or State Medical Councils can also deal with any other form of professional misconduct on the part of a registered practitioner.

- Any complaint with regard to professional misconduct can be made to the appropriate Medical Council for Disciplinary action. Upon receipt of any complaint, the appropriate Medical Council would hold an enquiry and give opportunity to the registered medical practitioner to be heard in person or by pleader.

- If the medical practitioner is found to be guilty of committing professional misconduct, the appropriate Medical Council may award such punishment as deemed necessary or may direct the removal altogether or for a specified period, from the register of the name of the delinquent registered practitioner. Deletion from the Register shall be widely publicized in local press as well as in the publications of different Medical Associations/Societies/Bodies.
- In case the punishment of removal from the register is for a limited period, the appropriate Council may also direct that the name so removed shall be restored in the register after the expiry of the period for which the name was ordered to be removed.
- Decision on complaint against delinquent physician shall be taken within 6 months. During the pendency of the complaint the appropriate Council may restrain the physician from performing the procedure or practice which is under scrutiny. Professional incompetence shall be judged by peer group as per guidelines prescribed by MCI.
- Where either on a request or otherwise the MCI is informed that any complaint against a delinquent physician has not been decided by a State Medical Council within 6 months from the date of receipt of complaint by it and further the MCI has reason to believe that there is no justified reason for not deciding the complaint within the said prescribed period, the MCI may—(i) Impress upon the concerned State Medical Council to conclude and decide the complaint within a time bound schedule; (ii) May decide to withdraw the said complaint pending with the concerned State

Format for Medical Record (See Regulation 3.1)

Name of the patient: .... Age: .... Sex: ....

Address: .... Occupation: ....

Date of 1st visit: ....

Clinical notes (Summary) of the case: ....

Provisional diagnosis ....

Investigations advised with reports: ....

Diagnosis after investigation: ....

Advice: ....

Follow-up: ....

Date: ....

Observations: ....

Signature in full ....

Name of treating physician

Medical Council straightaway or after the expiry of the period which had been stipulated by the MCI in accordance with para (i) above, to itself and refer the same to the Ethical Committee of the Council for its expeditious disposal in a period of not more than 6 months from the receipt of the complaint in the office of the MCI.

- Any person aggrieved by the decision of the State Medical Council on any complaint against a delinquent physician, can appeal to MCI within 60 days from the date of receipt of the order passed by the said Medical Council. If MCI is satisfied that the appellant was prevented by sufficient cause from presenting the appeal within the aforesaid 60 days, may allow it to be presented within a further period of 60 days.

REFERENCES

1. Theodore Roosevelt. The strenuous life: essays and addresses. Dover Publications; 2009.
2. Schloendorff v. Society of New York Hospital, 211 N.Y. 125, 105 N.E. 92.
3. Raanan Gillon. Medical Ethics: four principles plus attention to scope. BMJ. 1994;309:184-8.
4. Baile WF, Buckman R, Lenzi R, Glober G, Beale EA, Kudelka AP. SPIKES – A Six-Step Protocol for Delivering Bad News: Application to the Patient with Cancer. Oncologist. 2000;5(4):302-11.
5. Dana JL. The four principles of biomedical ethics: a foundation for current bioethical debate. J Chiropr Humnit. 2007;14:34-40.
6. Mathews E. Can paternalism be modernized? J Med Ethics. 1986;12:133-5.
7. Mill JS. On liberty. 1869. Library of economics and liberty. Available: http://www.econlib.org/library/Mill/mllbty.html
8. Rothman DJ (1991). Strangers at the Bedside: A history of how law and bioethics transformed medical decision making, 1992, Basic Books.
9. The Indian Medical Council (Professional Conduct, Etiquette and Ethics) Regulations, 2002. Issues Med Ethics. 2002;10(3):66-70. [online] Available at: https://ijme.in/articles/the-indian-medical-council-professional-conduct-etiquette-and-ethics-regulations-2002/. [Last accessed, March 2024].
10. Montgomery (Appellant) v. Lanarkshire Health Board. 2015 UKSC 11 On appeal from: [2013] CSIH 3; [2010] CSIH 104. Judgment of UK Supreme Court. [online] Available from https://www.supremecourt.uk/cases/docs/uksc-2013-0136-judgment.pdf. [Last accessed, March 2024].
11. Leng S. Who's in control? Why both doctors and patients are frustrated. [online] Available: http://www.kevinmd.com/blog/2013/11/control-doctors-patients-frustrated.html. [Last accessed, March 2024].
12. Blustein J. Doing what the patient orders: maintaining integrity in the doctor-patient relationship. Bioethics. 1993;7(4):290-314.
13. Charles C, Gafni A, Whelan T. Shared decision-making in the medical encounter: What does it mean? (or it takes at least two to tango). Soc Sci Med. 1997;44(5):681-92.
14. Charles C, Whelan T, Gafni A. What do we mean by partnership in making decisions about treatment? BMJ. 1999;319:780-2.
15. National Medical Commission Registered Medical Practitioner (Professional Conduct) Regulations, 2023. [online] Available at: https://www.nmc.org.in/rules-regulations/national-medical-commission-registered-medical-practitioner-professional-conduct-regulations-2023-reg/. [Last accessed, December 2024].
16. National Medical Commission Registered Medical Practitioners (Professional Conduct) (Amendment) Regulations, 2023. [online] Available at: https://www.nmc.org.in/ActivitiWebClient/open/getDocument?path=/Documents/Public/Portal/NmcGazette/248297.pdf. [Last accessed, December 2024].

SECTION 2

Legislations Related to Obstetrics and Gynecology

CHAPTER 4

Medicolegal Aspects of Abortion and Medical Termination of Pregnancy

Ashima Taneja, Muskan Soni

INTRODUCTION

Medical termination of pregnancy, a willful way of ending the pregnancy (by using medical or surgical methods), is regulated by the provisions of law. The Medical Termination of Pregnancy (MTP) Act is a legislation to provide for the termination of certain pregnancies by Registered Medical Practitioners and for matters connected therewith or incidental thereto.[1] This Act is an empowering legislation, and it has played a vital role in reducing the maternal mortality associated with illegal and unsafe abortions. '*Ignorance of Law is no excuse for its breach*,' and thus, it is imperative to understand medicolegal aspects of Medical Termination of Pregnancy.

OVERVIEW

WHO (2021)

- Approximately 73 million induced abortions occur worldwide annually. Globally 61% of all unintended pregnancies end up as induced abortions.
- Global estimates of 2010–2014 demonstrate that 45% of all induced abortions are unsafe.
- Developing countries accounted for 97% of all unsafe abortions. More than half of all unsafe abortions occur in Asia and Africa.[2]

India

- Around 6.4 million abortions occur annually, and 67% of abortions are unsafe. Each year 4.7–13.2% of maternal deaths are due to unsafe abortions. [3]
- Complications associated with unsafe abortion include incomplete abortion, hemorrhage, infection, uterine perforation, and damage to the genital tract and internal organs as a consequence of inserting dangerous objects into vagina or anus.[4]
- Barriers to access, safety, and respectful abortions include high costs, stigma for those seeking abortions, and refusal of health workers to provide an abortion based on personal conscience or religious beliefs.

THE MEDICAL TERMINATION OF PREGNANCY ACT

In India, until the early 1960s, abortion was considered illegal and, if not conducted in good faith, to save the life of the mother. It was in mid 1960s, when increasing maternal mortality rate, with unsafe abortions attributing as a prime cause, Dr Shantilal Shah Committee proposed the Medical Termination Bill in Lok Sabha and Rajya Sabha.[5] The Bill was passed by the Parliament in August 1971. The MTP Act 1971 came into force on April 1, 1972, for all of India, except Jammu and Kashmir. Subsequently, a few amendments were made based on Article 21 (right to choose) and Article 14 (right to equality) to extend the benefits equally to both married and unmarried women.

THE MEDICAL TERMINATION OF PREGNANCY ACT, 1971 (ACT NO. 34 OF 1971)[1]

An Act to provide for the termination of certain pregnancies by registered Medical Practitioners and for matters connected therewith or incidental thereto. Be it enacted by Parliament in the 22nd year of the Republic of India as follows:

Section 2: Definitions

In this Act, unless the context otherwise requires:

a. *Guardian:* Refers to a person caring for a minor or lunatic*.
b. *Lunatic*:* Meaning has been assigned to it in Section 3 of the Indian Lunatic Act of 1912 (4 of 1912).
c. *Minor:* Refers to a person who, under the provisions of the Indian Majority Act, 1875 (9 of 1875), is deemed not to have attained his majority.
d. *Registered medical practitioner:* This refers to a medical practitioner who possesses any recognized medical qualification as defined in clause (h) of Section 2 of the Indian Medical Council Act, 1956, (102 of 1956), whose name has been entered in a State Medical Register and who has such experience or training in Gynecology and obstetrics as may be prescribed by rules made under this Act.

Section 3: When a Registered Medical Practitioner Terminate a Pregnancy?

- *Section 3(1):* Notwithstanding anything contained in the Indian Penal Code (45 of 1860), a registered medical practitioner shall not be guilty of any offence under that Code or under any other law for the time being in force, if any pregnancy is terminated by him in accordance with the provisions of this Act.
- *Section 3(2): Section 3(2) of the principal Act has been amended* by the Medical Termination of Pregnancy (Amendment) Act 2021. The changes as per the amendment have been provided in the next heading of the MTP (Amendment) Act 2021.
- *Section 3(3):* In determining whether the continuance of a pregnancy would involve such risk of injury to the health as is mentioned in Section 3(2), account may be taken of the pregnant women's actual or reasonably foreseeable environment.
- *Section 3(4)(a):* No pregnancy of a woman, who has not attained the age of 18 years, or, who, having attained the age of 18 years, is a lunatic, shall be terminated except with the consent in writing of her guardian.
- *Section 4(b):* Save as otherwise provided in clause (a), no pregnancy shall be terminated except with the consent of the pregnant woman.

Section 4: Place Where Pregnancy may be Terminated

a. A hospital established or maintained by the Government, or
b. A place for the time being approved for the purpose of this Act by the Government.

Section 5: Sections 3 and 4 When not to Apply

1. The provisions of section 4, and so much of the provisions of sub-section (2) of section 3 related to the length of the pregnancy

*The Lunacy Acts 1890–1922 referred to "lunatics", but the Mental Treatment Act 1930 changed the legal term to "person of unsound mind", an expression which was replaced under the Mental Health Act 1959 by "mental illness".

and the opinion of not less than two registered medical practitioners, shall not apply to the termination of a pregnancy by a registered medical practitioner in a case where he is of opinion, formed in good faith, that determination of such pregnancy is immediately necessary to save the life of the pregnant woman.

2. Notwithstanding anything contained in the Indian Penal Code (45 of 1860), the termination of a pregnancy by a person who is not a registered medical practitioners shall be an offence punishable under that Code, and that Code shall, to this extent, stand modified.

Explanation: For the purposes of this section, so much of the provisions of clause (d) of section (2) as relate to the possession, by a registered medical practitioner, of experience or training in gynecology and obstetrics shall not apply.

Protection of action taken in good faith: No suit or legal proceedings shall lie against any registered medical practitioner for any damage caused or likely to be caused by anything, which is in good faith done or intended to be done under this Act.

THE MEDICAL TERMINATION OF PREGNANCY AMENDMENT ACT, 2002 (NO. 64 OF 2002)[6]

Amendment of Section 2

In section 2 of the MTP Act, 1971, (hereinafter referred to as the principal Act), -

i. In clause (a), for the word "lunatic", the words "mentally ill person" shall be substituted.
ii. For clause (b), the following clause shall be substituted, namely:

"(b) 'Mentally ill person' means a person who is in need of treatment by reason of any mental disorder other than mental retardation".

Amendment of Section 3

In section 3 of the principal Act, in sub-section (4), in clause (a), for the word "lunatic", the words "mentally ill person" shall be substituted.

Substitution of New Section for Section 4: Place where Pregnancy may be Terminated

For Section 4 of the Principal Act, the following section shall be substituted:

"4. No termination of pregnancy shall be made in accordance with this Act at any place other than:

a. a hospital established or maintained by the Government, or
b. a place for the time being approved for the purpose of this Act by the Government or a District Level Committee constituted by that Government with the Chief Medical Officer or District Health Officer as the Chairperson of the said Committee:

Provided that the District Level Committee shall consist of not less than three and not more than five members including the Chairperson, as the Government may specify from time to time:"

Amendment of Section 5

In section 5 of the principal Act, for sub-section (2) and the Explanation thereto, the following shall be substituted:

"(2) Notwithstanding anything contained in the Indian Penal Code, the termination of pregnancy by a person who is not a registered medical practitioner shall be an offence punishable with rigorous imprisonment for a term which shall not be less than 2 years but which may extend to 7 years under that Code, and that Code shall, to this extent, stand modified.

(3) Whoever terminates any pregnancy in a place other than that mentioned in section 4, shall be punishable with rigorous imprisonment for a term which shall not be less than 2 years but which may extend to 7 years.

(4) Any person being owner of a place which is not approved under clause (b) of section 4 shall be punishable with rigorous imprisonment for a term which shall not be less than 2 years but which may extend to 7 years.

Explanation 1: For the purposes of this section, the expression 'owner' in relation to a place means any person who is the administrative head or otherwise responsible for the working or maintenance of a hospital or place, by whatever name called, where the pregnancy may be terminated under this Act.

Explanation 2: For the purposes of this section, so much of the provisions of clause (d) of section 2 as relate to the possession, by registered medical practitioner, of experience or training in gynecology and obstetrics shall not apply".

MEDICAL TERMINATION OF PREGNANCY (AMENDMENT) ACT 2021 (FLOWCHART 1)[7]

Amendment of Section 2

In section 2 of the Medical Termination of Pregnancy Act, 1971 (hereinafter referred to as the principal Act):

i. after clause (*a*), the following clause shall be inserted, namely: (*aa*) "Medical Board" means the Medical Board constituted under sub-section (2C) of section 3 of the Act;
ii. after clause (*d*), the following clause shall be inserted, namely: (*e*) "termination of pregnancy" means a procedure to terminate a pregnancy by using medical or surgical methods.

Amendment of Section 3

In section 3 of the principal Act, for sub-section (2), the following sub-sections shall be substituted, namely:

Section 3, subsection (2): Subject to the provisions of sub-section (4), a pregnancy

Flowchart 1: Salient features of the MTP Act 2021.[7]

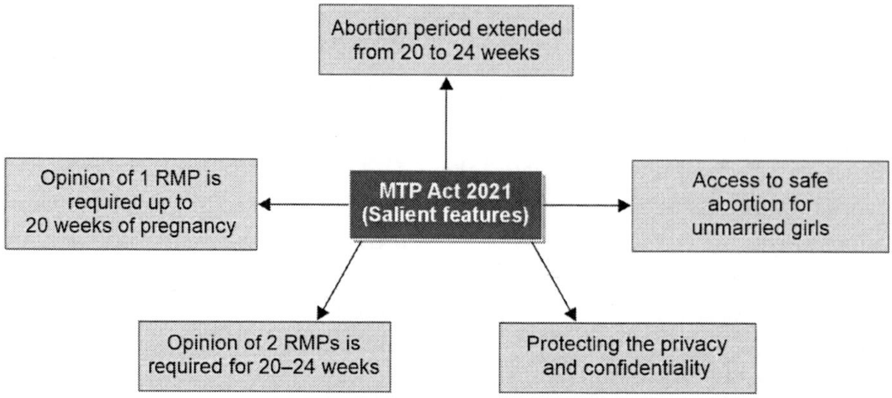

may be terminated by a Registered Medical Practitioner:

a. where the length of the pregnancy does not exceed 20 weeks, if such medical practitioner is, or
b. where the length of the pregnancy exceeds 20 weeks but does not exceed 24 weeks in case of such category of woman as may be prescribed by rules made under this Act, if not less than two registered medical practitioners are, of the opinion, formed in good faith, that:
    i. the continuance of the pregnancy would involve a risk to the life of the pregnant woman or of grave injury to her physical or mental health; or
    ii. there is a substantial risk that if the child were born, it would suffer from any serious physical or mental abnormality.

Explanation 1: For the purposes of clause (a), where any pregnancy occurs as a result of failure of any device or method used by any woman or her partner for the purpose of limiting the number of children or preventing pregnancy, the anguish caused by such pregnancy may be presumed to constitute a grave injury to mental health of pregnant women.

Explanation 2: For the purposes of clauses (a) and (b), where any pregnancy is alleged by the pregnant woman to have been caused by rape, the anguish caused by the pregnancy shall be presumed to constitute a grave injury to the mental health of pregnant women.

Section 3(2A)	The norms for the registered medical practitioner whose opinion is required for termination of pregnancy at different gestational age shall be such as may be prescribed by rules made under this Act

Section 3(2B)	The provisions of subsection (2) relating to the length of the pregnancy shall not apply to the termination of pregnancy by the medical practitioner where such termination is necessitated by the diagnosis of any of the substantial fetal abnormalities diagnosed by a Medical Board
Section 3(2C)	Every State Government or Union Territory, as the case may be, shall, by notification in the Official Gazette, constitute a Board to be called a Medical Board for the purposes of this Act to exercise such powers and functions as may be prescribed by rules made under this Act
Section 3(2D)	The Medical Board shall consist of the following, namely: a. Gynecologist, b. Pediatrician, c. Radiologist or Sonologist; and d. Such other number of members as may be notified in the Official Gazette by the State Government or Union Territory, as the case may be

Insertion of New Section 5A

Section 4	After section 5 of the principal Act, the following section shall be inserted, namely:
Section 5A (1)	No registered medical practitioner shall reveal the name and other particulars of a woman whose pregnancy has been terminated under this Act except to a person authorized by any law for the time being in force
Section 5A (2)	Whoever contravenes the provisions of subsection (1) shall be punishable with imprisonment which may extend to 1 year, or with fine, or with both

- *Medical Opinion for Termination of Pregnancy:*
  a. *Up to 20 weeks of gestation:* Opinion of a single RMP is required for the termination of pregnancy.
  b. *20 to 24 weeks of gestation:* Opinion of two RMPs is required for termination of pregnancy.
  c. *In cases of substantial fetal abnormalities:* If pregnancy needs to be terminated after 24 weeks of gestation, the opinion of a state-level medical board is mandatory. This medical board consists of a Gynecologist, a Sonologist, or Radiologist, a Pediatrician, and any additional members as notified by the respective state government.
- *Rule 3B of the Medical Termination of Pregnancy (Amendment) Rules, 2021:* Women eligible for termination of pregnancy up to 24 weeks—the following categories of women shall be considered eligible for termination of pregnancy under clause (b) of subsection (2) of Section 3 of the Act, for a period of up to 24 weeks, namely:
  i. Survivors of sexual assault or rape or incest.
  ii. Minors
  iii. Change of marital status during the ongoing pregnancy (widowhood and divorce)
  iv. Women with physical disabilities (major disabilities per criteria laid down under the rights of persons with Disabilities Act, 2016)
  v. Mentally ill women including mental retardation
  vi. The fetal malformation that has a substantial risk of being incompatible with life or if the child is born it may suffer from such physical or mental abnormalities to be seriously handicapped
  vii. Pregnant women in humanitarian settings, disasters, or emergencies may be decided by the government.
- The amendment raised the maximum gestational age at which a woman may obtain a medical abortion from 20 weeks under the MTP Act of 1971 to 24 weeks.
- *Confidentiality:*
  a. The confidentiality of information, including the identity of the woman whose pregnancy has been terminated, must be strictly maintained, except when authorized by the prevailing law.
  b. Failure to adhere to this directive may result in punishment for imprisonment for 1 year, with or without a fine as specified.

Failure of contraception as a ground for abortion until 20 weeks now available to a woman and "her partner:"

- Under the MTP Act 1971, failure of contraception as a ground for abortion was available only to a "married woman" or her "husband".
- The MTP Amendment Act 2021 expanded this to "any woman" or "her partner," Now, unmarried women in relationships can now invoke failure of contraception as a ground to seek abortion.

Medical Boards to decide abortions beyond 24 weeks under specific circumstances:

- The MTP Act, 1971 did not have the provision of such authorization.
- Although Medical Boards had been set up in post 20-weeks cases at the Court's direction.
- The MTP Amendment Act, 2021 provides for the constitution of Medical Boards which may "allow or deny termination of pregnancy" beyond 24 weeks **(Table 1 and Flowchart 2).**

TABLE 1: Quick comparison of the MTP Act 1971 and the MTP Amendment Act, 2021.

Gestational limits	*MTP Act 1971*	*MTP Amendment Act, 2021*
Until 12 weeks	Advice of one doctor	Advice of one doctor
12–20 weeks	Advice of two doctors	Advice of one doctor
20–24 weeks	Only to save the life of the pregnant woman	Advice of two doctors if the pregnant woman falls under categories prescribed
After 24 weeks	Only to save the life of the pregnant woman	Approval of Medical Board, and only if there is substantial fetal "abnormality"

Flowchart 2: Medical Termination of Pregnancy (As per the MTP Act).[7]

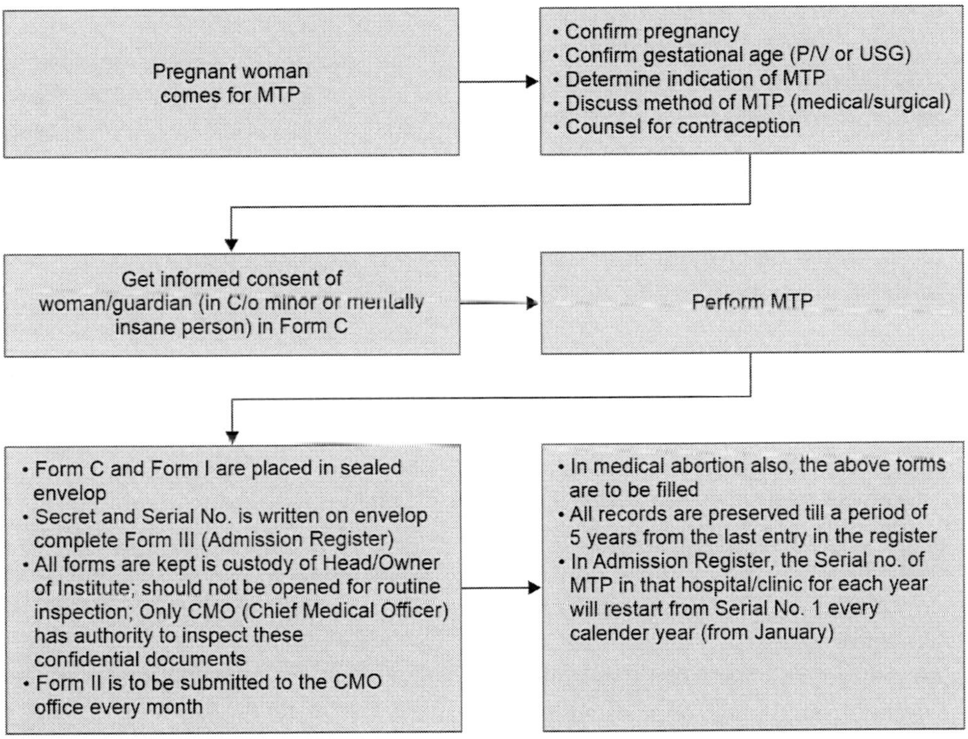

PROBLEMS WITH IMPLEMENTATION OF THE MTP ACT

Availability of Experts

The MTP Act states that abortions should be performed only by doctors specialized in Obstetrics and Gynecology. However, as per the 2019–2020 report on rural health statistics by the Ministry of Health and Family Welfare, there is a 70% shortage of obstetricians in India. This forces women to choose illegal and unsafe abortions, which leads to higher maternal mortality rates.

Availability of Over-the-Counter Drugs

The Federation of Obstetrics and Gynaecological Societies of India (FOGSI) and WHO recognize that, Mifepristone-Misoprostol administration for MTP up to 49 days from LMP (last menstrual period) is safe and effective as per the Drugs Controller of India. So, distribution of these drugs should be closely monitored to prevent unsafe abortions.[8]

Medicolegal Issues

a. The number of RMPs is relevant only for forming an opinion. Once the opinion has been formed, definite termination of pregnancy may be performed by one RMP. It is not necessary that more than one registered medical practitioner should act together to terminate a pregnancy.
b. Even during the "first trimester", the woman cannot abort at her will and pleasure. There is no question of "abortion on demand." Section 3 is only an enabling provision to save the RMP from the purview of the IPC.
c. The State Family Welfare Department of Maharashtra released a list of lethal congenital anomalies in January 2020. Screening tests are not sufficient to diagnose lethal congenital anomalies, and chromosomal defects should be confirmed by diagnostic tests such as Amniocentesis, chorionic villus sampling (CVS). The social and economic conditions of parents do not help to use fetal indications if the anomalies are nonlethal.

POCSO ACT: THE PROTECTION OF CHILDREN FROM SEXUAL OFFENCES 2012 [NO. 32 OF 2012] [19TH JUNE 2012]

- An Act to protect children from offences of sexual assault, sexual harassment and pornography and provide for establishment of Special Courts for trial of such offences and for matters connected therewith or incidental thereto.[9]
- The POCSO Act was legislated on 14th November 2012. It is gender-neutral and recognizes that young boys can also be victims of sexual violence.
- It defines a child as someone under the age of 18.
- It extended the definition of sexual assault to include nonpenetrative sexual assault as well as aggravated penetrative sexual assault. It also incorporated grave punishment for persons in positions of trust or authority like public servants, staff of educational institutions, hospitals, remand home, protection or observation home, police officer, any member of armed or security forces. Remarkably, this law recognizes sexual harassment of a child which involves touch, and also that which does not such as stalking, making a child expose themselves or exposing themselves to a child, and so on. The POCSO Act also specifically lays down rigorous punishments for exposing children to or using them to create child sexual abuse material (CSAM, also referred to as child pornography).
- This child protection law is also unique because it places the burden of proof on the accused, following "guilty until proven innocent," unlike the BNS.
- Under the provisions of the POCSO Act, a child is entitled to the following:
    - Getting their statement recorded at their residence or a place of their choice, and preferably by a woman police official or an official not below the sub-inspector rank, in civilian clothes.
    - The police official should ensure that during the investigation, the child should not come in contact with the accused.

- The child cannot be detained at the police station at night, and his/her identity should be protected from the public and media, unless directed otherwise by a Special Court.
- If the survivor is a girl, the medical examination should be performed by a woman doctor, and the examination can only be performed in the presence of a parent or a person the child trusts. If neither of the two are present, then the examination should be performed in the presence of a woman nominated by the head of the medical institution.

DOCUMENTATION AND CHECKLIST FOR LEGAL ABORTION

The documentation required as per the provisions of the MTP Act has been provided in **Box 1**.

Regulation 7 (MTP Regulations 2003)[10]

Entries in Registers Maintained in Hospital or Approved Place

No entry shall be made in any case sheet, operation theatre register, follow-up card, or any other document or register other than admission register, indicating that the name of the pregnant woman and reference to the pregnant woman shall be made therein by serial no. assigned to the women in the Admission Register.

BOX 1: Mandatory documentation as per the MTP Act.

Form C	Consent form
Form I	*Opinion form:* RMP shall certify this form within 3 hours from the termination of pregnancy
Form II	Head of the hospital or owner of the place shall send a monthly statement of cases to the CMO of the district in this form
Form III	*Admission register:* An approved site shall maintain case records in Form III. This register is kept for a period of 5 years from the date of last entry

Form III (Admission Register)

- An approved site shall maintain case records in Form III.
- This register is kept for a period of 5 years from the date of last entry.
- Admission Register shall be a secret document.
- Information contained therein as to the Name and other particulars of the pregnant woman shall not be disclosed to any person except under the "*authority of law*".

Form C (Consent for Termination of Pregnancy)

- If a woman is of the age 18 years or more then only her consent is required for the termination of her pregnancy.
- If a woman has not attained the age of 18 years, or is a mentally ill person, then consent of her guardian is required for the termination of her pregnancy.

FORM A: Application Form for Approval of a Private Place

This form is used by the owner of a private place to apply for approval for the establishment of MTP services. Form A has to be submitted to the Chief Medical Officer (CMO) of the district.

FORM B: Certificate of Approval

The certificate of approval of MTP for a "private" place issued by the district level committee chaired by the CMO shall be clearly displayed. The certificate of approval issued by the District Level Committee

FORM A

(See sub-rule (2) of rule 5)[10]

Form of Application for the Approval of a Place Under Clause (B) of Section 4 of the Act

Category of approved place:

(A) Pregnancy can be terminated up to 12 weeks

(B) Pregnancy can be terminated up to 24 weeks

(i) Name of the place (in capital letters): ....

(ii) Address in full: ....

(iii) Non-Government or Private or Nursing Home or Other Institutions:

(iv) State, if the following facilities are available at the place:

Category A

(i) Gynecological examination or labor table.

(ii) Resuscitation equipment.

(iii) Sterilization equipment.

(iv) Facilities for treatment of shock, including emergency drugs.

(v) Facilities for transportations, if required.

Category B

(i) An operation table and instruments for performing abdominal or gynecological surgery.

(ii) Drugs and parental fluids in sufficient supply for emergency cases.

(iii) Anesthetic equipment, resuscitation equipment and sterilization equipment.

Place: ....

Date: .... Signature of the owner of the place

FORM B

[See sub-rule (6) of rule 5]

CERTIFICATE OF APPROVAL

The place described below is hereby approved for the purpose of the Medical Termination of Pregnancy Act, 1971 (34 of 1971).

As read within upto..weeks

Name of the Place..

Address and other descriptions..

....

....

Name of the owner..

....

Place:......................................

Date:......................................

To the Government of the..

(DLC) does not require renewal. Each district must have a functional DLC for the approval and subsequent inspections of approved places.

CONSENT REQUIRED FOR TERMINATION OF PREGNANCY

- Consent is must in OPD as well as in IPD cases. Consent from husband/parent/guardian is not required if a woman is of or above 18 years of age and who is in sound state of mind.
- Only in cases of a minor and/or a mentally ill woman of any age, her guardian's consent is required.
- The MTP Rules, 2003 prescribe that consent needs to be documented on Form C.

FORM C
(Consent Form)

I...........................daughter/wife of.................. aged about .... Years, R/O............................*(here state the permanent address)* at present residing at .... do hereby give my consent to be termination of my pregnancy at .... *(state the name of place where the pregnancy is to be terminated)*.

Place : ....
Date :.. ....

Signature

(To be filled in by guardian where the woman is a lunatic or minor).
I .... son/daughter/wife of ....
aged about.......................... Years .... at present residing at ....
.... (permanent address) .... do hereby give my consent to the termination of pregnancy of my ward .... who is a minor/lunatic at ....(Place of termination of my pregnancy).

Place...............................
Date: ....

....

Signature

FORM D

(See sub-clause (ii) of clause (b) of rule 3A)

Report of the Medical Board for Pregnancy Termination Beyond 24 weeks

Details of the woman seeking termination of pregnancy:

1. Name of the woman: ....
2. Age: ....
3. Registration/Case Number:...
4. Available reports and investigations:

S. No.	Report	Opinion on the findings

5. Additional investigations (if done):

S. No.	Investigations done	Key findings

6. Opinion by Medical Board for termination of pregnancy:
   (a) Allowed
   (b) Denied
   Justification for the decision: ....
7. Physical fitness of the woman for the termination of pregnancy:
   (a) Yes
   (b) No
   Members of the Medical Board who reviewed the case:

S. No.	Name	Signature

FORM E

Opinion Form of Registered Medical Practitioners

(For gestation age beyond 20 weeks till 24 weeks)

[See sub-rule (2) of rule 4A]

I ....

(Name and qualifications of the Registered Medical Practitioner in BLOCK LETTERS)

....

(Full address of the Registered Medical Practitioner)

I ....

(Name and qualifications of the Registered Medical Practitioner in BLOCK LETTERS)

....

(Full address of the Registered Medical Practitioner)
hereby certify that we are of opinion, formed in good faith, that it is necessary to terminate the pregnancy of

....

(Full name of pregnant woman in BLOCK LETTERS)

resident of ....
(Full address of pregnant woman in BLOCK LETTERS)

Which is beyond 20 weeks but till 24 weeks under special circumstances as given below:

***Specify the circumstance(s) from (a) to (g) appropriate for termination of pregnancy beyond 20 weeks till 24 weeks:**

(a) Survivors of sexual assault or rape or incest
(b) Minors
(c) Change of marital status during the ongoing pregnancy (widowhood and divorce)
(d) Women with physical disabilities [major disability as per criteria laid down under the Rights of Persons with Disabilities Act, 2016 (49 of 2016)]
(e) Mentally ill women including mental retardation
(f) The fetal malformation that has substantial risk of being incompatible with life or if the child is born it may suffer from such physical or mental abnormalities to be seriously handicapped
(g) Women with pregnancy in humanitarian settings or disaster or emergency situations as declared by Government

We hereby give intimation that we terminated the pregnancy of the woman referred to above who bears the Serial No.................. in the Admission Register of the hospital/approved place.

Signature of the Registered Medical Practitioner

Place:..........................

Date:.......................... Signature of the Registered Medical Practitioner

Note: Account may be taken of the pregnant woman's actual or reasonably foreseeable environment in determining whether the continuance of her pregnancy would involve a grave injury to her physical or mental health.

OPINIONS REQUIRED FOR TERMINATION OF PREGNANCY

1. *Form I (Opinion Form):* RMP Opinion Form (For gestation age up to 20 weeks) RMP shall certify this form within 3 hours from the termination of pregnancy
2. *Form II:* Head of the hospital or owner of the place shall send a monthly statement of cases to the CMO of the district in this form.

FORM I—RMP OPINION FORM

I...(Name and qualifications of the Registered Medical practitioner in block letters)
....(Full address of the Registered Medical practitioner)
I...(Name and qualifications of the Registered Medical practitioner in block letters)
....(Full address of the Registered Medical practitioner) hereby certify that *I/We am/are of opinion, formed in good faith, that it is necessary to terminate the pregnancy of ....
....
(Full name of pregnant women in block letters) resident of..
(Full address of pregnant women in block letters)
for the reasons given below**.
* I/We hereby give intimation that *I/We terminated the pregnancy of the woman referred to above who bears the serial no. .... in the Admission Register of the hospital/approved place.

Place:..
Date:...

Signature of the registered Medical Practitioner

Signature of the registered Medical Practitioners

*Strike out whichever is not applicable,
**of the reasons specified items (i) to (v) write the one which is appropriate.

(i) In order to save the life of the pregnant women,
(ii) In order to prevent grave injury to the physical and mental health of the pregnant women,
(iii) In view of the substantial risk that if the child was born, it would suffer from such physical or mental abnormalities as to be seriously handicapped,
(iv) As the pregnancy is alleged by pregnant women to have been caused by rape,
(v) As the pregnancy has occurred as result of failure of any contraceptive device or methods used by married woman or her husband for the purpose of limiting the number of children

Note: Account may be taken of the pregnant women's actual or reasonably foreseeable environment in determining whether the continuance of her pregnancy would involve a grave injury to her physical or mental health.

Place:..
Date:...

Signature of the Registered Medical Practitioner

Signature of the Registered Medical Practitioners

FORM II

Refer Regulation 4(5)

1. Name of the State:
2. Name of Hospital/approved place:
3. **Duration of pregnancy:** (Give total number only under each sub-head)
   (a) Up to 9 weeks (Medical Methods of Abortion Only):
   (b) Up to 12 weeks (Surgical Methods of Abortion Only):
   (c) Between 12 and 20 weeks:
   (d) Between 20 and 24 weeks:
   (e) Beyond 24 weeks:
4. **Religion of woman:** (Give total number under each sub-head)
   (a) Hindu:
   (b) Muslim:
   (c) Christian:
   (d) Others:
5. **Termination with acceptance of contraception:** (Give total number under each sub-head)
   (a) Sterilization:
   (b) IUCD:
   (c) OCP/Injectable contraceptive:
   (d) Others:
6. **Reasons for termination:** (Give total number under each sub-head)
   A. Up to 20 weeks of gestation
      (a) Danger to the life of the pregnant woman:
      (b) Grave injury to the physical and mental health of the pregnant woman:
      (c) Pregnancy caused by rape:
      (d) Substantial risk that if the child was born, it would suffer from such physical or mental abnormalities as to be seriously handicapped:
      (e) Failure of any contraceptive device or method:

   B. Between 20 and 24 weeks of gestation
      (a) Survivors of Sexual Assault/Rape/Incest:
      (b) Minors:
      (c) Change of marital status during the ongoing pregnancy (widowhood and divorce):
      (d) Women with physical disabilities [major disability as per criteria laid down under the Rights of Persons with Disabilities Act, 2016 (49 of 2016)]:
      (e) Mentally ill women including mental retardation:
      (f) The fetal malformation that has substantial risk of being incompatible with life or if the child is born it may suffer from such physical or mental abnormalities to be seriously handicapped:
      (g) Women with pregnancy in humanitarian settings or disasters or emergency situations as declared by Government:

   C. Beyond 24 weeks of gestation
   (a) The fetal malformation that has substantial risk of being incompatible with life or if the child is born it may suffer from such physical or mental abnormalities to be seriously handicapped.

Signature of the Officer In-charge with Date

SECRECY OF MEDICAL RECORDS OF MEDICAL TERMINATION OF PREGNANCY CASES

No doctor, nurse or paramedical staff shall reveal the name and other particulars of a woman whose pregnancy has been terminated under the provisions of The Medical Termination of Pregnancy Act, 1977, The Medical Termination of Pregnancy Rules, 2003 and The Medical Termination of Pregnancy Regulations, 2003, except to a person authorized by any law.

Form III (Admission Register):

i. Every owner of the hospital/approved place shall maintain a register in form III for recording there in the details

FORM III Admission Register

Name of Facility............................ Month.................. Year..................

S. No.	Date of admission	Name of the Patient	Wife/daughter of	Age (in Year)	Religion	Address	Duration of pregnancy	Reasons for which pregnancy is terminated	Date of terminated of pregnancy	Date of discharge of patient	Result & remarks	Name of Registered Medical Practitioner (s) by whom the opinion is formed	Name of Registered Medical Prac-titioner (s) by whom the pregnancy is formed
1	2	3	4	5	6	7	8	9	10	11	12	13	14

of the admissions of women for the termination of their pregnancies and keep such register for a period of 5 years from the date of last entry.

ii. The entries in the Admission Register shall be made serially and a fresh serial shall be started at the commencement of each year and the serial number of the specific year shall be distinguished from the serial number of other years by mentioning the year against the serial number, for example, serial number 5 of 2022 and serial number 5 of 2023 shall be mentioned as 5/2022 and 5/2023.

iii. Admission Register shall be a SECRET document, and the information contained in that shall not be disclosed to any person.

Admission Register not to be open to inspection: The Admission Register shall be kept in the safe custody of the owner of the approved place, or by any person authorized by the owner and shall not be open for inspection by any person except under the authority of law.

Provided that the RMP on the application of an employed woman whose pregnancy has been terminated, grant a certificate for the purpose of enabling her to obtain leave from her employer;Provided further that any such employer shall not disclose this information to any other person.

Entries in registers maintained in hospital or approved place: No entry shall be made in any history-sheet, OT register, follow-up OPD card or any other document other than the Admission Register maintained at any hospital or approved place revealing the name of the pregnant woman and reference to the pregnant woman shall be made therein by the serial number assigned to the woman in the Admission Register.

Comprehensive abortion care (CAC): Comprehensive abortion care is one of the essential healthcare services published by WHO 2020. CAC includes pre and postabortion care, information and management of abortion.

WHO ABORTION GUIDELINES[2]

WHO abortion care guidelines provide access to quality abortion care and maintain sexual and reproductive health as an integral part. The new WHO guidelines include recommendations on many simple interventions at the level of primary care that:

- Improve the quality of abortion care provided to women and girls;
- Include task-sharing by a wider range of health workers;
- Ensure access to medical abortion pills, which mean more women can obtain safe abortion services; and
- Ensure that accurate information on care is available to all those who need it.

For the first time, the guidelines also include recommendations for the use of telemedicine where appropriate, which has helped support access to abortion and family planning services during the COVID-19 pandemic.

COMPREHENSIVE SEXUALITY CARE

Comprehensive sexuality education is a curriculum-based process of teaching and learning about the cognitive, emotional, physical and social aspects of sexuality.

Medical methods of abortion (MMA): Medical Methods of Abortion is a nonsurgical, noninvasive method for termination of pregnancy by using a combination of drugs.

VIOLATION OF MTP ACT[11]

Sections 88–92 Bharatiya Nyaya Sanhita 2023 (BNS) (previously Sec. 312-316 of the

Drug protocol for medical methods of abortion.		
Visit	***Day***	***Drug used***
First	One	200 mg Mifepristone oral; anti-D if Rh-negative
Second	Three	800 μg Misoprostol sublingual/vaginal/buccal; analgesics
Third	Fifteen	Confirm and ensure completion of procedure; offer contraception

The requisite documentation protocol for surgical abortions as under the MTP Act is also applicable to MMA.		
1st visit (Day 1/Day of mifepristone administration)	***2nd visit (3rd Day)***	***3rd visit (15th Day)***
• Detailed history • Counseling (*including general and method specific counseling*) • Physical and pelvic examination • Contraceptive options • Investigations (Injection anti-D 50 μg if Rh-negative) • Informed consent • Mifepristone 200 mg orally • Give contact address and phone number of the facility where woman can go in case of an emergency • Complete the follow-up card	• Note any history of bleeding/pain or any other side effects after mifepristone • Misoprostol 400 μg (two tablets of 200 μg) oral/vaginal • Observe for 4–6 hours in the clinic/hospital • Prescribe drug for pain relief • Perform bimanual examination just before discharging her from the facility, to rule out expulsion of POC • Inform the woman about warning signs • She must keep filling the card	• Note relevant history • Carry out pelvic examination to ensure completion of abortion process • Advise USG if pelvic examination does not confirm the expulsion of POC or completion of abortion process or if bleeding continues • Ask the woman to report back if there are no periods within 6 weeks • Reinforce contraceptive counseling and services

IPC) deals with miscarriage and death of an unborn child and depending on the severity and intention with which the crime is committed, the penalties range from 7 years to life imprisonment for 14 years and fine.

Section 88 BNS: Causing miscarriage (previously Sec. 312 IPC)

Whoever voluntarily causes a woman with child to miscarry, shall, if such miscarriage be not caused in good faith for the purpose of saving the life of the woman, be punished with imprisonment of either description for a term which may extend to 3 years, or with fine, or with both, and, if the woman be quick with child, shall be punished with imprisonment of either description for a term which may extend to seven years, and shall also be liable to fine.

Explanation: A woman who causes herself to miscarry, is within the meaning of this section.

Section 89 BNS: Causing miscarriage without woman's consent (previously Sec. 313 IPC)

Whoever commits the offence defined in the last preceding section without the consent of the woman, whether the woman is quick with child or not, shall be punished with [imprisonment for life] or with imprisonment of either description for a term which may extend to ten years, and shall also be liable to fine.

Section 90 BNS: Death caused by act done with intent to cause miscarriage (previously Sec. 314 *IPC)*

Whoever, with intent to cause the miscarriage of woman with child, does any act which causes the death of such woman, shall be punished with imprisonment of either description for a term may extend to 10 years, and shall also be liable to fine.

If act done without women's consent: And if the act is done without the consent of the woman, shall be punished either with [imprisonment for life] or with the punishment above mentioned.

Explanation: It is not essential to this offence that the offender should know that the act is likely to cause death.

Section 91 BNS: Act done with intent to prevent child being born alive or to cause it to die after birth (previously Sec. 315 IPC)

Whoever before the birth of any child does any act with the intention of thereby preventing that child from being born alive or causing it to die after its birth, and does by such prevent that child from being born alive, or causes it to die after its birth, shall, if such act be not caused in good faith for the purpose of saving the life of the mother, be punished with imprisonment of either description for a term which may extend to 10 years, or with fine, or with both.

Section 92 BNS: Causing death of quick unborn child by act amounting to culpable homicide (previously Sec. 316 IPC)

Whoever does any act under such circumstances, that if he thereby caused death, he would be guilty of culpable homicide, and does by such act cause the death of a quick unborn child, shall be punished with imprisonment of either description for a term which may extend to 10 years, and shall also be liable to fine.

LANDMARK JUDGMENTS

CASE 1: Mahima Yadav vs. Government of NCT of Delhi & Ors (2021)[12]

In this case, the petitioner has filed the petition to get permission to terminate her pregnancy. Although the petitioner's fetus was more than 24 weeks old, the counsel appearing on behalf of the appellant insists that she should be permitted to terminate the pregnancy because of anomalies of the fetus and risk to the petitioner, who is at present also suffering from severe hearing issues.

Judgment by the Court: According to the reading of section 3 of the amended MTP Act, the pregnancy can be terminated even after 24 weeks in case of substantial abnormalities.

The Medical Superintendent (MS) of AIIMS was directed by the court to designate a Board of Doctors to examine Mahima Yadav. Following the examination, the report was provided, and it found that continuing the pregnancy would harm both the mother and the child. It was found that the petitioner was a cardiac patient and had been prescribed blood thinners.

The court considered various similar matters and found that the recent amendments of the MTP are as per the decisions taken earlier in cases like *Shaikh Ayesha Khatoon vs. Union of India & Ors* (2018), *Nisha Suresh Aalam vs. Union of India & Ors* (2018), *Priyanka Shukla vs. Union of India & Ors* (2019), etc. in all these cases, the abortion was permitted beyond the set period of 20 weeks prevailing at that time. Hence, the court found the amendments confirming these cases and the precedents set in these cases.[11]

CASE 2: X vs. Principal Secretary Health and Family Welfare Department, 2022[13]

A 25-year-old single woman, approached the Delhi High Court for seeking permission for the termination of her 22-week pregnancy out of a consensual relationship. High court denied her permission by quoting the provisions of MTP Act, which allowed only married women to undergo abortion and she was not covered in any clauses under MTP Rules, 2003 on account of mental distress, rape, health complications

↓

Then she approached the Supreme Court on ground of social stigma pertaining to unmarried single parent and prolongation of unwanted pregnancy would involve a risk of grave and immense injury to her mental health

- On September 29, 2022, the Supreme Court bench declared that the Medical Termination of Pregnancy Act recognizes the reproductive rights of pregnant women, granting them the right to choose medical intervention for terminating pregnancies.
- The court emphasized that all women, regardless of marital status, are entitled to access legal and safe abortions up to 24 weeks of gestation.
- *In 2021 Amendment:* The words *'any married woman or her husband'* were replaced with the *'any woman or her partner'* bringing within the fold of the law pregnancies outside marriage institution but the main issue before the Supreme Court was to examine whether the *Rule 3B* of MTP Rules, 2003 is violative of Article 14 of the Indian Constitution, since it excludes an unmarried woman and deprives her the access to safe and legal abortion. According to the 2021 Amendment, all women are entitled to the benefit of safe and legal abortion.
- *Section 3B of MTP Rules, 2003 struck down* on the ground of being discriminatory against unmarried women, who may go through the same trauma and life situations as a married woman does. (Section 3B of Rules of MTP Act reads the categories of women considered eligible for termination of pregnancy: While the law recognizes change in circumstances of the relationship status between a pregnant woman and her spouse—in the case of divorce and widowhood, but it does not envisage the situation for unmarried women).
- The rights of reproductive autonomy, dignity and privacy under Article 21 give an unmarried woman the right to choose on whether or not to bear a child, on a similar footing of a married woman.
- *Incorporation of Marital Rape in the MTP Act:*
  a. The Supreme Court bench emphasized that the exception allowing abortions between 20 and 24 weeks of gestation should extend to married women, as it is not implausible for them to become pregnant as a result of marital rape.
  b. This ruling holds significance as it represents the initial legal acknowledgment of marital rape within the Indian Constitution, albeit solely within the specific context of abortion under the MTP Act and its accompanying rules and regulations.
- *Exemption for medical practitioners in disclosing the identity of minors:*
  a. The Protection of Children from Sexual Offences Act 2012 (POCSO) criminalizes any sexual activity involving individuals below the age of 18.
  b. The Apex Court recognized that minors under the age of 18 engaging in consensual sexual activity should also have access to safe abortions provided

by registered medical practitioners (RMPs).

c. Section 19(1) of POCSO imposes a mandatory obligation on RMPs to report to the investigation team when approached by a minor seeking an abortion.
d. However, the Supreme Court clarified that the MTP Act recognizes minors as a distinct category eligible for abortion up to 24 weeks.
e. RMPs, only upon the request of the minor and the guardian, are not required to disclose the minor's identity or other personal details in the information provided under Section 19(1) of the POCSO Act.

CASE 3: Suchita Srivastava & Anr vs. Chandigarh Administration[14]

- A three Judge Bench of the Supreme Court considered this case, where an orphaned woman suffering from a mental retardation, was impregnated as a result of rape. The Punjab & Haryana High Court determined, without the woman's consent, that it was in her best interests that the fetus should be aborted under Section 3 of the Medical Termination of Pregnancy Act, 1971 (MTP Act) as she did not have the capacity to take care of a child, nor did she have a parent or guardian to look after her.
- The Supreme Court stayed the order of the Punjab & Haryana High Court, and held that the right to reproductive choice flows from the Right to Liberty under Article 21 of the Constitution. It noted that taking away a woman's choice regarding her own body would amount to infringement of her right to privacy.
- It further distinguished between mental illness and mental retardation and considered that the woman's mental retardation did not take away her right to make a decision regarding her reproductive choices. Therefore, it held that a termination of her pregnancy without her consent could not be ordered.

REFERENCES

1. The Medical Termination of Pregnancy Act, 1971[cited 2023 June 28]. [online] Available from https://www.indiacode.nic.in/bitstream/123456789/1593/1/A1971-34.pdf [Last accessed, December 2024].
2. Abortion care guideline [Internet]. Abortion care guideline – Consolidated guidelines for clinical care, service delivery, and law and policy. Abortion care guideline; 2021 [cited 2023 June 21]. [online] (https://srhr.org/abortioncare/chapter-1/background-and-context) [Last accessed, December 2024].
3. Thelancet.com. [cited 2023 June 28]. [online] Available from https://www.thelancet.com/action/showPdf?pii=S2214-109X%2817%2930453-9[Last accessed, December 2024].
4. Abortion [Internet]. World Health Organization; [cited 2023 July 18]. [online] Available from https://www.who.int/news-room/fact-sheets/detail/abortion [Last accessed, December 2024].
5. Advances in Methods of Emergency Contraception, Experience with Liberalised Abortion Services– Dr V K Manchanda Commissioner, Maternal Health, MOHFW, GOI. [cited 2023 June 13]. [online] Available fromhttps://aiims.edu/aiims/events/Gynaewebsite/ma_finalsite/report/1_1_4.htm#:~:text=Government%20of%20India%20set%20up,related%20to%20abortion%20in%201966. [Last accessed, December 2024].
6. The Medical Termination of Pregnancy Act, 2002. [Internet]. Karnataka: Government of Karnataka; 2002 [cited 2024 Jul 18]. [online] Available from https://ekalyani.karnataka.gov.in/PdfDocuments/Gazette-MTP%20Act%202002.pdf [Last accessed, December 2024].

7. FOGSI Focus on Medical Termination of Pregnancy (MTP) Recent Update on clinical and legal aspects. [online] Available from https://fogsi.org/wp-content/uploads/fogsi-focus/medical-termination-of-pregnancy-2021.pdf [Last accessed, December 2024].
8. Abortion has been legal in India since the Medical Termination of Pregnancy Act (MTP Act) was brought into effect in April 1972. The MTP Act was a significant step forward in ensuring access to safe and legal abortion services for women under a broad range of conditions [Internet]. Pratigyacampaign.org. [cited 2023 June 21]. [online] Available from https://pratigyacampaign.org/wp-content/uploads/2019/09/abortion-in-india.pdf [Last accessed, December 2024].
9. Protection of Children from Sexual Offences Act, 2012 [Internet]. 1970 [cited 2023 July 18]. [online] Available from: https://www.indiacode.nic.in/handle/123456789/2079?sam_handle=123456789%2F1362#:~:text=India%20Code%3A%20Protection%20of%20Children%20from%20Sexual%20Offences%20Act%2C%202012&text=Long%20Title%3A,connected%20therewith%20or%20incidental%20thereto. [Last accessed, December 2024].
10. MTP Rules 2003. Tamil Nadu Social Welfare Department; 2003 [cited 2023 July 15]. [online] Available from https://tnsocialwelfare.tn.gov.in/website-345/sites/default/files/2022-01/MTP_Rules.pdf[Last accessed, December 2024].
11. The Bharatiya Nyaya Sanhita, 2023 NO. 45 OF 2023 [Internet]. [cited 2024 June 13] [online] Available from https://www.mha.gov.in/sites/default/files/250883_english_01042024.pdf[Last accessed, December 2024].
12. Mahima Yadav Vs Government of NCT of Delhi & Ors (2021) [Internet]. [cited 2024 January 10] [online] Available from https://indiankanoon.org/doc/129047686/[Last accessed, December 2024].
13. X vs. Principal Secretary health & Family welfare Dept, 2022. [online] Available from: https://indiankanoon.org/doc/134729746/ [Last accessed, December 2024].
14. Suchita Srivastava & Anr v. Chandigarh Administration [Internet]. [cited 2024 May 24] [online] Available from https://indiankanoon.org/doc/1500783/[Last accessed, December 2024].

CHAPTER 5

Medicolegal Aspects of the PCPNDT Act

Pradyumna Vaja, Nivedita Vaja, Mahesh C Jariwala

INTRODUCTION

Using diagnostic techniques for sex selection or sex detection of unborn baby and termination of pregnancy with female fetus is discriminatory and violates the fundamental right to equality of gender and is considered illegal as per the provisions of the PC & PNDT Act. Obsessive preference for sons and discrimination against the girl child and women, has spawned practices such as female infanticide by various cruel methods, bride-burning and sati and lead to the neglect of the girl child in terms of nutrition, education, health care and her overall development.

Prenatal diagnostic techniques have been used worldwide to detect genetic abnormalities and fetal malformations. However, in India, they are being misused for the past three decades for detection of the sex of the unborn child and subsequently for female feticide. The disturbing child sex ratios in the 1991 census and consistent campaigning on this issue by women's rights groups and other civil society groups all over the country led Parliament to enact the Pre-Natal Diagnostic Techniques (Regulation and Prevention of Misuse) Act (PNDT Act) in 1994 **(Fig. 1)**.[1]

This Act is legislation to curb the abhorrent practice of sex determination and female feticide, which has its roots in India's long history of strong patriarchal influence in all spheres of life. Thus, the "elimination" of girls and women is not entirely new to the Indian

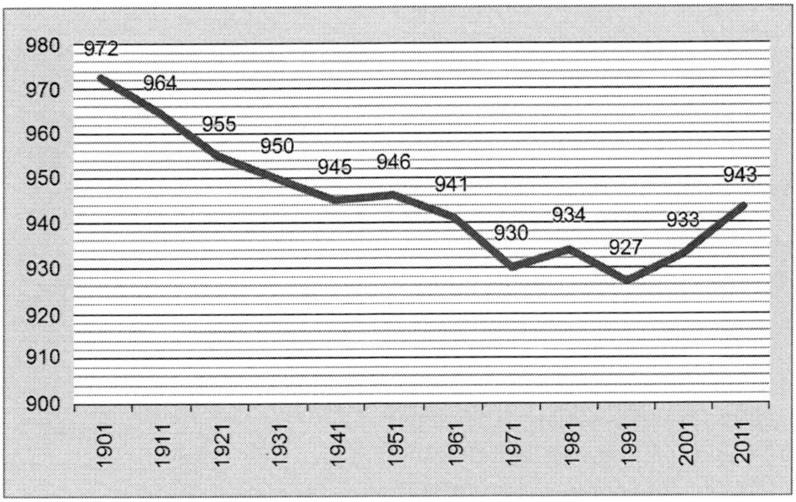

Fig. 1: *Census 2011:* Sex ratio in India since 1901 to 2011.

sociocultural fabric. The obvious result is that the sex ratio is increasingly adverse for women (The sex ratio is the ratio of females to thousand males in a population. According to the 2011 census, this ratio is 943 women for every 1000 men).

Sex ratio at birth (SRB) is one of the important indicators of NITI AYOG.

The situation could probably have been worse, but for the valiant efforts of some social reformers. However, they have been more successful in some parts of the country than others, as can be seen from the sharp variations in the child sex ratio across regions, with the north and west of India showing larger deficits of girls. The last few decades have seen the situation getting worse, despite the progress the country has been making in almost all other spheres and indicators.

With the advent of new sophisticated pre-conception sex selection technologies like sperm separation, the girl child's elimination started becoming more subtle, refined and probably also more socially acceptable. Not surprisingly, the 2001 census revealed a further drastic fall in the child sex ratio, signaling the precipitation of a demographic catastrophe on a nation-wide scale. Alarmed by these happenings, and in response to the directives of the Supreme Court (SC) in a PIL filed on this issue, the Government amended the Act to provide it more teeth and to cover the new pre-conception sex selection techniques. Thus, the Pre-Natal Diagnostic Techniques (Regulation and Prevention of Misuse) 1994, as amended in 2003, PC & PNDT (prohibition of sex selection) Act, 1994 came into effect from February 14, 2003.

The specific word *pre-conception* is added in heading and various provisions of law that means government of India had included any technique, before conception, used for sex selection is also blanket banned.

OBLIGATION OF AN OBSTETRICIAN/GYNECOLOGIST

It is the duty of every citizen to be law abiding, and doctors are no exception. Therefore, it is an obligatory duty of every gynecologist to abide by the relevant laws and implement the legal provisions in the true spirit. A cartoon shown in **Figure 2**[1] clearly depicts the consequences of not following the legal provisions. To fulfill this obligation in the best possible way, he/she must know:

- What are the rules?
- What are important regulations?
- What is right and what is wrong?
- What is legal and what is illegal?

In a nutshell, it is an obligation on his/her part to acquaint himself/herself with the basic knowledge of the Act and comply accordingly with the provisions of the Act. Government has focused all energy to enact and ensure implementation of the PC & PNDT Act, so that the medical professionals involved in the unethical practice of selective sex selection and sex detection of fetus and embryos must stop this cruel inhuman practice.

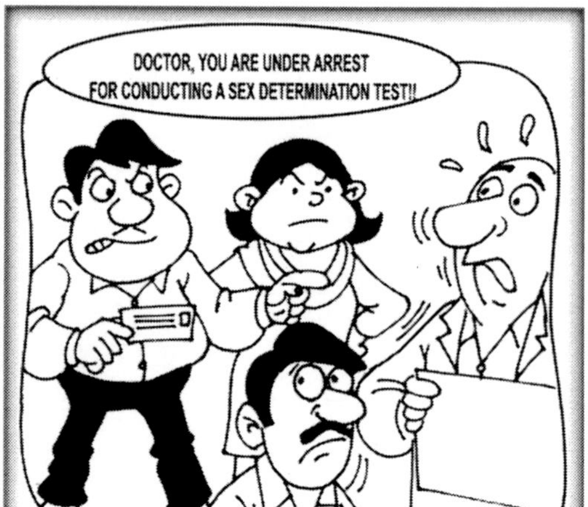
DOCTOR, YOU ARE UNDER ARREST
FOR CONDUCTING A SEX DETERMINATION TEST!!

Fig. 2: Cartoon depicting the consequences of not following the legal provisions.[1]

It is the moral as well as social duty of a doctor to assist the Government in its mission to fight this deadly social evil. For that, he/she must implement this act in his/her practice verbatim in the following way:

MEDICOLEGAL ASPECTS OF PC AND PNDT ACT [2–5]

Most of the practitioners are afraid of the PC and PNDT Act primarily due to lack of awareness related to the legal provisions of the Act. A genuine practitioner has no reason to be apprehensive, if he/she follows the guidelines laid down in the Act. Many a times, it is found that due to casual approach of the practitioners towards the legal provisions, results in medicolegal problems, specifically in the practice of obstetrics.

"We, the doctors, are highly criticized, not because of the treatment and medical management of the patients but because of the poor understanding of laws, unethical practices, and most of times, due to poor medical record maintenance. Our humble effort here is to make you aware of this Act and to pursue the practice as per the provisions of the Act which will relieve our mental stress.

The following are simple stepwise basic tips to avoid litigation in the case of PC and PNDT Act, an Act which every fellow of our fraternity must be aware of and implement them in their practice.

Registration of Place

- An institute, hospital, nursing home or any other place, by whatever name called, which provides genetic counseling irrespective of whether prenatal diagnostic procedures are carried out or not is to be registered as '*Genetic Counseling Centre*'.
- The place where prenatal diagnostic procedures are carried out, is to be registered as '*Genetic Clinic*', and a place for conducting analysis of or tests of samples received from genetic clinic is to be registered as '*Genetic Laboratory*'. This also includes a vehicle where a portable USG machine is used.
- The registration of a clinic also includes the registration of each and every mobile genetic clinic as a part of medical mobile unit. Such a vehicle has to be registered as a mobile genetic unit.
- *Prenatal Diagnostic procedures* include procedures such as USG, fetoscopy, taking or removing samples of amniotic fluid, chorionic villi, embryo, blood or any other tissue of a man or a woman before or after conception, for being sent to a Genetic lab or genetic clinic for conducting any type of analysis or prenatal diagnostic (PND) tests for selection of sex before or after conception. PND techniques include all PND procedures and tests. PND tests means USG or any test or analysis of amniotic fluid, chorionic villi, blood or any tissue or fluid of pregnant woman or conceptus conducted to detect genetic or metabolic disorders or chromosomal abnormalities or malformations or hemoglobinopathies or sex-linked diseases. All the places where these procedures are carried out must be registered to avoid litigations under this Act.
- Every application for registration shall be made to the appropriate authority, in duplicate, in Form-A in such form and in such manner and shall be accompanied by such fees as may be prescribed. It shall be accompanied by an affidavit containing:
  a. An undertaking to the effect that the center shall not conduct any test or procedure for sex selection

or detection except for the diseases mentioned in section 4 (2).

b. An undertaking that the center shall display prominently a notice that they do not conduct any such tests.

(Never forget to take acknowledgement after submission of Form A)

Certificate of Registration

The appropriate Authority grants a certificate of registration, in duplicate, in Form B. The details in all columns of Form B (license to practice sonography) must be checked for spellings and also the details of machines (*Criminal case no. 1212/2010, Ahmedabad metropolitan court).*

The certificate of registration must be displaced at a conspicuous place at the place of business. An inquiry for registration by the Appropriate Authority, including inspection at the premises, shall be carried out only after due notice is given to the applicant. Grant or rejection of certificate of registration shall be communicated to the applicant in Form B or C, respectively within a period of 90 days from the date of receipt of the application.

The certificate shall be non-transferable. In the event of a change of ownership or management of the place, the new owner or the manager of that place shall apply afresh for a certificate. Every certificate is valid for a period of 5 years from the date of issue.

Renewal, Cancellation or Suspension of Registration

Renewal

- An application for renewal shall be made in duplicate in Form A, to the Appropriate Authority 30 days before the date of expiry.
- Acknowledgement of receipt of such an application shall be issued by the Authority in specified manner.
- Fees payable for the renewal are one half the fees for new registration.
- On receipt of the renewed certificate or rejection of application for renewal, both copies of earlier certificates shall be surrendered immediately to the appropriate Authority.
- In the event of failure to renew the certificate or rejection of application within a period of 90 days from the date of receipt of the application, the certificate shall be deemed to have been renewed. *(MCA/3621/2016: Gujarat High Court)*

Cancellation or Suspension

- The appropriate authority may suo moto or on complaint, issue a notice to the center to show cause why its registration should not be suspended or cancelled for the reasons mentioned in the notice.
- After hearing the center and on the advice of the Advisory Committee, if the appropriate Authority is satisfied with the breach of the Act or the rules, it may cancel or suspend its registration for such a period it may think fit.
- Notwithstanding anything contained in above, if the authority is of the opinion that it is necessary or expedient so to do in the public interest, it may, for reasons to be recorded in writing, suspend the registration without issuing such a notice.

Public Information

- A notice in English and in the local language (in the prescribed color and size), to the effect that disclosure of sex of the fetus is prohibited under law and is a punishable offence, shall be displayed in the premises of the registered place.
- At least one copy each of the Act and the rules shall be available on the premises of

the registered place and made available to clientele on demand for perusal.

- All persons associated with the center shall display his/her name and designation prominently on the dress worn by him/her.
- Name and designation in full must be written under the signature.

Qualifications of the Persons

The qualifications of a person or employee shall be as under:

Qualification for Genetic Counseling Center

Any person being or employing, a *Gynecologist* or a *Pediatrician* having 6 months experience or 4 weeks training in genetic counseling or *Medical Geneticist*, having adequate space and educational charts/models/equipment may set up a '*Genetic Counseling Center*.'

Qualification for Genetic Lab

Any person having adequate space, and being or employing, a *Medical Geneticist*, and a *Lab Technician* having a BSc Degree in Biological Sciences or a degree diploma in medical lab course with at least 1 year experience may set up a '*genetic lab*'. Such labs should have necessary equipment for carrying out chromosomal studies, biochemical, and molecular studies.

Qualification for Genetic Clinic

Any person having adequate space and being or employing:

i. Gynecologist with experience of at least 20 procedures under supervision of an experienced gynecologist in these fields.
ii. A sonologist or imaging specialist (means a person having—medical qualifications recognized under the Indian Medical Council Act, 1956 (102 of 1956) or having a postgraduate qualification in USG or Imaging Techniques or Radiology) or a Registered Medical Practitioner having PG Degree or Diploma or six months training duly imparted in the manner prescribed in the "the PC and PNDT (Prohibition of Sex Selection) (Six Months Training) Rules, 2014".
iii. A medical Geneticist includes a person who possesses a degree or diploma in genetic science in the fields of sex selection and prenatal diagnostic techniques or has experience of not less than two years in such field after obtaining: (i) Any one of the medical qualifications recognized under the Indian Medical Council Act, 1956 (102 of 1956); or (ii) A postgraduate degree in biological sciences; may set up a *genetic clinic* which must acquire necessary equipment. Each person shall be permitted to be registered with a maximum of *Two* such clinics within a district. His consulting hours must be clearly specified for each clinic.

Sale of USG Machine

- No organization or a person shall sell, distribute, supply, rent, allow or authorize use of imaging machine or any other equipment capable of detecting sex of the fetus in any manner, whether on payment or otherwise, to any Genetic Counseling Center, Clinic or Laboratory or any other body or person unless such center is registered under this Act.
- The provider of such machines shall send to the concerned State/UT Appropriate Authority and to the Central Government, once in three months a list of those to whom the machine has been provided.
- Such a provider shall take an affidavit from the concerned purchasing center, clinic,

lab, person or both that the machine/ equipment shall not be used for detection of sex of fetus or selection of sex before or after conception.

Regulation of Portable Machines

Use of portable machines shall be permitted only in the following conditions:

i. The portable machine being used, within the premises it is registered, for providing services to the indoor patients.
ii. As a part of mobile medical unit, offering a Bouquet of other health and medical services like:
   a. Curative services like referral of complicated cases, early detection of some endemic communicable and noncommunicable diseases; minor surgical procedures
   b. RCH services (Reproductive and Child Health Services)
   c. Family planning services
   d. Diagnostic services like investigation of Hb, urine, clinical detection of leprosy and TB, screening of cancer, etc.
   e. Specialized facilities and services like X-ray, ECG, and ultrasound test, etc.
   f. Emergency services and care in times of disaster or epidemic or public health emergency or accident, etc.

Regulation of services to be offered by mobile genetic clinic:

- It shall operate only as a part of the Mobile Medical Unit offering a bouquet of other health and medical services in urban slums or rural or remote or hilly or hard to reach areas for improved access to healthcare services by underserved.
- The standalone mobile USG clinic offering only PND facilities are prohibited.
- The mobile unit shall have adequate space.
- The machine shall not be used for sex determination of fetus.
- A copy of certificate of registration shall be displayed inside the vehicle at a conspicuous place clearly specifying:
  a. The area of operation not exceeding the district wherein it is registered.
  b. Number of portable machines installed in the vehicle
  c. Make and model no of the portable machine
  d. Registration no of the vehicle
  e. Full address of the service provider
- In case of breakdown of the vehicle or for any other reason for which the registered unit cannot be used as a genetic clinic, the Appropriate Authority has to be informed within a period of seven days.

Purposes to Carry out PNDT Techniques

- PND techniques can be carried out for the detection of the following abnormalities:
  i. Chromosomal abnormalities
  ii. Genetic metabolic diseases
  iii. Hemoglobinopathies
  iv. Sex-linked genetic diseases
  v. Congenital anomalies
  vi. Any other abnormalities as specified by the Central Supervisory Board
- No genetic lab shall accept any sample for analysis unless referred by a Genetic Clinic.
- Every PND procedure shall be preceded by locating the fetus and placenta by USG and the procedure shall be done under direct USG monitoring.

Reasons for PNDT Techniques

Techniques shall be used only if the qualified person, to do so, is satisfied for reasons to be recovered in writing that any of the following conditions are fulfilled:

i. Age of the pregnant woman is >35 years
ii. History of two or > spontaneous abortions
iii. Exposure to potentially teratogenic agents
iv. Pregnant woman or her spouse has a family history of mental retardation or physical deformities or any other genetic disease.
v. Any other condition as specified by the CSB.

Counseling, Communication, and Consent

PND procedures (invasive) cannot be conducted unless:

i. All known sides and aftereffects of the procedures are explained.
ii. Written consent in the prescribed form G to undergo such a procedure is obtained in the language she understands.
iii. A copy of this consent is given to her.

A person conducting USG shall give a declaration that he has neither detected no disclosed the sex of the fetus. The pregnant woman shall declare that she does not want to know the sex of the fetus. Communication of sex of the fetus by words, signs or in any other manner to any person is prohibited.

Determination of Sex of the Fetus

No Genetic Center, Clinic or Laboratory or any person can conduct PND techniques for the purpose of determining the sex of the fetus or even selection of the sex before or after conception. The registered place shall on no account conduct or allow/cause to be conducted female feticide.

Maintenance Records

- Each and every registered place shall maintain a register showing in serial orders, names and addresses of the men or women given genetic counseling, subject to PND tests, the names of their spouse or father and the date on which they first reported.[1] Sample columns of the register are shown in **Table 1**.
- The record by Genetic Clinic shall be in Form F. It has been found that more than 90% of court cases are related with Form F, and thus it is advisable that Form F must be maintained diligently, and as per the legal requirements. Referral slips are to be preserved with Form F and in case of self-referral, note with indications and case papers are preserved with Form F.
- All case-related records, forms of consent, lab results, and microscopic pictures, USG plates, slides, recommendations and letters shall be preserved for a period of 2 years or for such a period as may be prescribed. All such records shall be made available to the Appropriate Authority or any other person authorized by the Appropriate Authority on his behalf.
- In case of legal proceedings against the center, the documents shall be preserved

TABLE 1: Register to be maintained at every registered place.[1]

Sr. No	*Name*	*Address*	*Spouse/father's name*	*Date of first reporting*

till the final disposal of the proceedings or for 2 years whichever is later.

- In the case of E records, a printed copy shall be taken and preserved after authentication.
- The report must be sent to the concerned Appropriate Authority in respect of each month by the 5th day of the following month.
- It is mandatory to submit the form online also. Online submission of Form F—not a procedural lapse but an independent offence *(full bench of Gujarat HC)*

Different Forms Under the Act[1] (Table 2)

TABLE 2: Forms to be maintained as per the legal provisions.[1]

Form No	*Purpose of the Form*
Form A	To be submitted in duplicate (with supporting documents) application for registration or renewal
Form B	is a certificate of registration (to be filled in duplicate)
Form C	Form for rejection of the application
Form D	For maintenance of records by the genetic counseling center
Form E	For maintenance of records by the genetic lab
Form F	Maintenance of record in case of PND test by genetic clinic
Form G	Consent for invasive techniques
Form H	(for Appropriate Authority) Form for maintenance of permanent record of applications under the PC PNDT Act

Intimation of Changes in Employees, Place or Equipment

The registered place shall intimate every change of employee, place, address and equipment installed to the Appropriate Authority at least 30 days in advance of the expected date of such a change and seek reissuance of certificate of registration with the changes duly incorporated.

Power and Procedure to Search and Seize Records, etc.

a. If the Appropriate Authority has the reason to believe that an offence under this Act has been committed at any place, he or the authorized officer may enter that place and search at all reasonable time in the presence of 2 or more independent witnesses and examine any record, register, document, book pamphlet or any other material found therein and seize and seal the same, if such Authority has reason to believe that it may furnish evidence of the commission of an offence. *(SCA21884/2018 Gujarat High Court)*
b. A list of documents/records/object materials so sealed shall be prepared in duplicate at the place of seizure. Both copies must be signed on every page by the Authority and by the witnesses unless it is not practicable to make the list at that place for the reasons to be recorded in writing.
c. One copy of the list shall be handed over to the person from whose custody the records/documents/object materials have been seized after due acknowledgement. If no person acknowledging the custody is available, the list may be sent by the registered post.
d. In the case of a perishable object, the authority shall make prompt arrangements for sealing, identification and preservation of material and also convey it to a facility for analysis or test, if required.
e. In case of non-completion of search and seizure operation, the Authority may make arrangements, by mounting a

guard or sealing of the premises, for safe keeping, listing and removal of records to be seized and to prevent any tampering.

The Authority shall maintain dignity and interest at all times and conduct their work in a just manner without any bias or perceived presumption of guilt.

Appeal

- Anyone aggrieved by the decision of the Appropriate Authority at sub-district level may appeal to the authority at district level within 30 days of the order of sub-district level authority.
- Anyone aggrieved by the decision of the Appropriate Authority at district level may appeal to the authority at state/UT level within 30 days of the order of district level authority.
- Each appeal shall be disposed of within 60 days of its receipt.
- If such appeal is not made within time, the appropriate Authority may condone the delay in case he is satisfied that the appellant was prevented for sufficient cause from making such appeal and may adjourn the hearing for reasons to be recorded in writing: Provided that more than 3 adjournments shall not be given.

Offences and Penalties

- Advertisement, in any form, and visible representation made by means of hoarding, wall painting, signal, sound, smoke or gas relating to sex detection or sex selection, is prohibited. Contravention is punishable with imprisonment up to 3 years and a fine up to ₹10,000.
- Any person who owns a genetic center, lab or clinic or is employed therein to render his services and who contravenes any of the provisions of the Act or rules shall be punishable with imprisonment up to 3 years and a fine up to ₹10,000 and on the subsequent conviction, imprisonment up to 5 years and fine up to ₹50,000.
- The name of the medical practitioner shall be reported to the concerned State Medical Council for taking necessary action.
- If any person seeks aid for sex selection or detection, he shall be punishable with imprisonment up to 3 years and a fine up to ₹50,000 for the first offence and on subsequent conviction, imprisonment up to 5 years and fine up to ₹1,00,000. But this shall not apply to the woman who was compelled to undergo such tests.
- Whoever contravenes any of the provisions of this Act or rules made thereunder, for which no penalty has been mentioned in this Act, shall be punishable up to 3-months' imprisonment or with fine up to ₹1,000 or with both. In the case of continuing contravention an additional fine may extend up to ₹500 for every day during which such contravention continues after the first conviction.

Offences by Companies

Where any offence, punishable under this Act, has been committed by a company, every person who was in charge at the time of commitment of the offence and was responsible to the company for the conduct of the business of the company, as well as the company, shall be deemed to be guilty of the offence unless such person proves that the offence was committed without this knowledge or that he had exercised all due diligence to prevent the commission of such offence.

Every offence under this Act shall be cognizable, non-bailable and non-compoundable and no court other than that of a Metropolitan Magistrate or a First Class Judicial Magistrate shall try any offence under this Act.

RELEVANT JUDGMENTS

1. *Vinod Soni and Ors vs. Union of India and CEHAT*[6]
    - The judgment states that 'the right to life or personal liberty cannot be expanded to mean that the right to personal liberty includes the personal liberty to determine the sex of the child which may come into existence. Right to bring into existence a life in future with a choice to determine the sex of that life cannot in itself be a right.'
    - Using diagnostic techniques for sex selection is discriminatory and violates the fundamental right to equality "balanced family". It is not a natural right, nor has it been bestowed on citizens by the political set-up apart from violating the PC and PNDT Act.
2. *Dr Pratikar Doshi vs. CDHO Ahmedabad*[7]
    - It is a landmark judgment of Gujarat high court on high-handed action of the Appropriate Authority of Ahmedabad.
    - Even if it is presumed that the petitioner has committed any wrong/ irregularity, then also, the respondent authority ought not to have sealed the consulting room without hearing the petitioner. Hence, it must be concluded that the action of the respondent authority is wholly illegal and improper.
    - In view of the aforesaid factual aspect, respondent no 3, who is present in court today, states that he will withdraw the order dated 16.03.2006 immediately."
3. *FOGSI vs. UOI and ORS*[8]
    - This petition was filed by FOGSI on 16.12.2016 for seeking following reliefs:
        - To strike down S.23 (1), 23 (2) of the Act as unconstitutional for violation of Article 14,19(1)(g) and 21 and interpret S.23(1), 23(2) to clarify exact nature of offence punishable for enabling the AA to take action only against cases of actual and proven sex determination and not for anomalies of paperwork/record keeping/clerical error.
        - To decriminalize and separate the anomalies in paperwork/record keeping/clerical errors from actual sex determination offence.
    - The Supreme Court in its judgment in this petition observed that non-maintenance of record is springboard for commission of feticide, not just clerical error. There is no substance in the submission that provision of Section 4(3) be read down. By virtue of the proviso to Section 4(3), a person conducting USG on a pregnant woman, is required to keep a complete record of the same in the prescribed manner and any deficiency or inaccuracy in the same amounts to contravention of Section 5 or Section 6 of the Act, unless the contrary is proved by the person conducting the USG. Section 23 of the Act, which provides for penalties of offences, acts in aid of the other sections of the Act is quite reasonable.
    - Therefore, dilution of the provision of the Act would only defeat the purpose of the Act to prevent female feticide and relegate the right to life

of the girl child under Article 21 of the constitution, to a mere formality.

- The Supreme Court further stated that, in view of the above, no case is made out for striking down the proviso for Section 4(3), provision of Section 23(1), Section 23(2) or to read down Section 20 or 30 of the Act.
- Complete contents of Form 'F' are held to be mandatory, and the writ petition is dismissed.

Do's and Don'ts given in **Table 3** must be followed by all the doctors for safe practice, and to prevent unnecessary litigations.[9] It is advisable to maintain a checklist **(Table 4)** so that all the legal requirements as per the PC and PNDT Act are fulfilled.[10]

TABLE 3: Do's and Don'ts for prevention of litigations.

Do's
• Service of qualified person only • Sell of machine to registered place only • Must register the place, person and equipment as an entire unit • Must observe the code of conduct • Must display the Certificate of Registration at a conspicuous place • Prominently display a notice in English and in the local language—disclosure of sex of the fetus is prohibited and is punishable offence • A copy of Act and Rules shall be available. • Maintain the records as specified. • Fill all the columns of Form F • Submission of reports by 5th and online too (Nil even if not done) • Renewal application—30 days before expiry • Declaration by patient before USG and consent, if required • Declaration by the doctor after USG • 1 month notice in case of change of person, place, equipment • Surrender registration, in case of change in ownership or management of the place • Use of portable machine in registered premises only • Cooperate with AA and respect • Advice of medicolegal expert
Don'ts
• Don't encourage or indulge in sex selection or detection • Don't advertise in any form for this • Never do USG at an unregistered place • Don't send the sample to an unregistered place or vice versa • Don't employ or take the services of unqualified person • Don't sell machines to unregistered place • Don't do PNDT except under the conditions and reasons specified • Don't make any sign or expression in any manner • Don't argue or misbehave with AA • Don't ignore any guidelines/instructions/circulars by AA • Don't use portable machines except conditions specified. • Don't change the place, person or equipment without informing the AA • Don't violate the code of conduct of rule 18 • Don't tamper the record • Never confess/admit your mistake to defend you later on in the court.

TABLE 4: PC and PNDT checklist.[9]

No	Point	Yes/No
1.	Registration of center	
2.	Employment of qualified staff	
3.	Maintain records scrupulously in the prescribed manner–5 column register records, lab reports, USG plates, recommendation letters, self-referral, forms, consents, all records	
4.	Filling the Form F as per the act accurately	
5.	Declaration by pregnant patient before USG	
6.	Written consent when necessary	
7.	Declaration by the doctor	
8.	Timely submission of records	
9.	Display of Board 3 * 2 blue and white—at conspicuous place	
10.	Certificate of Registration—at conspicuous place	
11.	Inform AA for change in place, person, or equipment—before 1 month of change and seek for reissuance of certificate with changes incorporated	
12.	Change in ownership or management—surrender the certificate	
13.	A copy of Act and rules, with amendment—available	
14.	E-records—take a print with authorized signature	
15.	Code of conduct—name and designation on dress	
16.	Submission of reports by 5th of following month	
17.	Online submission of Form F in the same month (Nil even if not done)	
18.	Application of renewal before 30 days of expiry of registration	
19.	Portable machines—use within the registered premises along with display or certificate	

Take Home Message

To conclude, in short, all persons including the owners, employees or any other person associated with the registered places under the Act should observe the code of conduct keeping in mind the above-narrated facts to avoid any further litigation and for safe and peaceful practice. They must ensure that no provision of the Act or the Rules mentioned above in this article is violated in any manner. So, knowledge of the Act and its implementation in practice will help us to avoid litigations or defend ourselves in court.

REFERENCES

1. The Pre-Conception and Pre-Natal Diagnostic Techniques (Prohibition of Sex Selection) Act, 1994. Answers to Frequently Asked Questions, A Handbook for implementing bodies. [cited 2024 June 12]. Available from: http://www.nhmmeghalaya.nic.in/programmes/pcpndt/pcpndt-faq-implementing-bodies.pdf
2. The Pre-conception & Pre-natal Diagnostic Techniques (Prohibition of Sex Selection) Act, 1994—BARE ACT [as amended by Act 14 of 2003, w.e.f. 14-02-2003 vide SO 175 (E), dt.14-02-2003] [cited 2024 June 11]. Available from: https://dhsfw.assam.gov.in/sites/default/files/swf_utility_folder/departments/dirfw_lipl_in_oid_5/menu/document/eng.pdf
3. The PC & PNDT (Prohibition of Sex Selection) Rules, 1996 [As amended vide GSR 599 (E), dt. 19-06-2017, w.e.f. 19-06-2017] [cited 2024 June 11]. Available from: https://rajswasthya.nic.in/PCPNDT%20%20Dt.27.06.2017.pdf.
4. The PC & PNDT (Regulation & Prevention of Misuse) (Advisory Committees) Rules, 1996. [cited 2024 June 10]. Available from: http://nhmmeghalaya.nic.in/acts-rules/advisory-pcpndt.pdf.
5. The PC & PNDT (Prohibition of sex Selection) (Six months Training) Rules, 2014. [cited 2024 June 15]. Available from: https://indiankanoon.org/doc/195755613/

6. Vinod Soni and Ors v. Union of India & CEHAT (2005 Cri LJ 3408) [cited 2024 June 25]. Available from: https://indiankanoon.org/doc/457104/.
7. Dr Pratikar Doshi v. CDHO Ahmedabad. SCA 5079/2006.
8. FOGSI v. UOI & ORS Writ Petition (C) no.129 of 2017 [cited 2024 June 25]. Available from: https://indiankanoon.org/doc/123238150/.
9. Thakker J, Jankharia B. PC-PNDT: Part I. Indian J Radiol Imaging. 2008;18(1):3. doi: 10.4103/0971-3026.38500.
10. Pre-Conception and Pre-Natal Diagnostic Techniques (PC-PNDT) Checklist. [Internet]. [cited 2024 Jul 20]. Available from: https://www.google.com/search?client=opera&q=PC+PNDT+Checklist&sourceid=opera&ie=UTF-8&oe=UTF-8.

CHAPTER 6

Medicolegal Aspect of Child Sexual Abuse and the Protection of Children from Sexual Offences (POCSO) Act 2012

BL Chaudhary

INTRODUCTION

Children contribute to more than one-third of India's current population, half of whom are deprived of basic education, nutrition, and health necessities. According to the 2011 Census, population of children across India during the measured time period was approximately 444 million, it means 19% of the world's children live in India and that makes India, the second child home of the world.[1] As per the survey conducted by Government of India, an estimate of more than 53% of Indian children are subjected to sexual abuse/assault.[2] The underreporting of child sexual abuse is today the biggest problem for the State as it is a suppressed fact in the name of family secrecy. Sharing private family matters is taboo, and the family is expected to deal with personal matters privately. To avoid shame, families must protect their reputation and remain within the community. Children's identities are rooted in the family's identity; thus, anything that would jeopardize their family's name is kept hidden, even from other family members. Secrecy about child sexual assault protects perpetrators instead of children and allows abuse to continue. The failure of parents or caregivers to believe and act to protect children increased their level of distress and prevented them from receiving mental health treatment.

The National Study on Child Abuse India 2007 was supported by the Government of India and was initiated so that a more accurate and comprehensive understanding of child abuse and neglect could be gained. Various forms of abuse, including child sexual abuse, were examined in two major states from each of the geographic regions of India (North, South, East, West, Central and Northeast) and the city of Mumbai. The study included children (5–18 years) and young adults (18–24 years). This report provides specific information about various forms and expressions of sexual abuse among children and youth in India.[2] The significant findings about child abuse and neglect emerged from the study on child abuse in India are: (a) Young children in the sample (ages 5–12) reported the highest levels of abuse; (b) There were no differences in incidence of physical abuse in boys compared to girls; and (c) Persons who committed sexual abuse were the trusted individuals who held positions of authority; 70% of victims of child sexual abuse (CSA) never disclosed their abuse.

DEFINITION: CHILD SEXUAL ABUSE AND NEGLECT[3]

According to the WHO, *child sexual abuse and neglect* involve the child in a sexual activity for which he or she is neither physically developed nor fully comprehended, and no informed consent is provided for the act. These are inducements or coercion of a child to engage in prostitution, drug crimes, or other unlawful sexual practices, such as pornographic performance for producing

TABLE 1: Indicators of child sexual abuse.[2,3]

• Running away from home frequently • Staying at school beyond class time • Threatening self-harm or suicide • Assaulting others • Trying to deny or hide signs of abuse • Verbalizing a poor self-image • Thumb-sucking or nail-biting • Poor relationships with other children • Verbal abuse of other children • Irrational fears • Overly compliant behavior • Being inattentive or absent from school frequently	• Hyper vigilance • Constant over activity • Aggressiveness • Rocking or uncontrollable crying • Excessive day dreaming • Perfectionism • Compulsive behavior • Never looking to caretaker (s) for comfort • Passivity, maintaining a "low profile" • Regression or delayed development • In-discriminant friendliness with strangers • Fearfulness when other children cry and are approached by an adult

adult sexual materials. In the United States, the Centers for Disease Control and Prevention (CDC) and the Department for Children and Families (DCF) define child maltreatment as any Act or series of acts of commission or omission by a parent or other caregiver that results in harm, potential for harm, or threat of harm to a child. Thus, child abuse includes physical, emotional, or sexual exploitation; any kind of threat of harm; or the neglect of a child. Child abuse is of the following types:

i. Neglect
ii. Physical abuse
iii. Psychological or emotional abuse (continuous or repeated exploitation of child, thus leading to re-victimization)
iv. Sexual abuse (including penetration or performing sexual act for transmitting images over the Internet)

Definition of a Child: Legal definition of child is adopted from the UN Convention on the Rights of the Child, 1989 (Article I) and is defined as any person below 18 years of age to be considered as child. India is a signatory to the UN resolution and charter. In India, according to the Juvenile Justice Care and Protection of Children Act and the POCSO Act 2012, child is defined as any person below 18 years.[4] For the purpose of medical facility or clinical aspect, the child is defined as any person who is less than 12 years of age.

POINTERS TO CHILD SEXUAL ABUSE AND NEGLECT[2,3]

The general signs and symptoms that might suggest child abuse and neglect include, but are not limited to, the list provided in **Table 1**.

According to India's Hell Holes report in 2013, more than 48,000 child-rape cases were recorded from 2001 to 2011, and India saw an increase of 336% in child-rape cases from 2001 (2,113 cases) to 2011 (7,112 cases). Child sexual abuse is rampant, indiscriminate and cuts across class, geography, culture and religion and it happens in cities and villages, by fathers, brothers, relatives, neighbors, teachers and strangers.[5]

Data recorded by the National Crime Records Bureau (NCRB):[6]

i. *Rise in Child Sex Abuse Cases:* There has been a rise in child sex abuse cases, with 969 cases registered in 2021, 842 in 2020, and 164 in 2019.
ii. *POCSO Act Cases:* In 2021, 53,874 cases were registered under the POCSO Act, accounting for 36% of all crimes against children.

iii. *Crimes Against Children:* In 2021, there were 1,49,404 cases of crimes against children, an increase of 16.2% from 2020.
iv. *Sexual Offences:* Sexual offences against children are steadily increasing, with 33,348 incidents registered under Sections 4 and 6 of the POCSO Act in 2021.
v. *Kidnapping and Abduction:* In 2021, 67,245 FIRs were registered under Kidnapping and Abduction, with 12,202 minor girls compelled for marriage.
vi. *Missing Children:* In 2021, 28,756 incidents of missing children were deemed kidnapped.

The WHO estimates that nearly three in four children or 300 million children aged 2–4 years regularly suffer physical punishment and/or psychological violence in the hands of parents and caregivers. One in 5 women and 1 in 13 men report having been sexually abused as a child aged 0–17 years. 120 million girls and young women under 20 years of age have suffered some form of forced sexual contact.[7]

CAUSE OF CHILD ABUSE BEHAVIOR

The root cause of action responsible for this abnormal sexual abuse behavior, especially towards children, cannot be explained in a few simple words, but it is the resultant action of the deep-rooted suppressed sexual desire coupled with contributing biological and psychological risk factors.

The contributing risk factors can be the following:

- Disabilities
- Mental retardation in children
- Social isolation of families
- Parents' lack of understanding of children's needs and child development
- Parent's history of domestic abuse
- Poverty and other socioeconomic disadvantages, such as unemployment, family disorganization, dissolution
- Violence, including intimate partner violence
- Lack of family cohesion
- Substance abuse in family
- Young and single non-biological parents
- Poor parent-child relationships
- Negative interactions
- Parental thoughts and emotions supporting maltreatment behaviors
- Parental stress and distress, including depression or other mental health conditions
- Community violence

Child abuse and neglect can occur at any place like Home, Public places, foster homes, schools, and even strects; all children can be at risk, whether they are normal children or a vulnerable group. Vulnerable group includes:

- Destitute children
- Orphans
- Abandoned children
- Street children
- HIV/AIDS affected children
- Child beggars
- Substance/drug abusers
- Child laborers
- Neglected children
- Children with a single parent
- Rape victims
- Sex workers
- Children of poor parents or with physical, mental or terminal illness
- Children of refugees, migrants, construction workers and of prostitutes

The key determinant factors that make individual children vulnerable to sexual abuse, are the following:

- Female sex
- Unaccompanied children

- Children in foster care
- Adopted children
- Stepchildren
- Physically or mentally handicapped children
- Children with history of past abuse, poverty, war/armed conflict
- Psychological or cognitive vulnerability
- single parent homes/broken homes
- Social isolation (lacking an emotional support network)
- Parent (s) with mental illness, or alcohol or drug dependency
- Street and working children
- Children of sex workers
- Abused, tortured and exploited children
- Substance abuse
- Children affected by natural calamities
- Emergencies and man-made disasters
- Children with disabilities
- Child beggars
- Children suffering from terminal/ incurable disease
- Orphans, abandoned and destitute children
- Missing or run-away children
- Children with STI/HIV/AIDS infection

RELATIONSHIP BETWEEN ABUSER AND VICTIM

Inappropriate Relationship Model

When an abuser is in a powerful position over the victim, the relationship could be physical, emotional, or financial. A victim is in the illusion that his/her relationship is pure, sincere, and loving, but the abuser continues to exploit it.

The Boyfriend Mode

When the abuser pretends to be a boyfriend and cares for her by offering gifts, dating, etc., at the same time, he takes gratification through manipulating or fondling her private parts, and with passing time, the abuser enters a sexual relationship with the victim.

Organized Exploitation and Trafficking

Children are abused by multiple adults on a network that moves victims across the country by exchanging their images of child abuse.

Dimensions

Its dimension is large and includes the following:

- Oral-genital
- Genital-genital
- Genital-rectal
- Hand-genital
- Hand-rectal
- Hand-breast contact
- Displaying or forced view of sexual anatomy
- Showing pornography
- Involving child for sexual materials, prostitution and spectrum of unlawful activities ranging from rape to exhibitionism and voyeurism
- Inappropriate sexual behavior such as fondling a child's genitals or making the child to fondle the adult's genitals and the sexual abuse (intercourse, incest, rape and sodomy)
- Intentionally engaging in sexual activity in front of a child or encouraging a child to engage in sexual activity with someone else or making a child strip or masturbate
- Meeting a child following sexual grooming
- With the mala-fide intention of abusing them, thus taking, making or allowing a stranger to take, distribute, show or advertise indecent videos or via webcams, the images or the photographs of the child
- Paying for the sexual services of a child

- Encouraging a child into prostitution or pornography

These are the acts, generally committed by persons responsible for the care and guardianship of the child or related to him (for example, a baby-sitter, parent, neighbors, relatives, peer, older child, friend, or a day-care provider) and have implied meaning of having no informed consent from the child; hence, the acts are termed as child abuse. When the acts are touching, any private part of the body, clothed or unclothed, either by using an object or by penetration, including rape or penetration of the mouth with an object or a part of the body, are termed sexual abuse.

INDICATORS

Consider the possibility of sexual abuse when the child:

- Has difficulty walking or sitting
- Suddenly, refuses to change to the gym or participate in physical activities
- Reports nightmares or bedwetting.
- experienced a sudden change in appetite.
- Demonstrates bizarre, sophisticated, or unusual sexual knowledge or behavior.
- Becomes pregnant or contract venereal disease, particularly under the age of 14.
- Reports of sexual abuse by a parent or another adult caregiver.

Consider the possibility of sexual abuse when the parent or other adult care giver:

- They are unduly protective of the child or severely limit the child's contact with other children, especially those of the opposite sex.
- They are secretive and isolated.
- They are jealous or controlling the family members.

Although no single behavior can be considered evidence of sexual abuse, a pattern of behaviors is a matter of concern. In practice, clear physical findings of sexual abuse are seldom seen in children, because child sexual abuse rarely involves physical harm.

CONSEQUENCES

Childhood is considered a developmental stage and prone to physical and psychosocial risks. Child abuse is a violation of a child's human rights and can develop both short- and long-term mental and emotional problems, apart from physical injuries such as internal lacerations, bleeding, damage to internal organs, and death.

As a result, children develop a disturbed personality with recurrence of depression, sadness, anger, low self-esteem, self-harm, anxiety, eating disorders, post-traumatic stress disorder such as difficulties in communication, school/learning problems or lower educational performance, tendency for substance abuse and suicide, disturbing emotional thoughts that cause distress or confusion, poor physical health such as obesity, aches and pains, and criminal behavior.

Abusers

There is no single type or community of child abusers. The abusers may be men, women, teenagers, or a near and dear person of any profession on whom the child reposes his trust or who he already knows. They come from all sections of society, with varied backgrounds. Abusers are quite normal, and people are in a position of trust and are often difficult to distinguish.

The abusers can be parents, caregivers, teachers, neighbors, family members, step-parents, siblings' frequent visitors, neighbors, strangers, employers, and childcare persons.

SCOPE OF A STANDARD OPERATING PROCEDURE FORMAT[8]

Currently, no uniform language exists for text to be adopted for conducting standard operating procedures, for making reports, method of carrying out the examination, or following the prescribed format for documentation in any of the hospitals or healthcare facilities. It is the high time that a manual of SOPs on the standard framework for taking informed consent, following the checklist for collection of evidences and the documentation while conducting the medical examination, providing intervention such as basic and emergency treatment, referrals such as counseling of child and parents, help of appropriate agency and help in opinion formation is drafted in order to guide the medical practitioners, healthcare providers, police, social service personnel's and the law officers dealing with such cases.

INVESTIGATION OF A CHILD SEXUAL ABUSE CASE[8]

Child sexual abuse victims are young and lack a policed way of giving testimony about sensitive and traumatic incidents, more so in an intimidating setting of the courtroom. This state of mind of the victim, with an overlapping trust relationship with the offender and his or her parent's siding with the offender (due to economic or loyalty burden), causes a delay in reporting the incident and thus in failure to preserve the physical evidence. Due to this child sexual abuse, cases are often difficult to prosecute successfully. Coupled with the poor level of interview of the child victim by the near and dear and the law enforcement officers who are not trained in forensic examination, collection and documentation of evidence of true facts leads to confusion and revictimization of the child by exposing him/her to emotional trauma brought about by the stress of being questioned time and again concerning the same unpleasant incident. Thus, the child victim in the process becomes so traumatized and exhausted that parents or caretakers develop a genuine fear that the pursuit of the case in court would cause more harm to the child victim than doing good to him or her. In addition, prosecutors also start fearing that the child victim may not be able to withstand the pressures of a courtroom trial, and thus will be unable to provide the testimony necessary to get a conviction.

For these reasons, forensic interviews are conducted, wherein the interviewer carries an enormous responsibility, as he or she can single-handedly determine the probability of disclosure and improve the disclosure rates, thereby increasing the likelihood of prosecution.

Approximately 90% of child victims of abuse do not show evidence of physical damage.[9] Therefore, forensic investigation based on interviews with a child is very important in disclosing the facts. Specific models can be developed and empirically examined with regard to legal system involvement (e.g., juvenile, domestic, criminal), age, gender, disability status, culture, and other variables such as relationship with the accused. The role of an appropriate forensic medical examination is of major importance in the full investigation of such cases and building an effective prosecution in the court. The physical examination included inspection of the whole body with special attention to the mouth, breasts, genitals, perineal region, buttocks, and anus, with the doctor performing the collection of biological evidence, provided that the alleged sexual abuse had occurred within the last 72 hours. Cultures and serological tests for STDs are decided by the doctor, and pregnancy tests should be mandatory in each case of a girl of reproductive age.

COMPREHENSIVE MEDICAL ASSESSMENT

The presence of a forensic nurse examiner was necessary for the assessment. Children may prefer to be examined by a doctor of the same sex. The details of the hymen and injuries should be noted. Recorded photographic evidence. It is important to note that in 70–85% of cases of documented sexual abuse, physical examination is normal.[9] Examination of clothes of victims for semen stains, struggle, tears, trace material, etc. should be performed. The assessment should be recorded with special performance. History taking from the child victim should be taken with a sensitive, empathic, and nonjudgmental attitude, and should be recorded verbatim. Child victims should be protected from any further emotional trauma by not exposing them to the accused during the physical examination; it is of great importance that the history taking from the parent or caretaker should be documented separately and must be done away from the child victim.

The child should be treated well with respect and dignity in a normal conducive environment that facilitates ease of comfort in the minds of sexually abused child victims. Points to be covered in history include place, time, witness, present and past history, noticeable behavioral change, developmental and immunization history, family history, pedigree chart, social history, psychosocial history including details regarding home, education, eating behavior, activities and peers, drugs, depression, suicide, sexual history, and sleep patterns. Any kind of resistance to examination: tip-to-toe general physical examination including vitals, sexual maturity, injuries, and examination of external genitalia. Forensic samples maintaining the chain of evidence, including skin, hair, clothing, saliva, and oral and genitourinary secretions, are preserved and sent to the forensic science laboratory for further evaluation, especially in acute cases of sexual abuse. Detailed hematological profile and imaging of body parts to evaluate the extent of injury The following investigations need to be done such as STD screening, including low and high vaginal (in post-pubertal girls) swabs and urethral swabs in boys and serology for HIV, hepatitis B and syphilis, pregnancy test, age estimation. To make a final conclusion after discussing the case with seniors, peers, psychologists, NGOs, and social workers.

One-Stop Centers

The one-stop center (OSC) facility is the initiation of The Ministry of Women & Child Development, Govt of India to provide support and assistance to victims of child sexual abuse.[10] OSC is a place where all facilities including medical, police, psychosocial counseling, legal aid, shelter, referral and facilities for videoconferencing, available under one place.

Safeguarding Sexually Active Children

In India, it has been the duty of the family to take care of and protect children. A strong-knit patriarchal family that is meant to look after its children well has seldom realized that children are individuals with their own rights. The constitution of India guarantees many fundamental rights to children, but the approach to ensure the fulfilment of these rights has been more needs-based rather than rights-based. Current child welfare schemes do not have sufficient budgetary allocations needed to create an enabling environment; thus, legislation is required to address issues of child abuse, make a policy on child protection, formulate interventions, welfare, outreach services, and create an information base on child protection.

Setting up a National Commission for the Protection of the Rights of the Child began with the process of drafting a bill to prevent offences against children and also to formulate a comprehensive national-level scheme to deal with child protection and welfare. The source of data presently available from the National Crime Records Bureau, though useful but constituted in miniscule numbers, as very often crimes against children are either not reported or cognizance is not taken, and some crimes against children are not covered under existing legislation.

Sexual offenses involving children are crimes against humanity, as they scare child victims for life. Child sexual abuse is considered to be one of the greatest threats to a child's well-being and safety. Prevention and dealing with this situation are difficult tasks. It requires a multidisciplinary approach with great effort and coordination among public administration, numerous professionals, families, victims, and society in general. Clinicians do not report all suspicious injuries to a child, even if the level of suspicion is high. The child, family, injury characteristics, and clinician's previous experience influenced the decisions to report. As child sexual abuse is a private and secretive crime, it is often difficult for law enforcement agencies to detect it without assistance. Any information, no matter how small or insignificant it may seem to the physician, could help protect a child. Pediatric academic programs must provide curricula on child abuse and neglect with far more internal training and resources for child abuse education than merely emergency medicine and family medicine programs. Decisions about reporting to child protective services must be made with a national duty to protect a child's tender life.

THE POCSO ACT 2012[10]

The Government of India promulgated (Protection of Children from Sexual Offences) Act 2012, w.e.f. 14th November, 2012. The POCSO Act, 2012, is a special law that governs and provides children protection from criminal offences of sexual assault, sexual violence, pornography, and safeguards the child victim's interests with child-oriented mandatory reporting, recording of evidence, and investigation with a speedy trial of offences through Special Courts.

It provides federal funding to states to support prevention, assessment, investigation, prosecution, and treatment activities. Additionally, it identifies the federal role in supporting research, evaluation, technical assistance, and data collection activities; establishes the District Child Protection Unit (DCPU) and mandates to sets forth a minimum definition of child abuse and neglect." This Act defines a child as a person below 18 years of age. Further it defines different forms of sexual abuse:

- Penetrative and non-penetrative assault on children
- Sexual harassment, sexual violence on children
- Pornography (Display via electronic media, images or videos of an sexual act involving children)

According to POCSO Act[11]

- All child abuse cases are mandartorily reported to the police, and a person with such knowledge is duty bound to report the case, failing which he may be punished with a six-month imprisonment or fine.

- Police shall act as child protectors during the investigative process with duty and responsibility to make arrangements for shelter home, medical treatment, care and protection of the said child, once reporting of sexual abuse case is received and matter is mandatorily brought to the Child Welfare Committee's (CWC) notice within 24 hours and CWC makes arrangements for safety and security, if in case needed).
- Medical examination of a child is meticulously conducted in a distress-free environment in the presence of a parent or any other person whom the child trusts. Medical examination was performed by a female doctor in the case of a female child victim.
- Special courts conduct trials in child-abuse cases under a camera without revealing the identity of the child. The child may have parents or a person of trust present during the trial or testifying and given an interpreter or other professional if needed for assistance.
- Child victims are allowed to testify via videoconferencing rather than by physical appearance in courtroom or for repeat appearance in court.
- Child abuse cases must be disposed of within a year from the date of the offences being reported.
- Courts are empowered to determine the amount of compensation given to the child for medical treatment and rehabilitation.
- State Government to frame guidelines (under section 39, POCSO Act 2012) for persons experienced in dealing with such cases, including NGOs, professionals, experts, or persons who are trained and have working knowledge of psychology, social work, physical health, mental health, and child development to assist the child at the time of the trial and pre-trial stage.
- Prompt and systematic multi-sectoral intervention and referrals that provide a conducive environment to children during medical examination, treatment, rehabilitation, and justice delivery process, and fast recovery of children from physical or mental trauma.

To achieve the above-mentioned objectives, a multidisciplinary response is warranted from police, medical institutes, the judiciary system, psychology counselors, etc. Therefore, medical professionals who are involved in providing medical examinations and treatment to the child need to foster an integrated response mechanism for enabling the last-mile holistic healing process and getting the child adopted by the whole community and integrating it back into the social fabric.

ROLE AND DUTIES OF MEDICAL PROFESSIONALS

Section 27 of the POCSO Act, 2012, provides guidelines for medical professionals providing treatment, medical examination, collecting forensic evidence, and later deposing the evidence in the courtroom.

Medical Examination of Victim

As per Section 27 of POCSO Act:

Section 27 (1): That the medical examination of a child in respect of whom any offence has been committed under this Act, shall, notwithstanding that a First Information Report or complaint has not been registered for the offences under this Act, be conducted in accordance with section 164A of the Code of Criminal Procedure, 1973 (Henceforth Section 184 Bharatiya Nagarik Suraksha Sanhita, 2023)

Section 27 (2): Medical examination is conducted by a lady doctor for a girl child victim.

Section 27 (3): Medical examination is conducted in the presence of a parent or a person of trust in the child victim.

Section 27 (4): Medical examination of the child victim shall be conducted in the presence of a female nominee of the head of the medical institution in case sub-section 3 conditions are not met.

The Protection of Children from Sexual Offences (Amendment) Act, 2019[12]

The Protection of Children from Sexual Offences (POCSO) Act, 2012, was amended in 2019 to strengthen laws related to child sexual abuse in India. The POCSO Act (2012) was enacted to protect children from sexual offenses, including sexual harassment, assault, and exploitation.

Key amendments were made in 2019:

1. Death penalty for aggravated penetrative sexual assault in children aged <12 years.
2. Increased minimum imprisonment for various offenses.
3. Mandatory reporting of sexual offenses by individuals and organizations.
4. Establishment of Special Courts for a Speedy Trial of POCSO cases.
5. Introduction to child-friendly procedures for recording statements and conducting trials.
6. Enhanced penalties for storage and possession of child pornography.
7. The inclusion of new offenses, such as using a child for pornographic purposes.

The POCSO Act, 2012, and its amendments aim to:

1. Protecting children from sexual exploitation and abuse.
2. Ensure prompt reporting and investigation of sexual offenses.
3. Provide child-friendly procedures for victims.
4. Punish offenders with stringent penalties.

Salient features of the POCSO Act 2012 are compared with the POCSO (Amendment) Act, 2019[10-12] in **Table 2**.

MEDICAL EXAMINATION OF CHILD UNDER SECTION 27 OF THE POSCO ACT 2012

A medical examination of a child was conducted as per the provisions of Section 27 of the POCSO Act, 2012 and Sec 184 Bharatiya Nagarik Suraksha (BNS) Sanhita 2023 (previously Sec. 164-A CrPC 1973). A medical examination of a child victim can be conducted before an FIR is filed or a complaint is registered. The medical examination shall be conducted in the presence of the parent or person of trust of the child by a registered medical practitioner in a government hospital or a hospital run by a local authority within 24 hours from the time of reporting of offence. Medical examination shall be conducted by a female doctor in the case of a girl-child victim. Medical examination of the child-abuse victim shall be conducted in the presence of a female nominee of the head of the medical institution, in case sub-section (3) conditions are not met. Once the medical examination of child abuse victim is over, its report should be immediately be sent by the doctor to the investigation officer who shall forward it to the Magistrate referred to in Section 193 BNS (previously Section 173 CrPC) as part of the documents referred to in clause: (a) of sub-section (5) of that section.

TABLE 2: Comparison between the POCSO Act, 2012 and the POCSO Act (Amendment) 2019.

	The POCSO Act, 2012	***The POCSO (Amendment) Act, 2019***
Salient Features	• Defined sexual offences against children, including penetration, touching, and exploitation • Made offences gender-neutral, applying to both boys and girls • Established Special Courts for trial of offences • Introduced the concept of "zero tolerance" for child sexual abuse • Prescribed punishment for offences, including life imprisonment	• The purpose of 2019 amendments is to strengthen the Act by introducing harsher punishments, expanding the scope of offences, and improving the reporting and trial mechanisms • Introduced death penalty for aggravated penetrative sexual assault on children under 12 years • Increased minimum punishment for certain offences, such as using children for pornographic purposes • Made punishment for certain offences, like storing or possessing child pornography, more stringent • Introduced a new offence: "administering hormones to a child to induce early sexual maturity" • Mandated the establishment of Special Courts for POCSO cases in every district • Introduced a provision for the mandatory reporting of sexual abuse by individuals and institutions
Offence	***The POCSO Act 2012***	***The POCSO (Amendment) Act, 2019***
i. Use of child for pornographic purposes	*Maximum:* 5 years	*Minimum:* 5 years
ii. Use of child for pornographic purposes resulting in penetrative sexual assault	• *Minimum:* 10 years • *Maximum:* Life imprisonment	• *Minimum:* 10 years (in case of child below 16 years: 20 years) • *Maximum:* Life imprisonment
iii. Use of child for pornographic purposes resulting in aggravated penetrative sexual assault	Life imprisonment	• *Minimum:* 20 years • *Maximum:* Life imprisonment, or death
iv. Use of child for pornographic purposes resulting in sexual assault	• *Minimum:* Six years • *Maximum:* Eight years	• Minimum: Three years • Maximum: Five years
v. Use of child for pornographic purposes resulting in aggravated sexual assault	• *Minimum:* Eight years • *Maximum:* 10 years	• *Minimum:* Five years • *Maximum:* Seven years

Contents of Medical Examination

Doctors and healthcare providers are the first point of contact, confirming that a child has been or is being abused. The following are the contents of medical examination of child-abuse case:

Consent

Firstly, doctors must take the informed consent of the child by exchanging details of the medical examination procedure and making the child aware about what is involved therein. The right to informed consent implies the right to informed refusal. Secondly, the child or her parent should be allowed enough time to understand and to clarify their doubts. Finally, the child and/or the parent/guardian should agree to the examination voluntarily. In the case of a toddler child or otherwise incapable of giving consent due to non-understanding or unconsciousness, consent should be obtained from the child's parent or a person of the trust of the child. Doctors should also inform the child or legal guardian that healthcare professionals may have a legal obligation to share the information with law enforcement agencies.

Medical History and Examination

Doctors should conduct examinations in a sensitive and empathetic manner and ensure that the examination is least disturbing to the child, should not be painful, obtain a detailed medical history of the child victim, conduct a detailed examination for physical or emotional symptoms, and prepare a complete medical report with diagnosis and treatment. Doctors should also examine and diagnose acute and chronic residual trauma and STDs with photographic/video documentation of all findings as a result of the offence. Make a differential diagnosis of emotional and behavioral complaints and physical signs of sexual abuse. The doctor's role becomes critical in diagnosing sexual abuse when a child-abuse victim complains; however, there is no direct allegation of sexual abuse. Complaint relates to:

- Vaginal discharge
- Abdominal pain or encopresis
- Has no complaint but an incidental finding of an enlarged hymeneal ring

Doctors should record the nature of the assault, such as anal or vaginal pain and bleeding, pain with voiding or defecation, or oral penetration, and any injuries such as bruises, burns, scars, or rashes on the skin and breasts. In addition, we checked for any signs of force and/or restraint, particularly around the neck and extremities. If the survivor is menstruating at the time of examination, a second examination is required to clearly record the injuries. Questions should be asked in the child's own and simple words, open-ended, non-leading questions like tell more or then what happened, etc. Encourage children to ask questions regarding the examination and show equipment to avoid fear. At a minimum, medical history should cover any known health problems (including allergies), immunization status, and medications.

Evidence Collection

Carefully collect and preserve forensic evidence, including clothing, especially underwear. This is positive evidence for DNA samples to testify in court whenever required.

Privacy

Examination should be least disturbing, never be painful to the child, and not be conducted in a labor room or else ensure patient privacy and be sensitive to the child's feelings of embarrassment. Allow it if the child chooses a trusted adult to be present.

Mandatory Reporting

Medical professionals have a legal obligation to report matters to law enforcement agencies. Failure to do this would result in imprisonment for up to six months, with or without fines.

Referral and Counseling

Wherever necessary, the child was referred to counseling to test for HIV and other STDs.

If the child resists the examination: Never force the examination. A rule of thumb is that the physical examination should not cause any trauma to the child, so if a child at any stage refuses the genital-anal examination, it may be wise to defer the examination. Doctors should address children's fears and anxieties, or potential sources of unease and utmost comfort, and care should be provided. Sedation or anesthesia is rarely needed but is considered only when the child refuses the examination and conditions requiring examination and evidence collection and medical attention, such as bleeding or a suspected foreign body. The speculum examination of a prepubertal girl should be performed under anesthesia.

Emergency Medical Care of the Child

On receipt of information under Section 19 of the POCSO Act about the offence and that police are satisfied that the child needs urgent medical care and protection, the child abuse victim is taken to a healthcare facility (government or private) for emergency medical care, as soon as possible, but not later than 24 hours of receiving such information. The standard operating procedure described in Section 397 BNS (previously Sec. 357C CrPC) states:

- The healthcare facility is to provide first-aid or medical treatment, free of cost, to the child abuse victims of a sexual offence with protection of privacy, in the presence of the parent or a person of trust of the victim, without demanding any legal, magisterial, or other documentation.
- Emergency medical care of child abuse victims should include treatment for cuts, bruises, other genital injuries, exposure to STDs, HIV, and their prophylaxis. In case of a possible pregnancy, the matter of giving emergency contraceptives can be discussed with the pubertal child, her parent, or a person of her trust.
- Referrals for mental or psychological health counseling should be performed, whenever necessary.
- Forensic evidences are collected in accordance with section 27 of the Act.

Compensation for Medical Expenses

The Special Court may award compensation to the child victim for the physical or mental trauma caused or for immediate rehabilitation under Section 33(8). As per Rule 7(1) of the Act, interim compensation may be paid to meet the immediate needs of the child after registration of the FIR. Furthermore, Rule 7(3) provides the criteria for fixing the award of compensation, including the severity of the mental or physical harm or injury suffered by the child, the expenditure incurred or likely to be incurred on his/her medical treatment for physical and/or mental health, and any disability suffered as a result of the offence.

ROLE OF MEDICAL PROFESSIONALS AS EXPERT WITNESSES

Child sexual abuse cases are often exceedingly difficult to prove based on no clear physical evidence. While many children are capable witnesses, they fail to give conclusive testimony; therefore, children's testimony becomes ineffective, and hence legally untenable in the court of law. In such cases, the testimony or opinion of an expert medical witness which is given on the basis of history, child's statements and findings of medical examination, becomes the basis for understanding the chain of evidence to build up a case for prosecution.

An expert medical witness in the present context, as understood from recent court judgements, is a person who has acquired special knowledge, skills, or experience in the medical profession branch dealing with forensic nursing examination of child sexual abuse cases. Such knowledge may have been obtained by practice, observation or careful study. Expert evidence is covered under Section 39-45 Bharatiya Sakshya Adhiniyam-BSA (previously *Sec. 45-51 of the Indian Evidence Act*). In general, the opinions of medical professionals are admissible upon questions such as insanity, the causes of diseases, the nature of the injuries, weapons that might have been used to cause injuries or death, medicines, poisons, and gestation conditions.

Regarding forensic examinations, medical professionals typically describe the process of examining the victim, the physical findings that were observed, and their interpretation. It is important to remember that the medical professional cannot be asked to testify to the diagnosis of sexual abuse, the degree of force used by the abuser, or the victim consented to any sexual activity. What he/she can appropriately conclude is whether there is evidence of sexual contact and/or recent trauma and whether the medical history and examination are consistent with sexual abuse. Opinions are also sought from mental health experts as to the psychological effects of child sexual abuse, such as PTSD and Child Sexual Abuse Accommodation Syndrome.

The legal representative who proposes the use of expert testimony to establish their credentials, preferably listings to their formal qualifications. The adequacy of the qualification of the expert and the admissibility of his/her testimony are within the discretion of the Special Court. Before providing evidence, the expert usually prepares a report, assessing either one or more parties to the case. His/her report should be reliable on the basis of the following criteria:

- It should provide a context in layman's terms from which to understand the basis of his/her opinion It should be clear when the expert is stating corroborated fact.
- The expert must review the information impartially before making assertions, rather than ignoring matters that are inconvenient to their conclusions.
- The report should focus on examining and analyzing the crucial issues of the case.
- The expert should demonstrate knowledge of the process and dynamics of child sexual abuse and help to make sense of the child's and non-abusing parent's experiences and perceptions.
- Victims and non-abusing partners of offenders often do not act rationally and can appear collusive with the offender, whereas their behavior results from control, the offender exercises over them. This can be explained in the expert report in language that the court, advocate, and parties can understand.

- The expert must not rely solely on quoted research to support his/her arguments and should also refer to clinical experience.
- Expert opinion must be premised at a reasonable degree of clinical certainty.

It is important to remember that while an expert's testimony may be deemed relevant, necessary, reliable and therefore admissible under the aforementioned guidelines, it is ultimately the prerogative of the judge to determine what weight should be afforded to the testimony. No matter how qualified the expert, the court is not bound by an expert's conclusions and can exercise its discretion in this regard, keeping in mind all other evidence presented to it.

CONCLUSION

Child sexual abuse is a violation of the chastity of a child's body, physically and emotionally, while still growing. This act of sexual abuse could not be comprehended by the victim because of its gravity and consequences, as it is perpetuated by a person close to him or her and entrusted with the responsibility for care and protection. It is potential harm to the child's health, survival, and development of child personality. It is a cruel and tragic occurrence in a child's life, and a serious infringement of a child's rights to health and protection.

This ignited the alarm in the government of the day in India for the need to immediately change the pace of convictions. Hence, the Govt of India promulgated the POCSO Act 2012, w.e.f. November 14, 2012, and it was amended in 2019 to strengthen the laws related to child sexual abuse in India. The POCSO Act, 2012 and its amendments aim to: (i) protect children from sexual exploitation and abuse, (ii) ensure prompt reporting and investigation of sexual offenses, (iii) provide child-friendly procedures for victims, and (iv) punish offenders with stringent penalties.

It should not be sufficient to rest on our laurels by bringing the POCSO Act, but it also needs better implementation of the Act at the grassroots level by making procedures and environment more child-friendly and ensuring sensitivity while dealing with and testifying to child abuse victims in the courtrooms. Ultimately, the burden of proving innocence must lie on the offender and not the child if we want to increase conviction in child sexual abuse cases. The focus must not be on the quantum of punishment, but on the certainty of its delivery. While we chase the law and policy for better implementation, the first order of our priority should be ensuring the safety, stability, and health of the child-abuse victim to better prevent and stop revictimization, along with immediate action with certainty in such cases.

REFERENCES

1. World Bank Open Data [Internet]. [cited June 10, 2024]. World Bank Open Data. Available from: https://data.worldbank.org.
2. Dr Loveleen Kacker, Srinivas Varadan, Parvesh Kumar (2007). Study on Child Abuse: India. Ministry of Women & Child Development, Government of India. Printed by Kriti, New Delhi. Available from: https://bettercarenetwork.org/sites/default/files/attachments/Study%20on%20Child%20Abuse%20-%20India.pdf.
3. Aggarwal K, Dalwai S, Galagali P, Mishra D, Prasad C, Thadhani A, et al. Recommendations on recognition and response to child abuse and neglect in the Indian setting. Indian Pediatr. 2010;47(6): 493-504.
4. World Health Organization. Child Sexual Abuse: A Silent Health Emergency. Report of the Regional Director. [Internet]. [Geneva]: WHO; [cited 2024 June 12]. Available from:https://apps.who.int/iris/bitstream/handle/10665/1878/AFR.RC54.15%20Rev.1.pdf?sequence=1&isAllowed=y.

5. Thangavelu SN. Assess the level of knowledge regarding child abuse among the mothers in selected areas at Latur. J Child Adolesc Behav. 2016;4:271. doi: 10.4172/2375-4494.1000271.
6. National Crime Records Bureau. Crime in India 2022. New Delhi: National Crime Records Bureau, Ministry of Home Affairs, Government of India; 2023. Available from: referencehttps://www.ncrb.gov.in/uploads/nationalcrimerecordsbureau/custom/1701607577CrimeinIndia2022Book1.pdf.
7. World Health Organization. Child Maltreatment [Internet]. Geneva: World Health Organization; 2022 [cited 2023 June 17]. Available from:https://www.who.int/news-room/fact-sheets/detail/child-maltreatment.
8. Kumar R, Chaudhary BL, Patel S, Mishra A. Child sexual abuse (CSA): India and the world. JIAFM. 2016;38(4):489-94.
9. Kumar A, Pathak A, Kumar S, Rastogi P, Rastogi P. The problem of child sexual abuse in india laws, legal lacuna and the bill PCSOB. JIAFM. 2012;34(2):170-5.
10. Ministry of Women and Child Development. One Stop Centres. Available from: www.wcdhry.gov.in/oscg.pdf. Accessed September 7, 2017.
11. Protection of Children from Sexual Offences Act, 2012. Act No. 32 of 2012. [Internet]. India: Ministry of Law and Justice; 2012 [cited 2024 June 17]. Available from: https://indiankanoon.org/doc/103108231/.
12. Ministry of Home Affairs. The Protection of Children from Sexual Offences (Amendment) Bill, 2019. [Internet]. New Delhi: Ministry of Home Affairs; 2019 [cited 2024 June 20]. Available from: https://www.mha.gov.in/sites/default/files/2022-12/20-11-2019%5B1%5D.pdf.

CHAPTER 7

Medicolegal Aspects of the Protection of Women from Domestic Violence Act, 2005

Madhurima Arora, Varun Modgil

INTRODUCTION

Domestic violence has become a global hazard because of the diversity of cultures, economy and beliefs all over the world. In India, it has taken a blasphemous form over the centuries. From the holy bibles to the Hindu mythologies, the patriarchy has been rooted in our culture which has somehow led to a belief that the males can dominate the society.

Even with the outnumbered educational qualifications and employments of the women in our country, they are still expected to sit at home and drown themselves into the social norms. Hence, the patriarchal society belief has downgraded the mind-sets of people to use their power over the weaker sex which can be seen in the forms of physical, sexual, emotional and financial abuse. In most countries, gender violence is punishable.

Domestic violence has drastically impacted the economy, mental health, physical health, social co habitation and the legal system. The global prevalence of physical/sexual intimate partner and non-partner violence is 35%. The prevalence of domestic violence in Southeast Asia is 37.7%, 29.8% in America, 25.4% in Europe and 36% in Africa. According to the data from National Family Health Survey-5, India, 29% of women aged 18–49 in India have experienced physical violence since age 15, and 22% have experienced physical violence in the 12 months preceding the survey. Among women aged 18–49 who have ever been pregnant, 3% have experienced physical violence during any pregnancy.[1]

WHAT CONSTITUTES THE DOMESTIC VIOLENCE?

- Domestic violence involves violence or abuse by one person against another in a domestic setting.[2]
- National Family Health Survey (NFHS) defines domestic violence to include violence by spouse, ex-spouse as well as other household members.[1]
- The Protection of Women from Domestic Violence Act, 2005 states that, any act, omission or commission or conduct of the respondent shall constitute domestic violence in case it:
  a. harms or injures or endangers the health, safety, life, limb or well-being, whether mental or physical, of the aggrieved person or tends to do so and includes causing physical abuse, sexual abuse, verbal and emotional abuse and economic abuse; or
  b. harasses, harms, injures, or endangers the aggrieved person with a view to coerce her or any other person related to her to meet any unlawful demand for any dowry or other property or valuable security; or

c. has the effect of threatening the aggrieved person or any person related to her by any conduct mentioned in clause (a) or clause (b); or
d. otherwise injures or causes harm, whether physical or mental, to the aggrieved person.[3]

Any form of behavior, actual or threatened, by a male member in the household to gain control or power over a woman who could be his wife, girlfriend, or any other female member constitutes Domestic Violence DV. Momentum for the policy intervention in this regard came after the *General Assembly of the United Nations* passed the *"Declaration on the Elimination of Violence against Women"* in 1993.[4]

BURDEN OF THE DOMESTIC VIOLENCE

In India, most of the married women have been physically abused by their husbands at some time in their lives. In a National Family Health Survey-5, during 2019–2021, women's experience of any spousal physical, sexual, or emotional violence varies greatly across states/UTs, from 1% in Lakshadweep to 10% in Goa and 11% each in Himachal Pradesh and Nagaland to 40–43% of women in Tamil Nadu, Telangana, Manipur, and Bihar, and to 48% in Karnataka. Bihar had reported maximum number of domestic violence cases accounting to high as 59% followed by Madhya Pradesh (45.8%), Rajasthan (46.3%), Manipur (43.9%), Uttar Pradesh (42.4%), Tamil Nadu (41.9%) and West Bengal (40.3%).[1]

National Crime Records Bureau (NCRB) stated a total of 89,097 cases related to crimes against women in 2018. The crime rate per lakh women population is 58.8 in 2018 in comparison to 57.9 in 2017.[5]

According to the global database on violence against women, lifetime physical and/or Sexual Intimate Partner Violence reported in India is: 28.8% and Physical and/or Sexual Intimate Partner Violence in the last 12 months in India accounts to 22%.[6] These figures may be under estimated given that violence within families is considered as a taboo and there may be any under reporting of such incidents.

Denial and unawareness that the victim is trapped in the Domestic Violence cycle **(Fig. 1)** leads to under-representation of

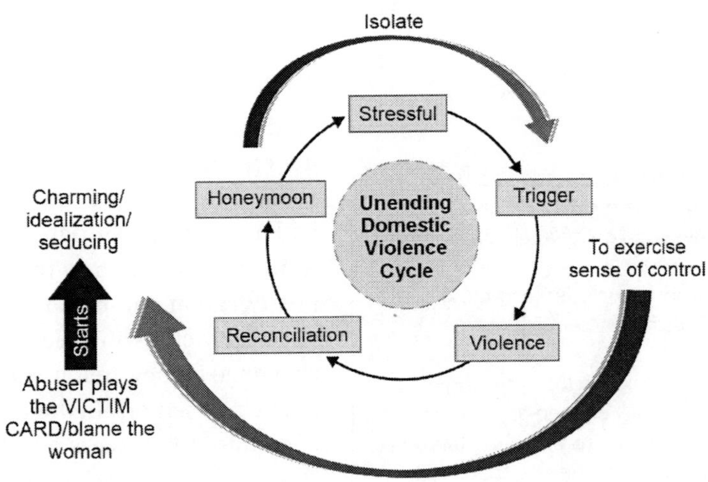

Fig. 1: Typical unending domestic violence cycle.[7]

this problem. The abuser will initially woo the victim and isolate her from her primary support system (parents or friends). This is followed by imposition of a sense of control as the abuser starts abusing, and subjects her to further violence. This is followed by a reconciliatory phase, aimed at continuation of incessant cycles of domestic violence. Abuser and the victim follow a course of interaction that ultimately ends up into domestic violence as depicted in **Figure 1**.[7]

Types of Domestic Violence (Box 1)

DV can manifest in the form of physical and/or emotional abuse, sexual abuse, economical abuse or it could be manipulative and controlling behavior.

Risk Factors for Domestic Violence

The causes of DV are multifactorial and can be divided into environmental, victim and perpetrator centric. Persons who are suffering from mental illness may suffer from domestic abuse.

Environmental factors include age-old redundant sociocultural traditions, lack of support from the community, patriarchal mindset, poverty and fragile legal justice system. Victim-related factors include young age, lack of formal education, and financial dependence on the perpetrator, separated or divorced marital status and broken families. Perpetrator factors include low income, lack of education, loss of job, antisocial personality, history of substance abuse or addiction, loneliness especially during the wake of COVID-19 pandemic, exposure to physical or sexual violence as a child.

BOX 1: Types of domestic violence.

i. Physical abuse includes hitting, slapping, or beating the victim without any reason. It may be a single incident or repetitive attempts at physical violence which may even cause death.
ii. Emotional abuse includes insulting or threatening behavior, stalking, falsely accusing the partner as infidel or intimidation.
iii. Sexual abuse includes coercive sexual act, refusing to use mechanical or oral contraceptives and deliberately passing on STI.
iv. Economical abuse includes restricting access to financial resources to which the victim is entitled.
v. Controlling behavior includes cutting off friend circles, family ties and depriving of one's support system, not allowing freedom and making the victim believe that she is unworthy.

HEALTH CONSEQUENCES OF DOMESTIC VIOLENCE

One in every three women in the world experiences sexual violence by a partner or a non-partner.[1] Due to the non-plummeting trends of the domestic violence around the world, mental health problems, emotional distress, and suicidal behavior are common among women who have suffered partner violence.[8]

MANAGEMENT OF THE VICTIMS OF DOMESTIC VIOLENCE

Medical professionals have a vital role in the management of the victims of domestic abuse. They can give advice, mental support and arrange appropriate referrals for them. A lack of adequate training about the identification and management of domestic violence victims in medical school poses a challenge in their treatment and may require the help of seniors. In the UK, the prevalence of domestic violence is reported to be around 30% and the doctors have to inform the social services in case of a suspicion of domestic violence even if it is refused by the patient. In India due to no set protocols regarding the report and records, neither the doctor goes into the cause of the injury inflicted on the victim, nor there is a willingness of victim to come forward.[9]

Although difficult, but utmost attention must be given to the history of the patient and her will to disclose the facts. Doctor, nurse or other para-medical staff in the healthcare facility can ask some leading closed-ended questions regarding gender violence.

All the healthcare centers should identify a nearby non-governmental organization (NGO) working for the women and send them to report their cases where further legal process could be initiated. It was identified that women were supportive of being asked about their experiences of domestic violence during voluntary counseling and testing (VCT sessions).[10]

SCREENING THE WOMEN FOR GENDER VIOLENCE

For an obstetrician-gynecologist, the domestic violence on a woman is very important because of its deleterious impacts on the lives of women and children. It may affect and complicate each and every aspect of women's health and well-being.[11]

Roelens K et al., threw a light on the protocol of care for victims of violence including partner violence during and outside pregnancy, was developed (Buylaert et al., 2004).[11] This protocol gives tools for acute medical care for victims, for referral to other facilities.

The aims of the protocol are:

- Immediate care to the victim, including psychological help.
- Prevention of consequences of violence such as unwanted pregnancy, sexually transmitted infections
- Adequate referral to psychosocial care facilities.
- Correct documentation of lesions, including forensic evidence collection.
- Referral to legal aid.
- Education and training of healthcare workers.

The management of the victim not only involves examinations that help in the assessment of the medical needs of victims but also collection of evidence for law enforcement purposes.[12,13] Concerns must be made to record the medical history and examination, description of the crime; collection, documentation, and preservation of evidence; treatment for medical needs; and referral for medical and psychological services.[14]

Gynecologists aim at providing primary obstetric care yet feel crippled with a routine intimate partner violence (IPV) screening policy due to the lack of knowledge and adequate training programs leading to underestimation of prevalence and unfamiliarity with signs and symptoms. Public health experts should be involved to conduct studies on the ideological and cultural aspects which give rise to and perpetuate the phenomenon of domestic violence. Similarly, proper policymaking and planning should be done including the health sector, education, legal and judicial, and social services.[15]

THE PROTECTION OF WOMEN FROM DOMESTIC VIOLENCE ACT, 2005[16]

The Protection of Women from Domestic Violence Act 2005 is an Act of the Parliament of India enacted to protect women from domestic violence which was brought into force on 26th October 2006. The Act provides protection to women from physical violence and other forms of abuses such as emotional/verbal, sexual, and economic. The Act contains five chapters and thirty-seven sections. Under this law, a Police Officer, Protection Officer, service provider or Magistrate who has received a complaint of domestic violence shall inform the aggrieved person of her rights to obtain a protection order, an order for monetary relief, a custody order, a residence order and a compensation order. Some of the salient features of the Act have been enumerated below:

1. It covers the women, who have been in relationship with the abuser, where both the parties have lived together in the same household and related by consanguinity, marriage, a relationship in the nature of marriage or adoption.
2. It defines domestic violence to include actual abuse or the threat of abuse that is physical, economic, emotional and sexual.
3. It confers on the aggrieved woman the right to reside in a shared household, whether or not she has any title or rights in the same. The respondent, not being the female can be directed under the act to remove himself from the shared household or to secure for the aggrieved woman the same level of alternate accommodation as enjoyed by her in the shared household.
4. The orders include protection orders, residence orders, monetary relief, custody orders and compensation orders.
5. It empowers the magistrate to pass protection order in favor of the abused to prevent the abuser from committing the act of domestic violence.
6. It provides for appointment of Protection Officers and recognizes and involves non-governmental organizations as service providers for providing help and assistance to the abused. The main areas which need to be taken into consideration are medical examination, legal aid and safe shelter.

The Act covers all women, who may be mothers, wives, sisters, widows, or partners living in shared households. The relationship may be marriage or adoption. In addition, the relationships with family members living together as joint family may be included. However, there is not any female relative of the husband or the male partner, who can file the complaint against the wife or the female partner. For example, mother-in-law cannot file a complaint against the daughter-in-law. But when she experiences domestic violence within homes, then she can file an application against the daughter-in-law as well as the son. In other words, when adult children mistreat and abuse their parents or conduct any forms of domestic violence against them, they have the right to file complaints against them or evict them from their homes (Chapter IV).

Any woman, who alleges to have been subjected to any act of domestic violence by the offender or any other person may file a complaint on her behalf. A child is also entitled to relief under the Domestic Violence Act. The mother of such children can make an application on behalf of her minor child (whether male or female). In cases where the mother makes an application to the court for herself, the children can also be added as co-applicants. The complaint can be filed against the adult male member, who has been in a domestic relationship with the woman, relatives of the husband or the male partners and includes both male and female relatives of the male partners (Chapter IV).

Duty of Protection Officers Under the Act

Protection Officers are assigned to make a domestic incident report to the Magistrate, upon receipt of a complaint of domestic violence and forward copies thereof to the Police Officer In-charge of the Police Station within the local limits of whose jurisdiction domestic violence is alleged to have been committed. The Protection Officers may get the aggrieved medical aid, offer shelter homes and free legal services to the victim.

Duty of Medical Officers Under the Act

If an aggrieved person or, on her behalf, a Protection Officer or a service provider requests the person in charge of a medical facility to provide any medical aid to her, such a person shall provide medical aid to the aggrieved person in the medical facility.

THE PROTECTION OF WOMEN FROM DOMESTIC VIOLENCE RULES, 2006[17]

1. *Qualifications and Experience of Protection Officers:*
    a. Preference shall be given to women belonging to Government or members of non-governmental organizations.
    b. Experience of at least three years in the social sector.
    c. The tenure of a Protection Officer shall be a minimum period of three years.
2. *Information to Protection Officers:*
    a. Any person who comes to know about any incident of domestic violence will have to report to the Protection Officer either in written form or verbally.
    b. The Protection Officer shall keep a record of the identity of the person giving such information.
3. *Domestic incident reports:* The Protection Officer shall prepare a domestic incident report in Form I and submit the same to the Magistrate and forward copies thereof to the Police Officer In-charge of the Police Station within the local limits of jurisdiction of which the domestic violence alleged to have been committed has taken place and to the service providers in that area.

Rule 17: Medical Facility to the Aggrieved Person[17]

1. The aggrieved person or the Protection Officer or the service provider may make a request under section 7 to a Person-in-charge of a medical facility in writing, clearly stating that the application is being made under section 7.
2. When a Protection Officer makes such a request, it shall be accompanied by a copy of the domestic incident report: Provided that the medical facility shall not refuse medical assistance to an aggrieved person under the Act, for her not having lodged a domestic incident report, prior to making a request for medical assistance or examination to the medical facility.
3. If no domestic incident report has been made, the person-in-charge of the medical facility shall fill in Form I and forward the same to the local Protection Officer.

CONCLUSION

To combat domestic violence, a well-planned multisectoral approach at local and national levels is a must. Doctors have a significant role in managing a case of domestic violence, and such cases have associated medicolegal issues. The issue of domestic violence must be tackled as per the provisions of the law. The doctors must be well aware about the relevant provisions related to the legislation dealing with Domestic violence (The Protection of Women from Domestic Violence Act).

REFERENCES

1. National Family Health Survey (NFHS-5), 2019–2021. Available on: https://dhsprogram.com/pubs/pdf/FR375/FR375.pdf. International Institute for Population Sciences, Deonar, Mumbai, 2022. Accessed on 15 October 2024.
2. Acharya NK Commentary on protection of women from domestic violence Act, 9th edition. Asia Law House; 2024.
3. India Parliament in the Fifty-sixth Year of the Republic of India, Protection of Women from Domestic Violence, Act 2005. Act No 43 OF 2005.
4. Doc.21_declaration elimination vaw.pdf [Internet]. [cited 2024 Jul 29]. Available from: https://www.un.org/en/genocideprevention/documents/atrocitycrimes/Doc.21_declaration%20elimination%20vaw.pdf.
5. Domestic violence tops crime against women in 2018: NCRB. [Internet]. National Herald; 2024 [cited 2024 June 13]. Available from: https://www.nationalheraldindia.com/national/domestic-violence-tops-crime-against-women-in-2018-ncrb.
6. Proportion of ever-married women aged 15–49 years experiencing intimate partner physical and/or sexual violence at least once in their lifetime. Source: International Institute for Population Sciences (IIPS) and ICF. 2017. National Family Health Survey (NFHS-4), India, 2015–2016: India. Mumbai: IIPS.
7. Forensic Psychiatry in India. Interface between Indian Laws and Mental Health. 1st edition. Bangalore: NIMHANS; 2021. NIMHANS Publication; No. 196. Chapter 14. Available from https://www.researchgate.net/publication/352544463_Protection_of_Women_from_Domestic_Violence_Act_PWDVA_2005#fullTextFileContent [Internet]. [2024 May 20].
8. Krug EG, Dahlberg LL, Mercy JA, Zwi AB, Lozano R, editors. World Report on Violence and Health. Geneva: World Health Organization; 2002.
9. Sugg NK, Inui T. Primary care physicians' response to domestic violence. Opening Pandora's box. JAMA 1992; 267:3157-60.
10. Christofides N, Jewkes R. Acceptability of universal screening for intimate partner violence in voluntary HIV testing and counseling services in South Africa and service implications. AIDS Care 2010;22: 279-85.
11. Roelens K, Verstraelen H, Temmerman M. Intimate Partner Violence. The gynaecologist's perspective. Ghent University Hospital, Department of Obstetrics and Gynaecology. Facts Views Vis Obgyn. 2009; 1(2):88-98.
12. Rockville MD. Agency for Healthcare Research and Quality. (2003, September). Medical examination and treatment for victims of sexual assault: vidence-based clinical practice and provider training (Report to Congress: AHRQ Publication No. 03-R210).
13. American College of Emergency Physicians. Evaluation and management of the sexually assaulted or sexually abused patient. Dallas, 1999. Available at: http://www.nhcadsv.org/uploads/ evaluationmanagementsapatient.pdf.
14. Littel K. Sexual assault nurse examiner (SANE) programs: Improving the community response to sexual assault victims (NCJ No. 186366). OVC Bulletin. Washington; 200
15. WHO. Multi country study on Women's health and domestic violence against women. Geneva: World Health Organization; 2007.
16. The Protection of Women from Domestic Violence Act, 2005. [Internet]. New Delhi: Government of India; 2005 [cited 2024 May 25]. Available from: https://www.indiacode.nic.in/bitstream/123456789/15436/1/protection_of_women_from_domestic_violence_act%2C_2005.pdf.
17. The Protection of Women from Domestic Violence Rules, 2006. [Internet]. New Delhi: Government of India; 2006 [cited 2024 May 24]. https://socialwelfare.tripura.gov.in/sites/default/files/Protection%20of%20Women%20from%20Domestic%20Violence%20Rules.pdf.

SECTION 3

Documentation and Checklists in Obstetrics and Gynecology

CHAPTER 8

Informed Consent in Obstetrics and Gynecology

Anupama Bhute-Anand

INTRODUCTION

Consent is a process where the healthcare provider discloses relevant and complete information to a competent patient so that he/she can easily understand the scenario and make a choice to refuse or accept the treatment. Informed consent is an agreement or permission to allow the physician to provide the proposed plan of care.[1,2] Informed consent has key medicolegal implications which includes ethical and legal obligations, and also requires that the treating doctor gives due importance to patient autonomy.[3] The goal of informed consent is to provide information to patients which are necessary for decision, making. It includes information related to the risks and benefits of accepting or refusing the proposed treatment, so that the patient understands and approves the suitable plan of care proposed by the treating doctor, as per the standards of practice.[4,5]

The ethical obligation of consent requires that a physician gives accurate and complete information to the patient, so as to understand and feel free to ask questions and make voluntary choices that include the refusal/approval to the proposed treatment.[6]

Ambiguities in the communication of medical information due to various languages and cultures between physicians and patients occur challenges in to informed consent process that affects people, migrants, and health disparities.[7] To avoid miscommunication related to languages difference, professional medical interpreters should be available in person, by phone through video remote technology to assist the consent process.[8]

According to ACOG documents, more information is related to racial and ethnic disparities in Obstetrics and Gynecology and the social determinants of health and cultural awareness. The consent conversation includes the basic requirement which is documented in the medical record and recommended testing, or treatment should be included in this documentation.[8,9]

It is the process where the healthcare provider gives information about risks and benefits and gives all alternatives for given procedure and treatment for easy access to a voluntary decision.

Informed consent is both an ethical and legal obligation of medical practitioners in the US and originates from the patient's right to direct what happens to their body. It gives complete information that includes:[9,10]

- Treatment plan
- Alternative medicine
- Risks and benefits of alternative medicine
- Assessment of the patient's understanding
- Decision-making process and avoid making the patient feel forced to accept the treatment

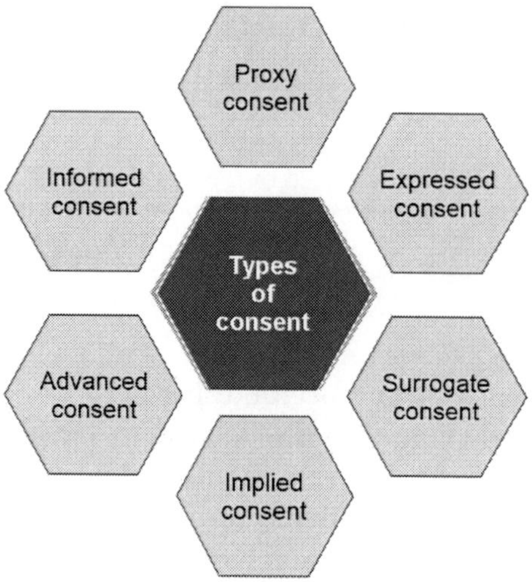

Fig. 1: Types of consent.[1,2]

TYPES OF CONSENT [1,2]

There are six types of consent forms as depicted in **Figure 1**.

1. *Informed consent:* Informed consent is to provide information to patients which are necessary and decision-making that includes the risk and benefits of accepting or refusing the treatments.[1,2]
2. *Expressed consent:*
   i. *Oral consent:* This consent is mainly required in cases, where the examination of females can be done by taking body fluids and radiological testing can be done after taking her concerns in form of oral consent.[1,2]
   ii. *Written consent:* This consent is mandatory for diagnostic procedures or any medical testing. It is given in the form of written with a valid signature. If a patient fails to signature on the consent form, it is invalid.[5,6]
3. *Implied consent:* Implied consent gives routine examinations or day-to-day treatment which is discussed with a doctor. It does not extend the intimate diagnosis.[1,2]
4. *Surrogate consent:* In this type of consent, the form is filled out by family members for minors or dead. Generally, courts have held that the consent of family members with the written approval of two physicians sufficiently protects a patient's interest.[1,2]
5. *Advanced consent:* It is the advanced process, which is given by the patient or concerned person in advance before death.[1,2]
6. *Proxy consent:* Proxy consent is given by an authorized person before /after death. If an unconscious patient is brought and an operation is done to save a life, more than two physicians are required to give consent by signing the consent form.[1,2]

CONCEPT OF CONSENT IN MEDICAL PRACTICE[11-13]

Taking consent from the patient before providing the proposed treatment/procedure is a legal requirement which must be followed in letter and spirit, so that it is accepted as legally valid. In case the patient/concerned person is not provided with sufficient information, the consent will be considered as legally invalid, despite the fact that the consent form was signed by then patient or the attendant.[1,2]

Medical Aspects of Consent

The main element of medical consent is one of the critical issues in medical treatment. The patient has a legal right to autonomy and self-determination enshrined within Article 21 of the Indian Constitution. Patients can also refuse treatment except in an emergency where the doctor need not get consent for treatment. It is important to understand the process of consent as an *opportunity to educate* the patient as well as to *clarify the doubts*, which goes a long way to suffice the patient's expectations and is also an essential component of good clinical practice.[11]

Legal Aspects of Consent

The legal principle related to informed consent is the expression of the basic right of every person to have self-determination. If the medical practitioner attempts to treat the person without valid consent, then they will be held liable under tort and criminal law. To standardize the medical practice, the National Medical Commission has drafted RMP Regulations 2022 and reiterated the importance of informed consent by stating that the doctor should obtain documented informed consent before performing any clinical, diagnostic, therapeutic or operative procedure.[12,13]

Contents of Informed Consent[1,2]

- Complete description of the proposed surgery or procedure.
- Information on the risks, benefits, and also exploring the risk of serious bodily, disability, or death
- Description of alternative treatments along with the risks and benefits of alternatives.
- The probable outcome, if no treatment is undertaken.
- Probability of successful results.
- Duration and challenges in recovery
- Any other relevant information is provided to the patients by another physician.

Tips for Valid Consent in Obstetrics and Gynecology

- The consent taken for any surgery or procedure should provide detailed information about the procedure/surgery that patient needs to know.
- For a consent to be legally valid it should include "procedure specific information".
- A consent form which includes "*procedure specific information*" as well as "*patient specific risk factors*" and "*undertaking*" signed by the patient, doctor and the

NATIONAL MEDICAL COMMISSION ETHICS & MEDICAL REGISTRATION BOARD NOTIFICATION,
New Delhi, 2nd August, 2023[14]

Chapter 1: Professional Conduct of RMPs

19. Informed Consent:

A. Before performing any clinical procedure, diagnostic or therapeutic, or operation, the RMP should obtain the signed documented informed consent of the patient. In case the patient is unable to give consent, the consent of the legal guardian or family member must be taken. The name of the operating surgeon must be mentioned in the medical records. In an operation that may result in sterility, the consent of both husband and wife is required. In case of an emergency, the doctor should try to obtain consent, but if this is not possible, he must act in the best interest of the patient. The medical records should describe the basis of decisions taken in an emergency No act of in-vitro fertilization or artificial insemination shall be undertaken without the informed written consent of the female patient and her spouse as well as the donor.
B. RMP shall not publish photographs or case reports of patients without their consent/permission in any medical or another journal in any manner by which their identity could be revealed.
C. Clinical drug trials or other research involving patients or volunteers must comply with ICMR guidelines and the New Drugs and Clinical Trials Rules, 2018. Consent taken from any patient or participant for the trial of drug or therapy which is not as per the guidelines shall be construed as misconduct.

witness is strong evidence that shows that the patient was genuinely given necessary information, and the patient consented for the same.

- During the counseling, written information (Information Leaflet) should be handed over to the patient and opportunity should be given to the patient to discuss and clarify the doubts. Once the patient is satisfied and willing to give consent, the patient has to sign the consent form as well as the information leaflet. The *information leaflet* signed by the patient becomes part and parcel of the Informed Consent.
- It is advisable to ask the patient to write in his/her own handwriting that:

> "I have read/I have been explained the above information and I have understood the same"......
> ....
>
> *Patient's Signature*

- In a *Procedure Specific Consent Forms*, there should be few lines available for write the individual/patient specific risks or specific concerns.
- If the patient cannot sign and wants to affix thumb or if the patient does not understand the language, it will be a good idea that it is documented that she was made aware of the draft of the consent.

Vaginal Delivery after Cesarean Delivery[15,16]

Vaginal birth after cesarean section (VBAC) describes a vaginal delivery in a woman who has given birth via cesarean section in a former pregnancy. Patients desiring VBAC delivery undergo a trial of labor (TOL), also called trial of labor after cesarean section (TOLAC). Many doctors believed that if women had one cesarean delivery, all the delivery is on the same way. But nowadays women ask for vaginal delivery even if they had C-section earlier. Many studies show that over the last 10 years, around 10–20% of women have had a prior cesarean section and attempted VBAC. From that 60–80% succeeded and gave birth to a child via vaginal delivery. Obstetricians need to counsel the patients with prior cesarean section regarding potential risks and benefits of TOL and the factors which affect the likelihood of successful vaginal delivery.

Informed Consent in VBAC

Healthcare professionals are responsible to provide additional inform in such patients, prior to trial of labor.

Salient points of informed consent in VBAC

- *Who will perform the delivery and his/her qualification?*
- *What is the patient's medical condition?*
- *Purpose of the proposed procedure*
- *Risk of complications involved*
- *Alternative procedure/treatment and associated risk of complications*
- *Chances of success of the proposed VBAC*

VBAC Safety

Regarding patient safety considering, VBAC should be informed about all the risks and alternatives before labor and delivery. In this case, a mother makes a good and well-educated decision to go ahead with a VBAC birth plan and to understand the potential condition where a C-section became necessary during labor and delivery. Mostly some important factors exist, the physician is obligated to make the mother aware of them and inform her that she is not having the capability of giving birth to VBAC delivery. If the patient has no information, then if the mother or baby is injured during VBAC it may come under malpractice case. If it happens, then you speak to an attorney as soon as possible. Reiter & Walsh ABC Law centers are birth injury attorneys who focus exclusively on birth injury cases.[15,16]

CONTRACEPTION[17–19]

Consent for the contraception process is a shared decision that guides a patient about birth control and prevents pregnancy. The physician should explain all the risks and benefits of contraception.

Part I of Consent (Information Leaflet)

INTRAUTERINE CONTRACEPTIVE DEVICE

Please read the information carefully, ask questions/doubts (if any) before you sign this leaflet and the consent form.

Name of Procedure: Insertion of an Intrauterine Contraceptive Device.

Description of the procedure: ....

Purpose/indications: ....

Benefits:..........

Alternatives if any:..........

Consequences of refusal of the procedure:..........

Risks associated with the Procedure:..........

This INFORMATION LEAFLET was received by the patient on..........

(Date):..........(Time)..........

Signature of the patient..........

Name of the patient..........

Signed copy of the INFORMATION LEAFLET is to be retained as part of the signed Consent form.

Part II of Consent (Undertaking)

INTRAUTERINE CONTRACEPTIVE DEVICE

I, Ms/Mrs.., aged......................years, female residing at............................give my free and valid consent for myself/ my...Ms/ Mrs... aged............................years residing at .... for the procedure of contraception.

I am aware that the procedure will be carried out under the directions of Dr...

I state that:

i. I have been explained about my medical condition.

ii. I have been given the information about the procedure as mentioned in *'Information Leaflet'* and I am aware of: (a) the nature of procedure, (b) its purpose, benefits and effect, (c) alternatives if any available, (d) an outline of substantial risks, (e) adverse consequences of refusing treatment

iii. I have been counselled about the nature of anesthesia, benefits, purpose, effects and alternatives and substantial risks.

iv. I give consent to observing, photographing, recording or televising of the surgery for medical, scientific or educational purpose provided my identity is not revealed.

v. I accept that medical science is not perfect and has its limitations. No guarantee can be given about the result or outcome.

vi. I agree to cooperate fully with my doctor and to follow instructions and recommendations about my care and treatment.

vii. I confirm that I have given all the details to the doctor about myself, including past medical history including previous ailments, surgeries and allergies to any drugs.

viii. Apart from the above-mentioned general information, I have been specifically informed about individual risks related to..

(*to be mentioned by doctor about any specific problems related to that patient*)

ix. I was encouraged to ask any question related to this operation and had been answered well all the questions asked, a way in which we could understood.

x. I have been explained that expected outcome in this treatment/procedure/operation is good/Fair/ Poor.

xi. I understand that I have a right to withdraw the consent and will inform the doctor in time (if needed)

By signing below, I indicate that I have understood the above information in language, I understand.

I am giving my free consent willingly with sound mind, without any undue influence, coercion, fraud, misrepresentation or mistake of facts.

I request Dr...to perform upon me the above-mentioned procedure.

* Interpreter, Mr/Ms. .... has read out above mentioned to me and explained everything to me in .... language. (If the *patient gave thumb impression or not understand the language of printed consent*)

Sign:	Sign/Thumb impression:............................
Dr.'s Name	Patient's Name ....
Reg. no:	Age: ....
Date:	Date: ....
Time: AM/PM	Time: AM/PM ....
Sign:	Sign: ....
Name of Witness..	Name of Witness.................................Age................
Age:..	Relation with Patient:..
Address..	Address:..
Date:......................Time: AM/PM	Date:......................Time: AM/PM ....

INFORMED CONSENT FOR ABDOMINAL HYSTERECTOMY[20,21]

Abdominal hysterectomy is a process to remove the uterus by a vertical or transverse incision in the abdominal wall, depending on the reasons for the hysterectomy. The main function of the uterus is to produce hormones by the ovary and carry a fetus in terms of pregnancy. Removal of uterus through the abdominal wall incision may be required for multiple and varied reasons like: Tumors/fibroids, bleeding problems, endometriosis, pelvic pain, cervix cancer, etc. After completion of this process, a woman cannot become pregnant, nor will she have a mensuration process. After the operation, they have pain in the pelvic area. Medications will be available for pain relief. [22,23]

The risk complications associated with abdominal hysterectomy are as mentioned hereinunder:

i. *Intraoperative complications* like accidental injury, side effects of medication, and side effects of medication, etc.
ii. *Postoperative complications* like Thrombophlebitis, Fallen vaginal, death, etc.
iii. *Anesthesia-related complications:*[24]
   a. Irregular heart rate
   b. Fluctuation in blood pressure
   c. Allergy
   d. Malignant hyperthermia

Part I of Consent (Information Leaflet)

ABDOMINAL HYSTERECTOMY

Please read the information carefully, ask questions/doubts (if any) before you sign this leaflet and the consent form.

Name of Procedure: Abdominal Hysterectomy

Description of the procedure:...

Purpose/ indications:...

Benefits:...

Alternatives if any:...

Consequences of refusal of the procedure:...

Risks associated with the Procedure:...

This INFORMATION LEAFLET was received by the patient on .... (Date)/........................ (Time)..

Signature of the patient ....

Name of the patient ....

Signed copy of the INFORMATION LEAFLET is to be retained as part of the signed Consent form.

Part II of Consent (Undertaking)

ABDOMINAL HYSTERECTOMY

I, Ms./Mrs.............................., aged ....years, female residing at ....give my free and valid consent for myself/ my ....Ms./ Mrs.............................. aged ...... years residing at .... for abdominal hysterectomy.
Additionally, following procedures may be done: *Salpingectomy*: Right/left/both; *Ovarian cystectomy:* Right/left/both; *Oophorectomy*: Right/left/both (Tick mark what is applicable/strike out what is not applicable)
I am aware that the procedure will be carried out under the directions of Dr..
I state that:

i. I have been explained about my medical condition.
ii. I have been given the information about the procedure as mentioned in 'Information Leaflet' and I am aware of: (a) the nature of procedure, (b) its purpose, benefits and effect, (c) alternatives if any available, (d) an outline of substantial risks, (e) adverse consequences of refusing treatment
iii. I have been counselled about nature of anesthesia, benefits, purpose, effects and alternatives and substantial risks.
iv. I give consent to observing, photographing, recording or televising of the surgery for medical, scientific or educational purpose provided my identity is not revealed.
v. I accept that medical science is not perfect and has its limitations. No guarantee can be given about the result or outcome.
vi. I agree to cooperate fully with my doctor and to follow instructions and recommendations about my care and treatment.
vii. I confirm that I have given all the details to the doctor about myself, including past medical history including previous ailments, surgeries and allergies to any drugs.
viii. Apart from the above-mentioned general information, I have been specifically informed about individual risks related to..
....
(to be mentioned by doctor about any specific problems related to that patient)
ix. I was encouraged to ask any question related to this operation and had been answered well all the questions asked, a way in which we could understood.
x. I have been explained that expected outcome in this treatment/procedure/operation is good/Fair/ Poor. I understand that I have a right to withdraw the consent and will inform the doctor in time (if needed)

By signing below, I indicate that I have understood the above information in language I understand.

I am giving my free consent willingly with sound mind, without any undue influence, coercion, fraud, misrepresentation or mistake of facts.
I request Dr..to perform upon me the above-mentioned procedure.
*Interpreter, Mr/Ms .... has read out above mentioned to me and explained everything to me in ....language. (If the *patient gave thumb impression or not understand the language of printed consent*)

Sign:	Sign / Thumb impression: ....
Dr.'s Name	Patient's Name ....
Reg. no:	Age: ....
Date:	Date: ....
Time: AM/PM	Time: AM/PM ....
Sign:	Sign: ....
Name of Witness....................................	Name of Witness....................Age..............
Age:....................................	Relation with Patient:....................................
Address....................................	Address:....................................
Date:....................Time: AM/PM	Date:....................Time: AM/PM ....

CONSENT FOR STERILIZATION

Informed Consent Form for Sterilization Operation/Re-sterilization

(For Female and Male Sterilization Services)

1. Name of client: Shri/Smt..
2. Name of spouse: Shri/Smt ....

   Address ....

   ....
3. Name of father: Shri ....

   Address ....

   ....
4. Religion ....
5. Educational Qualifications ....
6. Business / Occupation ....
7. Operating Centre ....

I, Smt/Shri..................................., hereby give consent for my sterilization operation. I am married and my husband/wife is alive. My age is ....years and my husband's/ wife's age is ....years. We have..........male and.........female living children. The age of my youngest living child is...........years.

I am aware that I have the option of deciding against the sterilization procedure at any time without sacrificing my rights to other reproductive health services.

a. I have decided to undergo the sterilization/re-sterilization operation on my own without any outside pressure, inducement or force. I declare that I/my spouse has not been sterilized previously (may not be applicable in case of re-sterilization).
b. I am aware that other methods of contraception are available to me. I know that for all practical purposes this operation is permanent. I also know that there are still he above information has been read out and explained to me in my own language, it has been explained to me that this form has the authority of a legal document. Some chances of failure of the operation for which the operating doctor and the health facility will not be held responsible by me or by my relatives or by any other, person whomsoever.
c. I am aware that I am undergoing an operation that carries an element of risk.
d. The eligibility criteria for the operation have been explained to me, and I affirm that I am eligible to undergo the operation according to the criteria.
e. I agree to undergo the operation under any type of anesthesia that the doctor/ health facility thinks suitable for me and to be given other medicines as considered appropriate by the doctor/health facility concerned.
f. If, after the sterilization operation, 1/my spouse experience (s) a missed menstrual cycle, then I/my spouse shall report within two weeks of the missed menstrual cycle to the doctor/health facility and may avail of the facility to get an MTP done free of cost.
g. In case of 'complications following the sterilization operation, including failure, I will accept the compensation as per the existing provisions of the Government of India Family Planning Insurance Scheme as full and final settlement.

h. If I/my wife get (s) pregnant after the failure of the sterilization operation and if I am not able to get the fetus aborted within two weeks, then I will not be entitled to claim any compensation over and above the compensation offered under the Family Planning Insurance Scheme from any court of law in this regard or any other compensation for the upbringing of the child.
I. I agree to come for follow-up visits to the hospital/institution/doctor/health facility as instructed, failing which I shall be responsible for the consequences, if any.

I understand that vasectomy does not result in immediate sterilization. *I agree to come for semen analysis three months after the operation to confirm the success of the sterilization surgery (azoospermia), failing which I shall be responsible for the consequences, if any.

(*Applicable in cases of male sterilization)

I have read the above information.

The above information has been read out and explained to me in my own language, it has been explained to me that this form has the authority of a legal document.

Name and signature/thumb impression of the acceptor

....

Signature of witness:....................................
Full name ....

Full address ....

(Only for those beneficiaries who cannot read and write)

Applicable in cases where the client cannot read and where the above information has been read out

Shri/Smt..................................has been fully informed about the contents of the Informed Consent Form in his/her own/local language.

Signature of counsellor**
Full name ....
Full address ....

I certify that I have satisfied myself that:

i. Shri/ Smt...is within the eligible age group and is medically fit for the sterilization operation.
ii. I have explained all clauses to the client and also explained that this form has the authority of a legal document.
iii. I have filled out the medical record-cum-checklist and followed the standards for sterilization procedures as laid down by the Government of India.

Signature of operating doctor | Signature of medical officer in-charge of the facility

(Name & address) Seal | (Name & address) Seal

Denial of Sterilization

Certify that Shri/Smt. .... is not a suitable client for re-sterilization/sterilization for the following reasons:

1...

2...

He/she has been advised the following alternative methods of contraception:

1...

2...

Signature of the counsellor** or doctor making the decision

(Name and full address) ....

....

....

The counsellor can be any health personnel, including a doctor.

CONCLUSION

Informed consent is the process by which the healthcare provider shares all the information with a patient or concerned person, for making their choice to accept/decline the prescribed treatment. Informed consent is a foundational bioethics principle of respect for the autonomy of patients. It is a shared decision-making framework where patients can take decisions by active participation in medical care to make a stronger therapeutic relationship with their physician. Some challenges that arise are more commonly in the practice of obstetrics and gynecology than in other specialty areas.

REFERENCES

1. Bhute A. Informed Consent in Obstetrics and Gynecology: Indian Scenario: International Journal of Recent Surgical and Medical Sciences; 2017;3(1):67-71.
2. Ethical Considerations for including Women as Research Participants. Committee Opinion No. 646. American College of Obstetricians and Gynaecologists. Obstet Gynecol. 2016;127:100-7.
3. Confidentiality in Adolescent Health Care. ACOG Committee Opinion No. 803. American College of Obstetricians and Gynaecologists. Obstet Gynecol 2020;135:171-7.
4. Appelbaum PS. Clinical practice. Assessment of patient's competence to consent to treatment. N Engl J Med. 2007;357(18):1834-40.
5. Faden RR, Beauchamp TL, King NMP. A history and theory of informed consent. Online edition. New York: Oxford University Press; 1986.
6. Burns, CR. Legacies in ethics and medicine. New York: Science History Publications; 1977. ISBN 9780882021669.
7. Annas GJ, Michael, AG. The Nazi doctors and the Nuremberg Code. New York: Oxford University Press Inc.; 1992.
8. Code of Ethics Regulations. Published in Part III, Section 4 of the Gazette of India; 2002 Apr 6.
9. Obtaining Valid Consent (Clinical Governance Advice No. 6) RCOG Published; 2015 Jan 28.
10. Katz AL, Webb SA. Informed consent in decision-making in pediatric practice. Committee on Bioethics. Pediatrics 2016;138:20161485.

11. Kumar A, Mullick P, Prakash S. Consent and the Indian medical practitioner. Indian J Anaesth. 2015;59(11):695-700.
12. Nandi math OV. Consent and medical treatment: The legal paradigm in India, Indian J Urol. 2009;25(3):343-7.
13. Shreekrishna HK, Rao AB. Consent in medical practice. International Journal of Preclinical & Clinical Research. 2021;2(1):13-7.
14. https://www.nmc.org.in/MCIRest/open/getDocument?path=/Documents/Public/Portal/LatestNews/NMC%20RMP%20Conduct%20Regulations%202023.pdf.
15. Malik MF, Awonuga AO, Iglesia CB. Informed consent for vaginal delivery: is it time to revisit the shared decision-making process? J Reprod Med. 2016;61(3-4):153-8. PMID: 27172638.
16. Tripathy S, Shubhashree T, Kumari S, Mohapatra S. Informed consent process before caesarean section: a study of patient's perspective regarding the adequacy of consent process. Indian Journal of Obstetrics and Gynaecology Research 2020;7(2):239-42.
17. https://www.csudh.edu/Assets/csudhsites/shs/docs/Hormonal%20Contraceptive%20Consent%20Form%202020.pdf
18. Hilger DJ, Raviele KM, Hilgers TA. Hormonal Contraception and the Informed Consent. Linacre Q. 2018;85(4):375-84. Available at https://www.ncbi.nlm.nih.gov/pmc/articles/PMC6322130/.
19. Larimore WL, Stanford JB. Post-fertilization effects of oral contraceptives and their relationship to informed consent. Arch Fam Med.2000;9:126-33. Cited at https://onemoresoul.com/contraception-abortion/risks-consequences/what-awoman-should-know-about-birth-control.html.
20. Meeks GR, Harris RL. Surgical approach to hysterectomy: abdominal, laparoscopy-assisted, or vaginal. Clin Obstet Gynecol. 1997;40:886.
21. Harris WJ. Complications of hysterectomy. Clin Obstet Gynecol. 1997;40:928.
22. Carlson KJ, Miller BA, Fowler FJ Jr. The Maine Women's Health Study: I. Outcomes of hysterectomy. Obstet Gynecol. 1994;83:556.
23. https://www.uptodate.com/contents/abdominal-hysterectomy-beyond-the-basics.
24. Jain M, Singh M. Assisted Reproductive Technology (ART) Techniques. [Updated 2022 Nov 28]. In: StatPearls [Internet]. Treasure Island (FL): Stat Pearls Publishing; 2022. Available from: https://www.ncbi.nlm.nih.gov/books/NBK576409/.

CHAPTER 9

Medicolegal Aspects of Documentation in Obstetrics and Gynecology

Utsav Parekh, Kunjan Modi, Ronakben Modi

India witnessed a drastic increment in medical negligence cases following the inclusion of medical practitioner under the Consumer Protection Act. Physician-patient relationship, communication, damage, duty, standard of care and documentation are few among important aspects in negligence suits. Obstetrics and Gynecology is one of the specialties of medicine with higher number of litigation cases in India as well as abroad.[1,2] About 26% of medical negligence cases were reported in the field of obstetrics and gynecology.[2] The purpose of this chapter to highlight various medicolegal issues regarding the documentation in obstetrics and gynecology practice.

Medicolegal issues are always higher in the field of obstetrics and gynecology. Problems related to pregnancy and childbirth attract more lawsuits as pregnancy is believed to be a physiological process, and any deviation from normal is considered to be abnormal. In fact, there is a raise every year when it comes to the medicolegal issues in obstetrics and gynecology. One of the most common reasons for the rise is due to the increasing amount of compensation each day.

Back in 1995, the case of V Chandrasekar against Apollo Hospital, Chennai, became the most awarded one with ₹19 lakh as the compensatory amount. In 2009, in the case of Prashant Dhananka versus Nizam Institute of Medical Sciences, Hyderabad became the next such case with the compensatory amount being shot up to ₹1 crore.[3]

DOCUMENTATION RELATED ISSUES IN PROVED NEGLIGENT CASES[1]

- Documentation has inadequate information about the diagnosis, nature of treatment, intervention, prognosis and the risks involved.
- Documentary failure to detect internal hemorrhage or diagnose intestinal injuries while laparoscopic procedure.
- Documentary failure to diagnose major congenital anomalies in fetus.
- Documentary failure to show adequate resuscitation measures for the newborn.
- Documentary evidence of delay in conducting cesarean resulting in irreversible brain damage in hypoxic fetus.
- Failure to monitor postpartum hemorrhage.

LACUNAE IN DOCUMENTATION LEADS TO MEDICOLEGAL ISSUES

- Particulars of the patients and must-to-have contents are incomplete in prescription.
- *Alteration/changes in the record afterwards:* Sophisticated technology can detect alteration of records. Again, in

India fabrication with the evidence is an added offense.

- *Time and date is not written in the record*: Chronicity is very important to reconstruct what happened.
- Records lack any mention of history, or references to history are illegible.
- Records are illegible.
- Laboratory findings are not written in the record.
- Not providing detail and rationale as to your plan.
- Failed to show necessity of required procedure
- The consent is missing.
- Professional secrecy is not maintained.

CONSENT

Major factors which have been considered by the court of law in proving negligence by physicians in Obstetrics and Gynecology field are incomplete consent, i.e., lack of 'informed' essence. In the UK, the current law of consent is a result of judgment of Montgomery.[2] It emphasizes on counseling of the patient.

The consent form presented to a patient and filled just before the interventional procedure does not fulfil the criteria of a complete informed consent which amount to professional misconduct provided that the patient was not being in position to understand all the facts.

Communication and counseling have a vital place in informing the details pertaining to the consent of the patient. How and when the details of consent were explained would be more emphasized as compared with consideration of description of all risks and benefits of the intervention. In the future, it will only be reflected in documentation. From first contact to the patient, history taking, examination, prescription, interventions, and future actions, the physician should be patient-oriented, empathic, maintaining patient autonomy and encouraging the patient for making shared decisions.

OBSTETRICS ANESTHESIA

It is a significant area of the field where large number of litigations have been focused. Standard and valid checklists will be mandatory to ensure the standard of care and prevention of omissions. Obstetric anesthesia is a particularly high-risk subspecialty of anesthesia and may lead to serious morbidities and even mortality. Good doctor-patient relation from the time of admission till discharge is the most important factor to avert future litigations. Any procedure done or planned should be clearly documented. Documentation should start with a valid consent in the patient's own language, and have all three components of voluntariness, capacity and knowledge. A 'Surgical Safety' checklist is particularly helpful in documentation and decreasing errors.[4] Safety of the mother (and her child) is paramount. Both regional as well as general anesthesia, either inadvertently or if not administered properly, may be associated with morbidities like headache, pain and emotional distress. However, deaths do occur and general anesthesia is associated with care should be routine practice and inculcated by everyone involved in patient care.

Apart from the consent of the patient, records of the relevant history of the patient and clinical examination done at admission should be properly documented at all times deemed necessary for the particular patient. For operative procedures a detailed preoperative evaluation, intraoperative management (anesthesia and surgical procedures, blood product and drugs administered) including details of any critical incidents, as well as a detailed postoperative care and advice should be diligently noted.[5] For labor analgesia details of the analgesic procedure, record of continuous maternal and fetal and any critical incidents should be documented in a concise but complete manner.[5,6] Proper documentation is invaluable for medicolegal purpose and serves as an essential form of communication between health care professionals.[7]

THE MTP ACT

As per the legal provisions envisaged in the Medical Termination of Pregnancy Regulations, 2003, Ministry of Health & Family Welfare (Department of Family Planning) Notification, we have to obey the following rules regarding documentation:

Maintenance of Admission Register

1. Every head of the hospital or owncr of the approved place shall maintain a register in *Form-III* for recording there in the details of the admissions of women for the termination of their pregnancies and keep such register for a period of *five years* from the end of the calendar year it relates to.
2. The entries in the Admission Register shall be made serially and a fresh serial number shall be started at the commencement of each calendar year and the serial number of the particular year shall be distinguished from the serial number of other years by mentioning the year against the serial number, e.g., serial number 5 of 1972 and serial number 5 of 1973 shall be mentioned as 5/1972 and 5/1973.
3. Admission register shall be a secret document, and the information contained therein as to the name and other particulars of the pregnant woman shall not be disclosed to any person.

Admission Register not to be Open to Inspection

The Admission Register shall be kept in the safe custody of the head of the hospital or owner of the approved place, or by any person authorized by such head or owner and save as otherwise provided in sub-regulation (5) of Regulation 4 shall not be open for inspection by any person except under the authority of law:

i. In the case of a departmental or other enquiry, the Chief Secretary to the Government of a Union Territory;
ii. In the case of an investigation into an offence a Magistrate of the First Class within the local limits or whose jurisdiction the hospital or approved place is situated;
iii. In the case of a suit or other action for damages, the District Judge, within the local limits of whose jurisdiction the hospital or approved place is situated:

Provided that the registered medical practitioner on the application of an employed woman whose pregnancy has been terminated, grant a certificate for the purpose of enabling her to obtain leave from her employer; Provided further that any such employer shall not disclose this information to any other person.

Entries in Registers Maintained in Hospital or Approved Place

No entry shall be made in any case-sheet, operation theater register, follow-up card or any other document or register other than the admission Register maintained at any hospital or approved place indicating therein the name of the pregnant woman and reference to the pregnant woman shall be made therein by the serial number assigned to the woman in the Admission Register.

Destruction of admission register and other papers: Save as otherwise directed by the Chief Secretary to the Union Territory Administration or for in relation to any proceeding pending before him, as directed by a District Judge or a Magistrate of the First Class, every Admission Register shall be destroyed on the expiry of a period of five years from the date of the last entry in that Register and other papers on the expiry of a period of three years from the date of termination of the pregnancy concerned.

THE PC AND PNDT ACT

As per the Pre-Natal Diagnostic Techniques (Regulation and Prevention of Misuse) Act, 1994, Chapter viii, Miscellaneous stats:

Maintenance of Records

1. All records, charts, forms, reports, consent letters and all other documents required to be maintained under this Act and the rules shall be preserved for a period of two years or for such period as may be prescribed: Provided that, if any criminal or other proceedings are instituted against any Genetic Counseling Center, Genetic Laboratory or Genetic Clinic, the records and all other documents of such Centre, Laboratory or Clinic shall be preserved till the final disposal of such proceedings.
2. All such records shall, at all reasonable times, be made available for inspection to the Appropriate Authority or to any other person authorized by the Appropriate Authority on this behalf.
3. *Power to search and seize records, etc.:* If the Appropriate Authority has reason to believe that an offence under this Act has been or is being committed at any Genetic Counselling Centre, Genetic Laboratory or Genetic Clinic, such Authority or any officer authorized thereof in this behalf may, subject to such rules as may be prescribed, enter and search at all reasonable times with such assistance, if any, as such authority or officer considers necessary, such Genetic Counseling Centre, Genetic Laboratory or Genetic Clinic and examine any record, register, document, book, pamphlet, advertisement or any other material object found therein and seize the same if such Authority or officer has reason to believe that it may furnish evidence of the commission of an office punishable under this Act.

The Pre-Natal Diagnostic Techniques (Regulation and Prevention of Misuse) Rules, 1996

Maintenance and Preservation of Records

1. Every Genetic Counseling Center, Genetic Laboratory and Genetic Clinic shall maintain a register showing, in serial order, the names and addresses of the women given genetic counseling, subjected to pre-natal diagnostic procedures or pre-natal diagnostic tests, the names of their husbands or fathers and the date on which they first reported for such counseling, procedure or test.
2. The record to be maintained by every Genetic Counselling Centre, in respect of each woman counseled shall be as specified in *Form D.*
3. The record to be maintained by every Genetic Laboratory, in respect of each woman subjected to any prenatal diagnostic test, shall be as specified in *Form E.*
4. The record to be maintained by every Genetic Clinic, in respect of each woman

subjected to any prenatal diagnostic procedure, shall be as specified in *Form F.*

5. The Appropriate Authority shall maintain a permanent record of applications for grant or renewal of certificate of registration as specified in *Form H.* Letters of intimation of every change of employee, place, address and equipment installed shall also be preserved as permanent records.
6. All case-related records, forms of consent, laboratory results, microscopic pictures, sonographic plates or slides, recommendations and letters shall be preserved by the Genetic Counseling Center, Genetic Laboratory or Genetic Clinic for a period of *two years* from the date of completion of counseling, pre-natal diagnostic procedure or pre-natal diagnostic test, as the case may be. In the event of any legal proceedings, the records shall be preserved till the final disposal of legal proceedings, or till the expiry of the said period of *two years,* whichever is later.
7. In case the Genetic Counseling Center or Genetic Laboratory or Genetic Clinic maintains records on computer or other electronic equipment, a printed copy of the record shall be taken and preserved after authentication by the person responsible for such record.

ANTENATAL CARE AND DELIVERY

Required documentation must be fulfilled for each patient immediately at the time of examination or any procedure which includes but not restricted to maternal–fetal assessment before delivery, findings during labor, augmentation required if any during labor, blood loss of any during and after the delivery, complications, new-born status, etc.

Antenatal record Documentation: Must include following information

1. Patients' information like name, age address and contact number
2. Her gestational history like gravida, parity, live-children and abortion
3. History of tetanus toxoid injections
4. Reports of blood investigations especially HIV, HbsAg, blood group and cross-matching, Hemoglobin, VDRL, blood glucose level, sickle cell anemia, thalassemia
5. High risk factors like diabetic or hyper-tensive
6. Past history of any medical condition like status of respiratory/hepatic/renal/cardiac functioning
7. Special remarks like allergy as well as, history of intake of other medicines
8. Sonography details with its findings

Delivery related Documentation: Must include following information

1. Date, time and day of birth
2. Weight and gender of child
3. Mode of delivery
4. Any special intervention
5. If delivered by cesarean section than indications of it.
6. Operative notes in detail with each and every step-in chronology
7. Baby cried or not immediately after birth
8. Pediatric assessment details
9. Referral details (if patient is referred)

PRESCRIPTION WRITING

Prescription order is an important therapeutic transaction between physician and patient, as it brings into focus the diagnostic acumen and therapeutic proficiency of physician with instructions for restoration of patient's health. The most carefully conceived prescription orders may become therapeutically useless, however, unless it communicates clearly with pharmacist and adequately instructs patient on how to take prescribed medication.[8] Prescriptions are medicolegal documents which need to be written legibly, accurately and completely.[9] Moreover, a good quality prescription is an extremely important factor for minimizing errors in dispensing medication and it should be adherent to guidelines for prescription writing for benefit of the patient.[10]

These are the points one should always incorporate without fail to avoid future litigation for prescription writing.

Prescription Documentation: Must include following information

1. Date and time of prescription
2. Name of doctor (with Qualifications)
3. Address with contact no, if any error is detected by a pharmacist, then the RMP can be contacted for needful correction, or an instruction not clearly understood by patient can be clarified if contact number of the RMP is documented on the prescription slip.
4. *Medical Council Registration Number:* Doctors are required to mention their registration number on all medical prescriptions, reports, documentation and records; whether in paper or electronic format relating to their medical practice. It is advisable that a doctor should put his rubber stamp bearing his full name, qualification and registration number on the prescription slip.[11,12]
5. *Doctor's signature:* If prescriptions do not carry doctor's sign, then the validity and authenticity of prescriptions can be questioned, thereby raising major legal issues.
6. *Date of issue of prescription to the patient:* The mention of date signifies the fact that a medical consultation was sought, and action was taken by clinician for ailment. Since treatment protocols follow a certain set of algorithms, the mention of date is essential to access the prognosis as well. It is important for legal matters in case of mortality. This can have serious implications in medicolegal cases since the prescription is a legal document and not mentioning date can be taken as negligence even in non-medicolegal cases.
7. *OPD number:* A lack of serial case recording for future easy access to old case records if required.
8. *Patient's name:* It is imperative to mention full name of the patients as it restores the correct identity of the recipients and helps in reducing medication error, because there can be more than one person with same name.
9. *Patient's age:* According to WHO the inclusion of weight is recommended and should be included in prescription especially at the extremes of ages.[9,13] Weight is an important piece of information since it has implications on pharmacokinetics and pharmacodynamics.
10. *Address of patient:* The name and contact number of patients can help in reminding follow-up and at times even to make corrections if errors of omission or commission are noticed by the clinicians before an unwanted event occurs.
11. *Drug name and dosage*: Write down generic name instead of brand name. It is important for clinicians to remember that mention of dose or dosage form of medicines in prescriptions, is very important and particularly needed when a pharmaceutical product exists in more than one strength/dosage form.
12. *Direction for drug use:* Numerous studies have demonstrated a patient's difficulty in recalling or understanding basic directions for taking the medicines. If the

medication is to be taken at a specific time of the day, if a particular dosage interval is desired or if there are any additional directions for use, those should be noted on the prescription and precisely explained to the patient in simple terms. The presence of this information is of help to prevent dispensing errors. Observance of prescription standards could avoid medication errors. A rational prescription is the one in which all mentioned standards are observed and clear information regarding the prescribed medications and the order of their use is provided.[13]

13. *Details like allergy, mention of medical condition like status of respiratory/hepatic/renal/cardiac functioning as well as, history of intake of other medicines:* Clinicians should have the habit of mentioning all these important points in prescriptions.
14. *Mention of revisit details*: This is an interesting observation and perhaps partially explained by the fact that most clinicians are either uncomfortable with the patient taking medicines for long periods of time without regular follow-up checks as doses and drugs may need to be altered with changing patient physiology, prognosis and additional factors or perhaps have financial considerations not to mention refills.

The computer-generated prescriptions were less prone to errors than handwritten ones. Almost all computer-generated prescriptions contained 100% information on clinician details like name, qualification, address, registration number, esoteric symbol and the patient details like OPD number, name, age, sex of the patient. Similarly, in the drug item-related prescriptions errors there was a marked reduction in the errors in areas like dose, unit, frequency of drug administration, duration of treatment, quantity, signs and legibility of prescriptions.

On the other hand, the use of computer software for prescription writing was a very tedious job. Doctors need separate skilled person for the same since they got dissociated from the patient while entering data themselves.

Poor handwriting is a serious problem and is a matter of concern for pharmacist especially, if he is unable to read the name of drugs prescribed.

HARMFUL DRUGS DURING PREGNANCY

Physician must be vigilant in his prescription about the drugs if consumed during the pregnancy causing harm either maternal or fetal, as it would be prima facie evidence. In cases where it requires to prescribe certain drugs during pregnancy which may have a minimal or theoretical risk, the disclosure must be evident in the case papers being informed to the patient in detail.

PRECAUTIONS IN PRACTICE

Standard Treatment Guidelines in Obstetrics and Gynecology prescribed by the Ministry of Health and Family Welfare, India should be followed and documented accordingly. One must be cautious while practicing.

Some examples of obstetric negligence are:

- Administering incorrect medications or treatments during pregnancy
- Wrong advice or medical treatment regarding gestational diabetes
- Various types of medical misdiagnosis during pregnancy or childbirth
- Errors that result in premature birth
- Medical errors resulting in birth injuries or birth defects

- Negligence during labor, such as negligence with regards to anesthesia
- Surgical negligence concerning a cesarean section operation
- Special cases, such as those resulting in wrongful conception or birth

TELEMEDICINE

Telemedicine has been widely prevalent in the recent pandemic situation at such an extent that the government had to formulate guidelines regarding it. Its advantages and disadvantages are debatable, however, in cases where the telemedicine and tele-consultation are being perused by the physician utmost care and vigilance should be demonstrated in documentation which has been emphasized in guidelines too.

HOW TO PREVENT MISTAKES IN DOCUMENTATION?

- *Don't destroy evidence*: In India, destroying a record is an added offense.
- *Don't ever change the record:* Sophisticated technology can detect alteration of records. Again in India, fabrication with the evidence is an added offense.
- *Do time and date your entries in the record*: Chronicity is very important to reconstruct what happened.
- *Don't rely on memory*: Recall is faulty.
- *Do include significant positives and negatives from the patient's history and physical examination:* Many records lack any mention of history, or references to history are illegible.
- *Do make your notes legible:* You will not look credible in court if an unreadable phrase has meaning to you and no one else.
- *Do indicate that you reviewed the laboratory data, etc.:* Physicians frequently neglect to note these things in the record.
- *Do describe your management plan well:* Provide detail and rationale as to your plan.
- *Don't editorialize about your patient or anyone else:* Personal comments are recipe for legal disaster!
- *Don't add risk management comments:* There were not enough beds available.
- *Don't include peer-review comments:* Dr Yadav failed to arrive in a timely fashion.
- The service(s) performed must be sufficiently documented to show medical necessity. This is the most important.

It all comes down to documentation. You can be a highly credentialed physician who does great work, and you are honest and bill exactly what you perform. However, if you don't document sufficiently for the services rendered, it is as if you did not perform the work at all.

JUDGMENTS RELATED TO DOCUMENTATION IN OBSTETRICS AND GYNECOLOGY

CASE 1: Federation of Obstetrics vs. Union of India on 3rd May 2019[14]

It is submitted that the record keeping provide information on individual patients who could have potentially undergone sex selection/determination techniques, which is an offence under this Act. If record keeping is diluted or exempted from the mandatory requirement of the Act, the probable involvement in sex determination and sex selection in the guise of use of diagnostic techniques would continue unbated.

The way in which the non-maintenance of record can be used for violating the provisions of the Act, is apparent from the aforesaid example. The aforesaid facts that have been mentioned in the show cause notice that had been issued. In many Form 'F', female patients with wrong phone numbers were mentioned. In other Form 'F' patients with wrong identity, proof of address and no identity proof were found. In another set of Form 'F' wrong obstetric and abortion history was mentioned. The signature of patient was also found missing in the consent forms. Thus, the non-filling of information cannot be termed to be clerical error, but in case it is kept vague that itself facilitates an offence. It would definitely a blatant and intentional violation of the provisions of the Act in order to prevent the mischief which is intended to by maintenance of record, filling up details of the forms is mandated by Sections 4 and 5. The wholesome social legislation would be defeated in case Form is not filled which is sine qua non toto undertake tests/ procedures if such condition does not exist, no such procedure can be performed and diluting the provisions would be against the gender justice. It is in order to create equality that the provisions have been enacted, not those unequals are being treated equally. The non-maintenance of form/not reflecting correct medical condition is offence, not mentioning it would also be an offence or keeping it vague.

CASE 2: Dr (Mrs) Indu Sharma vs. Indraprastha Apollo Hospital on 22nd April 2015[15]

The Opponent Parties produced three expert opinions from doctors in own hospital, namely Prof (Dr) Kamal Buckshee, Senior Consultant with Department of Obstetrics and Gynecology of Hospital, Dr (Mrs) Urmil Sharma and Dr (Mrs) Harmeet Malhotra, all have examined the treatment papers, opined that the treatment given to the patient was correct, and that there was no deficiency or negligence on the part of the treating doctors.

CASE 3: Justice KS Puttaswamy (Retd) vs. Union of India on 26th September 2018[16]

The applicant submits that the women's clinic's submission of copies of her medical records to the Social Insurance Office without her knowledge or consent interfered with her right to respect for her private life. She maintains that the information contained in these records were of a highly sensitive and private nature. Allegedly, she could not anticipate, when she claimed compensation from the Office, that information on the abortion performed several years after alleged back injury would be forwarded to the Office. She further refers to the fact that the information in question is not protected by the same level of confidentiality at the Office as at the clinic.

CASE 4: Smt. Gayatri Alias Gadigevva vs. Vijay S/o Siddappa Hadimani on 3rd December 2021[17]

Whether, it is permissible for a Family Court to summon the medical records of a spouse on the request of the other spouse, especially when it pertained to records relating to any procedures relating to the reproductive choices of the spouse?

In order to get over the bar imposed on the medical practitioners to disclose the secrets of the patients to which they are privy, the Courts should not be asked to exercise their power to secure medical records. If this is permitted, it would mean the medical practitioner is required to divulge the secrets that the patient has disclosed to him contrary to his professional ethics only because an adversary in litigation wishes to use it to non-suit the other.

It is to be kept in mind that the medical records of an individual are very private and are not for public consumption. If the medical record of a person is private to him, a direction to his medical practitioner to produce the medical records or divulge any secret that he is privy to it would essentially amount to infringing the fundamental right of privacy guaranteed to an individual, which emanates from the Right to Life granted under Article 21 of Constitution of India.

It is therefore clear that Courts cannot as a matter of course summon medical records or direct the Doctors to give evidence about the medical condition of a litigant.

CASE 5: Maharaja Agrasen Hospital vs. Master Rishabh Sharma on 16 December 2019[18]

The Delhi Medical Council vide order dated 14.12.2007 issued a warning to the Appellant No 1—Hospital for the delay in supplying the medical records of the Respondent No 1—baby to the Complainant.

Regulation 1.3.2 of the IMC Regulations casts a statutory obligation upon every doctor/hospital to provide medical records within 72 hours of the request being made by the patient.

Regulation 1.3.2 of the Indian Medical Council (Professional Conduct, Etiquettes and Ethics) Regulations, 2002 provides as under:

1.3 Maintenance of medical records:

1.3.1 Every physician shall maintain the medical records pertaining to his/her indoor patients for a period of 3 years from the date of commencement of the treatment in a standard proforma laid down by the Medical Council of India.

1.3.2. If any request is made for medical records either by the patients/authorized attendant or legal authorities involved, the same may be duly acknowledged and documents shall be issued within the period of 72 hours.

As per Regulation 7, if the doctor refuses or fails to provide the medical records within 72 hours when the patient or his/her authorized representative makes a request as per Regulation 1.3.2, the said act of commission or omission would constitute professional misconduct rendering him/her liable for disciplinary action and punishment under Regulation 8.

We find that withholding the medical records of Respondent No 1, who was a premature baby, for a period of over 2 years, would constitute grave professional misconduct under Regulation 7, apart from being a gross deficiency in service on the part of the Appellant No 1—Hospital and its management.

CASE 6: Mrs Anuja Chaudhary vs. Shivam Hospital and Research... on 18th March 2020[19]

It is pertinent to note that, that regular antenatal care, identification of high-risk factors, close monitoring of labor, active management of the third stage of labor, and to avoid difficult vaginal delivery the timely decision to do cesarean can reduce the incidence of EOH. In the instant case, on the basis of medical record, it is evident that the patient was under the care of OP No 3 during antenatal period and as per standard protocol patient was monitored. In our view the OP No 3 Dr Sarika Roy adopted conservative measures till the patient was hemodynamically stable. Patient was transfused about 10 units of blood, but the intractable obstetrical hemorrhage of the patient was unresponsive to all measures and, thus, to save the life of patient from obstetric shock, OP No 3 performed an emergency subtotal hysterectomy.

Diagnosis-related negligence: Medical negligence can occur when incorrect diagnosis is made in spite of the glaring presence of the signs and symptoms attributable to the ailment, e.g., the inability of a medical practitioner to diagnose pre-eclampsia in a pregnant patient with obvious signs of hypertension, edema, and significant proteinuria, or when a woman with three previous cesarean sections, ordinarily requiring another C-section is allowed to go into labor-probably rupturing her uterus and dies. Advice/counseling-related negligence may occur when a patient has not been sufficiently advised or counseled on his/her medical condition to prevent harm from occurring, e.g., a patient who had a minor operation and requiring to stay in bed over a period of time, may if not counseled to do so, fall down from dizziness and sustained injuries, the hospital is liable of counseling-related negligence. Treatment-related negligence can occur when harm occurs from treatment given without obtaining the consent of the patient or when a wrong medication has been administered for an ailment or even when a patient needing protection is neglected, e.g., a woman who has had a minor gynecological surgery under anesthesia falls off from the theater table and injured herself, because she was unattended to.

REFERENCES

1. Gowda SL, Bhandiwad A, Anupama NK. Litigations in obstetric and gynaecological practice: can it be prevented? A probability to possibility. J Obstet and Gynecolog Ind. 2016;66:541-7.
2. Glaser L, Alvi F, Milad M. Trends in malpractice claims for obstetric and gynecologic procedures, 2005 through 2014. American J Obstet Gynecolog. 2017; 217(3):340.e1-340.e6.
3. Nizam's Institute of Medical Sciences vs. Prasanth S Dhananka and Ors. on 14 May 2009. Civil Appeal No. 4119 of 1999.
4. Chattopadhyay S, Rudra A, Ray M, Sengupta S, Goswami S. (2016). Legal Aspects in Obstetric Anaesthesia. Nepal Journal of Obstetrics and Gynaecology. 10.3.10.3126/njog.v10i2.14327.
5. American Society of Anesthesiologists Task Force on Obstetric Anesthesia. Practice guidelines for obstetric anesthesia: an updated report. Anesthesiology. 2007; 106:843-63.
6. Williams MS. Davies JM, Ross BK. Medico-legal Issues in Obstetric Anesthesia. In: Chestnut DH, Polley LS, Tsen LC, Wong CA (Eds). Obstetric Anesthesia Principles and Practice, 4th edition. Philadelphia, USA: Elsevier Mosby; 2009. pp. 727-46.
7. Palmer SK, Gibbs CP. Risk management in obstetric anesthesia. Int Anesthesiol Clin. 1989;27:188-9.
8. Benet LZ. Principles of prescription order writing and patient compliance instructions In Appendix-1: Goodman and Gilman's. The Pharmacological Basis of Therapeutics. New York: McGraw-Hill. 1996; pp. 1697-706.
9. De Vries TPGM, Henning RH, Hogerzeil HV, Fersle DA. Guide to good prescribing: a practical manual. Geneva, World Health Organization. 1995; pp. 51-5 (WHO/DAP/94.11).
10. Meyer TA, Improving the quality of the order writing process for inpatient order and outpatient prescriptions American Journal of Health System Pharmacy. 2000;57(4):18-22.
11. Jaykaran, Bhardwaj P, Chavda N, Yadav P, Panwar A. Prescribing knowledge of the intern doctor in India. The Internet Journal of Epidemiology. 2009;7(1):1-3.
12. Medical Ethics. Text of Medical Council of India Regulations [cited 14 July 2009]. Available from: http//www.medclic.comIndia
13. Lofholm PW, Katzung BG, Rational prescribing and prescription writing. In: Katzung BG (Ed). Basic and Clinical Pharmacology. New York: McGraw-Hill. 2001; pp. 1104-12.

14. Federation of Obstetrics vs. Union of India on 3 May 2019. SC Writ Petition (Civil) No. 129 of 2017. Available from: https://indiankanoon.org/doc/123238150/
15. Dr. (Mrs.) Indu Sharma vs. Indraprastha Apollo Hospital on 22 April 2015. Available from: https://indiankanoon.org/doc/64183895/.
16. Justice KS Puttaswamy (Retd) vs. Union of India on 26 September, 2018. Available from: https://indiankanoon.org/doc/127517806/.
17. Smt Gayatri Alias Gadigevva vs. Vijay s/o Siddappa Hadimani on 3 December 2021. Available from: https://indiankanoon.org/doc/54113030/.
18. Maharaja Agrasen Hospital vs. Master Rishabh Sharma. on 16 December 2019. Available from: https://indiankanoon.org/doc/35792279/.
19. Mrs Anuja Chaudhary vs Shivam Hospital & Research on 18 March 2020. Available from: https://indiankanoon.org/doc/164209365/.

SECTION 4

Forensic Gynecology

CHAPTER 10

Medical Laws Related to Sexual Offences Against Women

Prateek Rastogi

INTRODUCTION

Crime against women is prevalent in every society since time immemorial. Issues like prohibition on girl education, triple talaq, *sati pratha*, child marriage, prohibition on widow remarriage, dowry demands, acid attacks, marital rapes, denial of inheritance rights, sexual crimes, physical and psychological abuse, to name a few. One or the other women related crime is present or was present in almost every country involving either one or other religion although presently few of them have been either abolished or prohibited by law. Of all the crimes sexual offences are considered most grievous as they are directed towards not only physical but also social and psychological abuse and humiliation of the victim.

Regulations to prevent or prohibit sexual offences and provisions for punishing the offender are present in our legislature. After infamous Delhi rape case of 2012 (Nirbhaya case) the traditional definition of sexual offences against women was modified to give a wider coverage and hence there was even a revision in existing laws against sexual crimes and penal provisions against sexual offenders.

In India, numerous acts have been drafted and implemented to prevent above mentioned crimes against women:

- The Child Marriage Restraint Act, 1929
- The Immoral Traffic (Prevention) Act, 1956
- The Dowry (Prohibition) Act, 1961
- The Indecent Representation of Women (Prohibition) Act, 1986
- The Commission of Sati (Prevention) Act, 1987
- Protection of Women from Domestic Violence Act, 2005
- The Sexual Harassment of Women at Workplace (Prevention, Prohibition and Redressal) Act, 2013
- Muslim women (Protection of Rights on Marriage) Act, 2019

TABLE 1: Offences commonly known to target women.[1]

• Rape including marital rape, custodial rape, gang rape, etc. • Unnatural sexual offences • Molestation • Voyeurism • Stalking • Immoral trafficking • Kidnapping and abduction • Outraging the modesty	• Sexual harassment • Disrobing • Child marriage • Dowry harassment • Pornography • *Sati pratha* • Triple talaq and halala • Acid attacks

Even as per the Bharatiya Nyaya Sanhita/ BNS (previously Indian Penal Code 1860 and subsequent amendments), Indian Law recognizes and penalizes following offences which can involve women:[1]

1. Murder, Dowry death, Abetment of Suicide, etc. (Sections 103 (1), 80 and 108 BNS respectively)

2. Acid Attack—Sections 124 (1) and 124 (2) BNS
3. Kidnapping and abduction for different purposes (Sections 137 and 138 BNS)
4. Outraging the modesty of women (Section 74 BNS)
5. Sexual harassment (Section 75 BNS)
6. Assault on women with intent to disrobe a woman (Section 76 BNS)
7. Voyeurism (Section 77 BNS)
8. Stalking (Section 78 BNS)
9. Rape (Sections 63 to 71 BNS)
10. Cruelty done by husband or his family (Section 85 BNS)
11. Words, gestures or any other act with a motive to damage a woman's modesty (Section 79 BNS)

OUTRAGING MODESTY OF A FEMALE: SECTION 74 BNS (PREVIOUSLY SECTION 354 IPC)[1]

- If a person does any act against a woman with an intention or knowledge that it may outrage her modesty, can be penalized with imprisonment of up to 2 years, with or without fine.
- According to Supreme Court in "State of Punjab vs. major Singh (1967 AIR 63, 1966 SCR (2) 286)" modesty of a woman lies in her gender, i.e., by being born as a woman she possesses modesty.[2] This means anything which a woman considers outrageous for her gender comes under purview of this section.
- In "Rupan Deol Bajaj and Anr. vs. Kanwar Pal Singh Gill & Anr.", or the "Butt Slapping Case", Mr KPS Gill a decorated police officer slapped Mrs Bajaj an IAS officer on her buttocks during a party. Court decided that the action of Mr Gill amounted to 'outraging of her modesty'.[3]

SEXUAL HARASSMENT: SECTION 75 BNS (PREVIOUSLY SECTION 354 A IPC)[1]

This law covers acts constituting sexual harassment, i.e., unwanted advances (physical or verbal) of any kind, showing pornography against will, demand for sexual favors punishable with prison sentence up to 3 years with or without fine and making sexually colored remarks punishable with imprisonment for up to 1 year with or without fine.

ASSAULT OR USE OF CRIMINAL FORCE TO WOMAN WITH INTENT TO DISROBE: SECTION 76 BNS (PREVIOUSLY SECTION 354 B IPC)[1]

An assault or using force against a female with motive of disrobing her is punishable with prison sentence from 3 to 7 years and fine. Any person helping in perpetration of such act is also eligible to get same punishment.

In case of "Raju Pandurang Mahale vs. State of Maharashtra and Anr. (AIR 2004 SC, 1677)", victim was brought to the house of an accomplice by the accused, where she was held and compelled to consume alcohol. She was disrobed and photographed in nude. The Supreme Court pronounced the accused guilty as their acts violated female decency.[4]

VOYEURISM: SECTION 77 BNS (PREVIOUSLY SECTION 354 CRPC)[1]

Voyeurism is an act wherein a man sees or clicks the picture or video of any female engaged in a personal task in situations where she will not expect the perpetrator or any other person to observe her. This is punishable with a sentence of 1–3 years with fine. For repeat offences imprisonment of 3–7 years along with fine is detailed. If woman consents to be photographed in any such acts with the understanding that it will be kept private and if that person shares the same image, then he is also liable.

STALKING: SECTION 78 BNS (PREVIOUSLY SECTION 354 D IPC)[1]

If a male continuously follows or contacts a female or attempts to contact, her to develop terms even after display of lack of interest by her or even monitors her electronic conversation the offence amounts to stalking. First offence is punishable with imprisonment of up to 3 years with fine whereas for repeat offence term extends up to 5 years with fine. Stalking as a part of legal obligation for detecting and preventing crime is not a punishable offence.

KIDNAPPING: SECTION 87 BNS (SECTION 366 IPC)[1]

Kidnapping/abducting any woman with the intention or knowledge that such woman may be compelled, for illicit intercourse or marriage is punishable offence with imprisonment of up to 10 years and fine.

HUMAN TRAFFICKING: SECTION 143 BNS (PREVIOUSLY SECTION 370 IPC)[1]

Human trafficking is defined as illegally transporting people or transporting them without their consent mainly for use in commercial sex industry or in labor. It is regulated by Immoral Traffic (Prevention) Act, 1956 in India.

RAPE: SECTION 63 BNS (PREVIOUSLY SECTION 375 IPC)[1]

A man causing penetration of penis or insertion any other object into woman's mouth, vagina, urethra or anus or manipulating any of her body part to commit such act or if he applies his mouth to her vagina, urethra or anus or makes her do so either with him or someone is said to commit rape.

Such acts amount to rape if done against her will, without her consent or if consent is obtained by fear, fraud, impersonation, by virtue of intoxication or unsoundness of mind if she is above 18 years of age or by any means including consent if she is below 18 years of age or in cases where woman is unable to express her consent.

Mere absence of injuries does not suggest consent for sexual act, medical procedures or interventions done as required following prescribed protocols do not fall under purview of rape. Earlier, Marital rape, i.e., forceful sexual intercourse by husband was not considered rape for woman aged above 15 years however, in October 2017 Supreme Court have raised this age bar to 18 years. Sexual intercourse by spouse of his wife if they are under living separately by law Sec 67 BNS (previously Section 376 B IPC) constitutes rape and punishment of 2–7 years with fine is prescribed in law.

According to Sec 64 BNS (previously section 376 IPC), whoever except in the cases provided for in subsection 2 of Sec 64 BNS, commits rape shall be punished with rigorous imprisonment of 10 years to life with fine. Criminal law (amendment) act 2013[5] provides special provisions under section 64 BNS (previously section 376 IPC) for cases of aggravated rape. Rape is considered aggravated if it committed by someone in position of authority due to legal status over women (police officer or army personal) Sec 68 BNS (previously Section 376 C IPC), by someone whom the victim trusts (family members, hospital staff), in certain cases like rape on pregnant female, a mentally ill woman, woman incapable of consenting, a female less than 16 years of age, rape during communal riots, repeated rape, accused is punishable with imprisonment of 10 years to life with fine.

In case of gang rape (Sec 70 (1) BNS—previously Section 376 D IPC) or if, the woman dies or is lead into to a persistent vegetative state (Sec 66 BNS —previously Section 376 A), offender can be sentenced to prison for a duration of 20 years to life or death penalty.

INSULTING THE MODESTY OF A WOMAN: SEC 79 BNS (PREVIOUSLY SECTION 509 IPC)[1]

Anyone who speaks any word, makes any noise or action, or displays any object, with the motive of making such words heard, or actions and objects seen by a woman or invades her privacy with intention of insulting her modesty is punished with imprisonment up to one year, with or without fine.

THE INDECENT REPRESENTATION OF WOMEN (PROHIBITION) ACT, 1986[6]

This act prohibits representation of women in advertisements, publications, writings, paintings, figures, etc. in an indecent way. "Indecent representation of women" is defined as the "depiction in any manner of the woman form or body or any part as to have the effect of being indecent, or derogatory to, or denigrating, or is likely to deprave, corrupt or injure the public morality or morals."

THE SEXUAL HARASSMENT OF WOMEN AT WORKPLACE (PREVENTION, PROHIBITION AND REDRESSAL) ACT, 2013[7]

- It was enacted to prevent, prohibit and redress the issues related to the female harassment at workplace irrespective of government or private setup.
- The Act defines sexual harassment to include unwelcome acts such as physical contact and sexual advances, a demand or request for sexual favors, making sexually colored remarks, showing pornography, and any other unwelcome physical, verbal, or non-verbal conduct of a sexual nature.
- The Hon'ble Supreme Court of India in a landmark judgment in the Vishakha and others vs. State of Rajasthan 1997[8] case gave 'Vishakha guidelines'. These guidelines formed the basis for the Act [*Sexual Harassment of Women at Workplace (Prevention, Prohibition and Redressal) Act, 2013*].
- The Act places a legal obligation on employers to prevent and prohibit sexual harassment in the workplace.

Internal Complaints Committee (ICC): Employers are required to constitute an ICC at each workplace with 10 or more employees to receive and address complaints of sexual harassment. The Complaints Committees have the powers of civil courts for gathering evidence. Employers must undertake awareness programs, provide a safe working environment, and display information about the Act at the workplace.

- *Complaint mechanism:* The Act lays down a procedure for filing complaints, conducting inquiries, and providing a fair opportunity to the parties involved.
- *Penalties:* Non-compliance with the Act's provisions can result in penalties, including fine and cancellation of business licenses.

ROLE OF OBSTETRICIANS AND GYNECOLOGISTS IN HANDLING SEXUAL ASSAULT SURVIVORS[9]

In cases of sexual offences especially rape, unnatural sexual offences or sometimes when any other sexual offence have taken a physical overturn, medical examination of the victim is of prime importance. This may be required sometimes either to prove or disprove the allegation or else to treat the victim. In dealing with survivors of sexual assault health care providers need to:

a. Provide medical and psychological support
b. Ensure meeting medicolegal requirements like evidence collection, documentation and reporting for safeguarding patient's as well as their own interests.

As per Sec 184 BNSS-previously Section 164 (A) CrPC there are few legal liabilities for the doctor such as:[10]

1. Examination of victims should be conducted by a doctor in a government hospital or by any other doctor in the absence of such a practitioner.
2. Examination to be conducted at the earliest and detailed report to be prepared.
3. Due consent for examination to be taken and recorded.
4. Recording of the time of start and end of examination is required.
5. The RMP shall forward the report to the investigating officer within a period of 7 days, who shall forward it to the Magistrate.

As per Sec 397 BNSS—previously Section 357 CrPC, doctors in private and government set up should provide treatment to a victim of sexual assault and refusal of treatment is culpable in Sec 200 BNS—previously Section 166 B IPC with imprisonment up to one year or fine or with both.[1,10]

Doctors need a comprehensive approach while dealing with victims of sexual offence including:

1. Necessary medical support
2. Uniform method of examination and evidence collection using Sexual Assault Forensic Evidence (SAFE) kit,
3. Obtaining proper consent (informed) for examination
4. Collection of evidentiary material, preservation and police intimation.
5. Maintaining chain of custody for evidence at each level.

While dealing with victim, care needs to be taken to:

1. Refer victim to appropriate agencies for legal and shelter services
2. Develop a good rapport with victim
3. Avoid unsympathetic remarks and behavior.
4. Avoid blaming the survivor for the incident
5. Appreciate her strength in coming for treatment.
6. Explain that all steps taken are required for her treatment and also to punish the perpetrator.
7. Explain in simple language the rationale for various procedures including genital examination.
8. Confidentiality should be ensured at all levels so that survivor can repose her trust in doctor.

Examination of victim less than 18 years has to be done by female doctor only. In case the victim is aged more than 18 years still preference to be given for female doctor. If due to unavoidable circumstances male doctor need to examine such a victim, then examination should compulsorily be done in presence of female attendant only ensuring full privacy and confidentiality. Examination of victim cannot be done without her consent or without the consent of her parents or guardians in case victim is a minor.

Detailed history should be elicited regarding timing, place and nature of act along with details of changing dress or washing the private parts after the act.

At the end of the examination, the doctor needs to opine on:

1. If a sexual act has been attempted or completed.
2. If such a sexual act is recent or remote.
3. If any harm has been caused to the victim in terms of injury or disease.
4. The age of the survivors is especially in the case of adolescent girls.
5. If any intoxicant has been administered to the victim.
6. Mental status of the victim

CONCLUSION

Sexual offences are considered serious not only due to the physical nature of crime but also because such acts leave a long-lasting scar on body, mind, soul as well as reputation of victim and family. Healthcare providers, especially doctors and nurses, play a vital role in the treatment, support and rehabilitation of victims. In addition, health professionals need to handle legal, social and ethical responsibilities while discharging their medical duties in treatment of sexual assault survivors. Awareness of law, sense of ethical and social responsibilities in addition to medical knowledge is the key in sexual assault examination cases.

REFERENCES

1. The Bhartiya Nyaya Sanhita, 2023. Available online at https://www.mha.gov.in/sites/default/files/250883_english_01042024.pdf.
2. State of Punjab vs. Major Singh (1967AIR 63, 1966 SCR (2) 286) https://main.sci.gov.in/jonew/judis/2651.pdf.
3. Rupan Deol Bajaj and Anr. vs. Kanwar Pal Singh Gill & Anr. Available online at https://en.wikipedia.org/wiki/Rupan_Deol_Bajaj_case.
4. Raju Pandurang Mahale vs. State of Maharashtra and Anr. (AIR 2004 SC 1677). Available online at: https://www.legalserviceindia.com/legal/article-3994-sexual-assault-and-rape.html.
5. Crimal law Amendment (2013) Act. Available online at https://www.iitk.ac.in/wc/data/TheCriminalLaw.pdf
6. The Indecent Representation of Women (Prohibition) Act, 1986. Available online at: https://thc.nic.in/Central%20Governmental%20Acts/Indecent%20Representation%20of%20%20%20Women%20(Prohibition)%20Act,%201986.pdf.
7. The Sexual Harassment of Women at Workplace (Prevention, Prohibition and Redressal) Act, 2013. Available online at https://legislative.gov.in/sites/default/files/A2013-14.pdf.
8. Vishaka and others vs. State of Rajasthan. Available online at https://en.wikipedia.org/wiki/Vishakha_and_ others_v._State_of_Rajasthan
9. Guidelines and Protocols: Medicolegal care for survivors/victims of sexual assault. Available online at: https://main.mohfw.gov.in/sites/default/files/953522324.pdf.
10. The Code of Criminal Procedure, 1973. Available online at: https://prsindia.org/files/bills_acts/bills_parliament/2023/Bharatiya_Nagarik_Suraksha_Sanhita,_2023.pdf.

CHAPTER 11

Medicolegal Examination of Survivors of Sexual Offences

Jagadeesh Narayanareddy

INTRODUCTION

Sexual violence is a public health emergency. Among one of the fastest growing crimes in India is Rape. The numbers reported according to National Crime Records Bureau (NCRB) are alarming. On an average every day, India reports 67 cases that means three cases of Rape reported every hour.[1] The whole country was shaken by the Nirbhaya incident in December 2012 and took to streets to protest against the undeterred increase in sex crimes, which forced the government to constitute Justice Verma Commission to advise on the measures to be taken in this regard. The Criminal Law Amendment Act 2013, which brought several legal changes in the approach of investigating and adjudicating of sexual violence was one such measure.[2]

But the actual numbers of sexual violence are more and the NCRB statistics only capture the cases which have reached the criminal investigation; and these numbers are just the tip of the iceberg. Due to social concerns, poor conviction rate, stigma and biases attached in society, victim blaming, male dominated society—several cases of survivors of sexual violence silently suffer and not reach the criminal investigation. And all of these survivors postsexual violence have health concerns, and this adds to the health burden of society. The health sector has to prioritize its actions in this regard.

Lot of criticism was against health sector for insensitive practices of two finger test, denial of treatment, insistence of police complaint before medical examination, incomplete opinions, violation of privacy and confidentiality during medical examination procedures, psychological counseling being undermined, basically not following uniform procedures, sensitivity and good clinical practices in many healthcare settings. In the year 2014, the Ministry of Health and Family Welfare, Government of India brought uniform guidelines for medical examination of sexual violence survivors, which is another measure towards gender sensitive approach of health sector towards combatting sex crimes and overcoming much of the criticism against the health sector.[3] The only problem being 'Health' is a subject in State list, and thus these guidelines issued by the Central government needs to be adopted by each State government for implementation in that State.

STEPS IN MANAGEMENT OF SURVIVORS OF SEXUAL OFFENCES

Sexual violence will often result in health consequences to the survivor. But there are many cases of sexual violence who may not have any health concerns, and those individuals would not require to approach any hospital/doctor. Every doctor should thus remember it is only a section of sexual violence survivors who reach the hospital for their health concerns. And in addition, we should also recognize that every case of sexual violence would have psychological consequences which require psychological first aid and several sessions of counseling to overcome them.

Thus, medical management of survivors of sexual offences for a comprehensive care includes after informed consent and along with proper documentation for care for injuries, psychological disturbances, sexually transmitted illness, contraceptive advice, pregnancy advice, drug deaddiction program (if needed), disability care (if needed) along with evidence collection. This requires multidisciplinary approach for better management. Every medical establishment caring for survivors of sexual violence should have a separate room for medical examination and counseling with availability of human resources, material resources and management of all health concerns at the same place preferably for better and effective management of these cases to overcome privacy and confidentiality issues.

For comprehensive medical management[3] of survivors of sexual violence, based on the Guidelines from Ministry of Health and Family Welfare, the steps are as follows **(Flowchart 1)**:

MEDICOLEGAL DUTIES OF A DOCTOR (STEP-BY-STEP APPROACH)

Below is a detailed step-by-step approach to be adopted by a doctor, whenever a survivor of sexual violence reaches a hospital/doctor.[3] There are three ways a survivor of sexual violence reaches a hospital/doctor. One—Voluntary approach, wherein the

Flowchart 1: Step-by-Step approach for management of survivors of sexual violence.

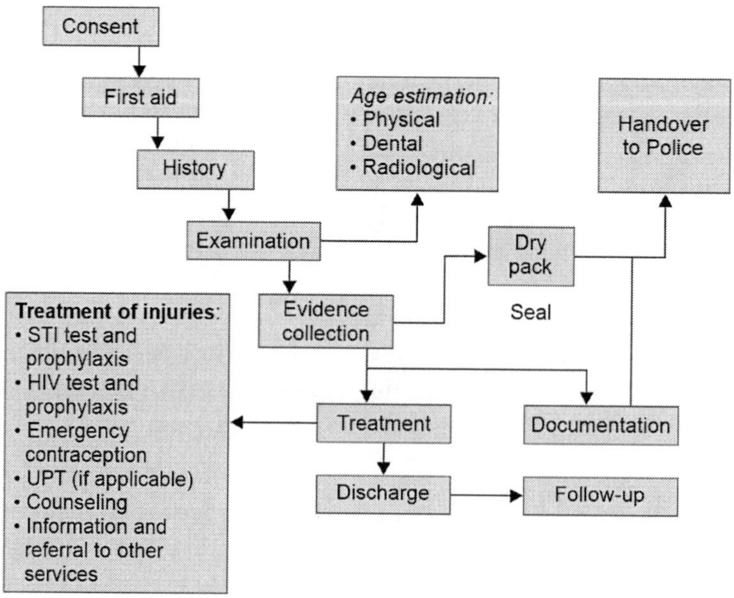

Source: Adopted from Guidelines and Protocols from Ministry of Health and Family Welfare, Government of India for Responding to Victims/Survivors of Sexual Violence[3])

survivor of sexual violence may reach to the trusted hospital/doctor for management of health consequences. Another—with Police requisition, wherein the survivor of sexual violence has already lodged a police complaint, and the police forwards a requisition to the nearest/jurisdictional hospital/doctor to conduct medical examination as a part of procedure of criminal investigation. Another—with Court order, wherein the survivor of sexual violence has lodged a complaint with the Court (could be due to no faith with the Police or accused is influential or powerful) and then the court orders to the hospital/doctor to conduct medical examination.

First Aid

Every survivor postsexual violence has psychological consequences, fear of accused, social stigma, shyness, self-blame, etc. Hence, every survivor needs reassurance, and a firm statement that it was never the survivor's fault. The person responsible and to repent is the accused. Every healthcare provider has to provide psychological first aid, treatment of bleeding injuries and other acute trauma. Assessment of pregnancy risk and providing emergency contraception within 5 days but more effective if provided earlier than this duration post-assault.[3]

History Seeking

This is an art and has to be sensitively probed particularly in these cases of sexual violence. Doctor has to provide both auditory and visual privacy and ensure confidentiality so as to enable the survivor to share much of the information, which they might have not shared with even parents/spouse/friends. History of sexual violence should be sought and documented verbatim. The use of probing questions should be done with caution not to cause revictimization of the survivor. History of any physical violence, emotional abuse, verbal threats, use of weapons, luring with sweets, chocolates, money, job, etc. should be probed and documented. Whether the violence occurred under the influence of drug and/or alcohol; whether survivor was sleeping or unconscious at the time of violence has to be probed and documented. History of penetrative sex or nonpenetrative sex; which orifice (s) penetrated, penetrated by penis/object/body part; history of emission of semen; post-assault activities like changing clothes, bathing, douching, urination, defecation, rinsing of mouth, brushing, vomiting; use of condom; use of lubricant has to be sought and documented.[3]

History of menstruation either at the time of assault or post-assault or at the time of examination should be sought and documented; this information has a bearing on the interpretation of presence/absence of trace evidence. History of presence of pregnancy and its duration at the time of assault or post-assault or at the time of examination should be sought and documented; this information has a bearing on the award of increased punishment along with health consequences for the survivor.

Survivors could add information to the history already given, change information given earlier, or even give information any number of times. The doctor has to document the history given chronologically with the date and time, information on who gave the information, informant is conscious or not and obtain signature in addition after explaining what is being documented.

Informed Consent

Before the medical examination every doctor has to seek and document informed consent. Complete information about medical examinations, and treatment is provided to the survivor in a language understood by the survivor and to the parents/guardian if the survivor is less than 12 years of age. Consent is sought separately for medical examinations for treatment; medicolegal examination; sample collection for clinical and forensic examination; and for revealing information to police. If survivor refuses to consent, then informed refusal is documented.[3]

Survivor always has the right to withdraw consent at any point of time of examination and this withdrawal will not affect survivor's right for treatment. For non-invasive examination or routine medical examination survivor above age of 12 years can consent. For invasive examination or medical termination of pregnancy survivor above age of 18 years can consent. In both situations if survivor's age is below the legal permissible age of 12 years/18 years respectively then consent is sought from parents/guardian.

In the absence of parents/guardian then consent can be sought from the panel of doctors (who are not part of therapeutic care in the hospital— administrative heads in hospital-like medical superintendent, resident medical officer, head of the department) who would act in the best interest of patient (Survivor). In case of absence of panel of doctors to consent in case of child survivor, then consent is sought from the guardian, who is appointed by Child Welfare Committee who has the responsibility of care and protection of children. Only in those cases wherein the termination of pregnancy is warranted beyond the provisions of the Medical Termination of Pregnancy Act, Amendment Act, 2021, then the advocate can apply to the jurisdictional Court to intervene and seek Court permission for MTP for the gestations beyond 24 weeks of gestational age.

Mandatory Reporting to Police

Whenever any doctor/hospital sees or cares or examines a survivor of sexual violence, then as per section 397 BNSS (previously Sec 357 C CrPC) and section 19 of POCSO Act, they are required to compulsorily inform the police/special juvenile police unit. The legal provisions only require to mere inform the police of care of such survivors by doctor/hospital. There is no need for the doctor/hospital to wait for the police arrival before carrying out therapeutic care. Both events can parallelly occur.

Failure to do this mandatory reporting to police will attract 1-year imprisonment with fine under section *200 BNS* (previously Sec 166 B IPC) to the doctor; and 6 months for individual doctor and 1 year for administrative doctor of the hospital under section 21 of the POCSO Act. There is no time limit for this mandatory reporting clause. Hence all cases which even reporting on a later date for medical termination of pregnancy or pregnancy and delivery, or for psychiatric disturbances later on as a consequence of sexual violence have to be mandatorily reported to the police. But this mandatory reporting has problems in those cases of survivors who are yet to make up their mind to join criminal investigation. They may avoid in reaching the hospital to obtain therapeutic care in the fear of joining the unwanted criminal investigation by the process of mandatory reporting. Thus, there may be no therapeutic care obtained or MTP avoided or done by quacks or report in advanced stages of pregnancy seeking abortion or suffer sexually transmitted infections or psychological disturbances in advanced stages; overall the morbidity and mortality risks are increased adding to the health burden of the society.

Physical and Genital Examination

Ensuring privacy, confidentiality and gender sensitive practices for examination of physical and genital findings of injuries or lesions or stains is to be done.[3] This examination has to be done based on history obtained of sexual violence. Head-to-toe examination may not be required in all cases unless informed consent is obtained from the survivor. If sexual violence is only restricted to a particular part of the body/orifice, then restricting the examination to that part of the body/orifice will ensure trust and confidence of the survivor; unless the doctor feels/is of the opinion that the survivor is not able to understand the nature of sexual violence or part of the body/orifice violated or penetrated. This may be a case in young children who may not be able to distinguish from introitus to anal opening, ejaculation, etc.

Good clinical practices based on scientific approach should be the basis for physical and genital examination. Documenting gaits may not be required in every survivor as it stereotypes that every survivor should have an abnormal gait. The pattern of injuries sustained during sexual violence shows considerable variation from complete absence of injuries (more commonly) to presence of grievous injuries (rarely). Injuries if present should be documented including description of number, type, site, size, shape, swelling, color, stage of healing. Similarly, lesions corresponding to a disease process and description of stains—type, site, size, shape, color, possible cause should be described.

Two finger test performance, interpretation, and documentation are banned by the Supreme Court of India and is not warranted. Per vaginum examination and per speculum examination should not be done unless required for detection of injuries or for medical treatment. Anus and oral cavity examination is also done if history warrants and checked for any bleeding, tear, discharge, edema, tenderness, etc.

Evidence Collection

Based on current medical understanding of sexual violence, we can have five types of medical evidence—trace evidence, injuries, sexually transmitted infections, pregnancy and its complications, and evidence of treatment.

Based on Locard's Principle of Exchange, we can have exchange of trace evidence between survivor and accused or vice versa. Trace evidence could be like semen, spermatozoa, blood, hair, cells, dust, paint, grass, lubricant, fecal matter, body fluids, saliva, entirely based on type and place of sexual violence. Delay in medical examination puts the detection of much of these trace evidence to a minimal. Much of this evidence is based on time limitation. Detection of motile spermatozoa is possible for 12–24 hours post-assault, detection of spermatozoa for 24–48 hours and detection of sperm heads is possible till 72–96 hours. Use of Wood's lamp to detect the fluorescence of seminal stain has limited role as there are many false positive results due to the presence of fluorescence to other body fluids, antibiotic ointments, lubricants, etc. Post-assault activities like washing, douching, bathing, urination and defecation may further diminish the presence of trace evidence. Hence prioritization of this medical examination in the doctor's busy schedule is warranted. Use of condom by the accused and if such condom is not detected/found will further reduce the detection of semen/spermatozoa. Use of condom by the accused and if such condom is detected/found, then the inner surface of condom will have trace evidence to connect to the accused (epithelial cells of shaft of penis); and the outer surface of condom will have trace evidence to connect to the survivor (vaginal or anal or oral epithelial cells depending on the site of penetration). This is similar to accused leaving his visiting card at the scene of crime! DNA evidence is found from trace evidence on genitals or body or clothes or from sexual violence scenes, or nail clippings or products of conception or fetus. DNA evidence is evidence to compare. Positive match of DNA profile helps prosecution in convictions but the negative match of DNA profile does not give clean chit/acquittal of the accused. Non-matching of DNA could be due to extraction of DNA from improper sample (maternal sample instead of fetal sample in dilatation and curettage procedure); or denatured sample (formalin-fixed tissue or exposure to heat or sunlight or loss of cold chain); or contaminated sample (Touch DNA or absence of pretested swabs devoid of DNA). Moist swabs after swabbing the stains must be air-dried in shade before packing. Dry stains can be swabbed by moistening the stain with the use of distilled water or water for injection.

Injuries could be on the skin or mucosal surfaces of body or genitals. It could be of abrasions or contusions or lacerations or incised injuries or stab injuries or chop injuries or even firearm injuries or thermal injuries or electric injuries. The injury documentation acts as medical evidence; but the absence of injuries does not rule out the possibility of the occurrence of sexual violence. The presence of injuries is limited to only one third of cases of sexual violence. Delayed medical examination may not detect presence of injuries due to possibility of healing of injuries. Even immediate medical examination may also not detect all the injuries caused due to sexual violence, as mucosal injuries are reported to heal within hours. Injuries are possibly produced on the survivor due to the resistance offered. Now the Indian law also does not require the survivor to offer resistance in sexual violence as absence of resistance injuries does not construe that the survivor consented for the sexual act (Sec 63 BNS—previously explanation 2 to Sec 375 IPC). Use of Colposcopy and Toluidine blue dye test have limited or no role today as detection of microinjuries is not necessary. Because microinjuries are possible even with consented sexual activity and also with iatrogenic medical procedures.

If either of the survivor or accused is harboring a sexually transmitted infection at the time of assault, then based on Locard's Principle of Exchange, there is possibility of transmission of microorganisms from one person to another. By examining at least twice, one as early as possible and then another examination after the lapse of incubation period of the infection (3–4 days for gonococcal infection, 1 week for *Chlamydia*, weeks to months for HIV and Hepatitis) detection of sexually transmitted infection is possible. This is one of the best corroboration possible, if proper examination and detection is done as it connects the assault/sexual violence.

Presence of pregnancy and its complications also acts as medical evidence. But this is possible only in those cases of unprotected sex corresponding to ovulation time and circumstances conducive to conception in those females. Products of conception retrieved from abortion and fetus are proof of pregnancy and by DNA profiling we can connect to the accused of sexual violence.

All the above, four types of medical evidence have its own limitations in detection in every case of sexual violence. But evidence of treatment is present in every case due to compulsory treatment being provided in every case of sexual violence. Documentation of history of pain post-assault, documentation of tenderness at the same site in examination findings, prescription of analgesics by doctor, proof of consumption of analgesics or prescription slip/pharmacy bill for analgesics will be indirect proof of pain post-assault. Documentation of history of infection post-assault, documentation of infection at the same site in examination findings, prescription of antibiotics by doctor, proof of consumption of antibiotics or prescription slip/pharmacy bill for antibiotics will be indirect proof of infection post-assault. Documentation of history of depression post-assault, documentation of depression in examination findings, prescription of antidepressants by doctor, proof of consumption of antidepressants or prescription slip/pharmacy bill for antidepressants will be indirect proof of depression post-assault. Similarly, counseling notes will also be a proof of psychological disturbances post-assault.

A ready-reckoner to remember which swab to take in which type of sexual violence, the rationale for the same and the limitations is given in **Table 1**.[3]

Medical Opinion

The law expects the doctor to give a reasoned opinion immediately after the medical examination. The doctor can provide medical opinion with regard to any evidence of penetrative or non-penetrative sexual violence; evidence of any mental incapacity to give consent due to the consequence of any disease or consumption of any ethyl alcohol/ narcotic drug/ psychotropic substance; evidence of age which may be important to decide whether the survivor has incapacity to give legal consent for sexual intercourse or whether the age at the time of sexual violence increases the punishment for the accused; any evidence to identify assailant(s).

Opinion on penetrative sexual violence should have details of whether it is vaginal or anal or oral penetration by penis or objects or body parts, whether there are signs of use of any force, whether sexual intercourse is recent or not. Detection of semen and/ or spermatozoa and/or injuries at vagina or anus or oral cavity helps in opining whether it is vaginal or anal or oral sexual intercourse. Presence of injuries and/or lubricant helps in opining penetration by objects or body parts (fingering). Use of force can be opined if there are physical and/or genital injuries. Time since injuries and detection of motile or non-motile spermatozoa helps in timing the sexual violence. Determination of medical age is done as the mean/average of physical age determination, dental age determination and radiological age determination. Medical opinion should be gender sensitive, scientifically correct and ethically and legally correct.

Provisional Medical Opinion Drafting

After the medical examination procedure, the doctor should draft a provisional medical opinion if there are presence of injuries, time since injuries, presence of motile or non-motile spermatozoa on wet smear examination. Care should be taken to document the duration elapsed between the alleged sexual violence and the current medical examination. If the doctor fails to provide a provisional medical opinion the Investigating Officer may get stranded in the criminal investigation and then the benefit of doubt may help the accused in procuring bail from the Courts. Doctors should avoid such defensive practices of not providing provisional opinion wherever it was feasible. Below are the templates of provisional

TABLE 1: Type of swab to be taken based on the type of sexual violence.

History of sexual violence	*Type of Swabs*	*Purpose*	*Any other points to consider?*
Penovaginal	Vaginal	• Semen/sperm detection • Lubricant • DNA	• Whether ejaculation occurred inside vagina or outside • Use of condom
	Body	• Semen/sperm detection • Saliva (in case of sucking/ licking)	If ejaculation occurred outside
Penoanal	Anal	• Semen/sperm detection • Lubricant • DNA • Fecal matter	• Whether ejaculation occurred inside anus or outside • Use of condom
	Body	• Semen/sperm detection • Saliva (in case of sucking/ licking)	If ejaculation occurred outside
Peno-oral	Oral	• Semen/sperm • detection • DNA • Saliva	• Whether ejaculation occurred inside mouth or outside • Use of condom
	Body	• Semen/sperm • detection • Saliva (in case of sucking/ licking)	If ejaculation occurred outside
Use of objects	Swab of the orifice (anal, vaginal, oral)	Lubricant	Detection of lubricant used if any
Use of body parts (Fingering)	Swab of the orifice (anal, vaginal, oral)	Lubricant	Detection of lubricant used if any
Masturbation	Swab of the orifice or body part	• Semen/sperm detection • DNA • Lubricant	• Whether ejaculation occurred or not • If ejaculated in orifice or body parts

Source: Adopted from Guidelines and Protocols from Ministry of Health and Family Welfare, Government of India for Responding to Victims/Survivors of Sexual Violence.[3]

opinion possible in different case scenarios, which would equip the doctor in drafting provisional opinions[3] in actual case scenarios **(Table 2)**.

Final Medical Opinion Drafting

Once all the laboratory reports (from hospital laboratories and forensic science laboratory) of all the tests of swabs, slides, body fluids, body cells /tissues are done, then the doctor is expected to draft the final opinion incorporating all the test reports. Below are the templates of final opinions possible in different case scenarios, which would equip the doctor in drafting final opinions[3] in actual case scenarios **(Table 3)**.

TABLE 2: Templates of provisional opinion possible in different case scenarios.

Genital injuries	*Physical injuries*	*Opinion*	*Rationale why forced penetrative sex cannot be ruled out*	*What FSL can detect?*
Present	Present	There are signs suggestive of recent use of force/forceful penetration of vagina/ anus. Sexual violence cannot be ruled out	Evidence of semen and spermatozoa are yet to be tested by laboratory examinations in case of penile penetration	Evidence of semen except when condom was used
Present	Absent	There are signs suggestive of recent forceful penetration of vagina/anus	Evidence of semen and spermatozoa are yet to be tested by laboratory examinations in case of penile penetration. The lack of physical injuries could be because the survivor, being unconscious, was under the effect of drug/alcohol, overpowered or threatened. It could be because of fingering or penetration by object with use of lubricant which is also an offence under Sec 63 BNS (previously Sec 375 IPC)	Evidence of semen or lubricant except when condom was used
Absent	Present	There are signs of use of force, however vaginal or anal or oral penetration cannot be ruled out	The lack of physical injuries could be because the survivor, being unconscious, was under the effect of drug/ alcohol, overpowered or threatened or use of lubricant	Evidence of semen or lubricant
Absent	Absent	There are no signs of use of force; however, final opinion is reserved pending availability of FSL reports. Sexual violence cannot be ruled out	The lack of genital injuries could be because of the use of lubricants. The lack of physical injuries could be because the survivor, being unconscious, was under the effect of drug/alcohol, overpowered or threatened. It could be because of fingering or penetration by object with use of lubricant which is also an offence under Sec 63 BNS (previously Sec 375 IP C)	Evidence of semen, lubricant and drug/alcohol

Source: Adopted from Guidelines and Protocols from Ministry of Health and Family Welfare, Government of India for Responding to Victims/Survivors of Sexual Violence.[3]

TABLE 3: Templates of final opinion possible in different case scenarios.

S No.	*Genital*	*Physical injuries/ diseases*	*FSL report injuries/diseases*	*Final opinion*
For penile penetration				
1.	Present	Present	Positive for presence of semen	There are signs suggestive of forceful vaginal/anal intercourse
2.	Present	Absent	Positive for presence of semen	There are signs suggestive of forceful vaginal/anal intercourse
3.	Absent	Present	Positive for presence of semen	There are signs suggestive of forceful vaginal/anal intercourse
4.	Absent	Absent	Positive for presence of semen	There are signs suggestive of vaginal/anal intercourse
5.	Absent	Absent	Positive for drugs/alcohol and semen	There are signs suggestive of vaginal/anal intercourse under the influence of drugs/alcohol
For nonpenile penetration				
6.	Present	Present	FSL report is negative for presence of semen/alcohol/ drugs/ lubricant	There are no signs suggestive of vaginal/anal intercourse, but there is evidence of physical and genital assault
7.	Present	Absent	FSL report is negative for presence of semen/alcohol/ drugs/lubricant	There are no signs suggestive of vaginal/anal intercourse, but there is evidence of genital assault
8.	Absent	Present	FSL report is negative for presence of semen/alcohol/ drugs/ lubricant	There are no signs suggestive of vaginal/anal intercourse, but there is evidence of physical assault
9.	Absent	Absent	FSL report is negative for presence of semen/alcohol/ drugs/lubricant	There are no signs suggestive of penetration of vagina/anus
10.	Absent	Absent	FSL report is positive for presence of lubricant only	There is a possibility of vaginal/ anal penetration by lubricated object
Non-penetrative Assault				
S No.	***Findings***			***Final opinion***
11.	Bite marks present and/or FSL detects salivary stains			There are signs suggestive of evidence of bitemark (s) on .... Site (time of injury)
12.	Sucking marks (discoid, subcutaneous extravasation of blood, with or without bitemarks) present and/or FSL detects salivary stains			There are signs suggestive of sucking mark (s) on .... Site (time of injury)

Contd...

Contd...

S No.	Findings	Final opinion
13.	Forceful fondling, with presence of bruises or contusions with or without fingernail marks	There are signs suggestive of forceful physical injuries on .... Site (time of injury) (which may be due to fondling)
14.	Only forceful kissing and FSL detects salivary stains	There are signs suggestive of salivary contact (which may be due to kissing)
15.	If history suggests forced masturbation of the assailant by the survivor and if there is evidence of seminal stains detected on the hands	There are signs suggestive of the survivor in contact with the seminal fluid (which may be due to masturbation)
16.	In case there are no signs of sucking, licking...... detected but history suggests some such form of assault	*It is still important to document a good history because the survivor may have had a bath or washed him/herself*

Source: Adopted from Guidelines and Protocols from Ministry of Health and Family Welfare, Government of India for Responding to Victims/Survivors of Sexual Violence.[3]

Chain of Custody

The evidence collected and documentation done on sexual violence should be under lock and key secured and handed over to police. Handing over of custody from doctor to medical records department or to police must be duly documented by way of writing the name, police constable number, police station, contact phone number and signatures in writing. Any breach in this process may lead to questioning of tampering of chain of custody in judicial proceedings.

Follow-up

The follow-up medical examination is warranted for examination of deep-seated injuries (deep bruises), sexually transmitted infections, compliance of counseling sessions. It should also be documented. A proper explanation of the need for follows-up examination which is in the interest of the survivor's health status, would help the survivor in following the doctor's advice of complying for follow-up medical examination.

Treatment

The doctor should treat physical injuries, treat sexually transmitted infections including HIV, assess risk of pregnancy and advise either continuation of pregnancy or emergency contraception or medical termination of pregnancy, psychological counseling, advise about drug deaddiction program, disability assessment and management. Proper prescription and advice on medical procedures to be explained along with proper documentation of the same.

Psychosocial Care

Psychosocial care is a must in every case of survivors of sexual violence. No doctor should lose the opportunity in providing the same. Every first responding doctor can provide psychological first aid. Not all cases of survivors need professional counselor support. Assessment should be made of very severe psychological disturbances in the survivor and referred to professional counselor for counseling.

Psychological first aid being provided to survivor of sexual violence by first responding doctor[3] has the following steps: Creating an enabling atmosphere and establishing trust; Facilitation and demystification of medical procedures; Addressing survivor's emotional wellbeing; Safety assessment; and positive supportive role of family, friends and community.

Documentation

All the medical examination procedure carried out, treatment advised and provided has to be documented in writing (computerized e-records are also acceptable if facilities exist). Injuries are better documented in writing in words or on pictograms. Photographs and videographs of injuries cannot be done unless survivor has given informed consent. The number of pages in the survivor medical examination report should be serially numbered along with the signature of the doctor on every page. A copy of the survivor's medical examination report is to be handed over to the survivor free of cost immediately after the completion of the medical examination. Multiple number of copies (four) of medical examination report to be made to hand over one each to police, survivor, forensic science laboratory and hospital copy. A detailed format to be used as medicolegal examination report of sexual violence has been provided below in **Performa 1**.

PREVENTION

The government's ambitious project of one-stop centers or Nirbhaya centers/Sakhi centers/Gelathi centers are supposed to address the medical management issues including counseling at one-stop/place and in addition providing legal aid, documentation, shelter and also addressing rehabilitation concerns.[4]

Awareness about legal changes in investigation and adjudication of sexual offences, advocacy of programs like Childline number 1098, Women help line; safety gadgets—mobile phone emergency button, pepper sprays; Cyber-crimes and Cyber/Online safety protocols; Women police station, Special juvenile police units, PCR vans/Mobile police patrols; Safety and life skill sessions in schools; mandatory awareness of POCSO Act provisions; Adolescent health programs covering sexual hygiene—secondary sexual characteristics, menstruation, contraception, pregnancy, sexually transmitted infections; Internal Complaints Committee; or POSH committees to address sexual harassment at workplace are the need of the hour.

Gender sensitive practices[5-7] to overcome gender discriminative issues like sex selection, female fetus abortions, child abuse, child sexual abuse, child labor, girlchild illiteracy, child marriage, malnutrition, eve-teasing, dowry harassment, domestic violence and intimate partner abuse, gender-based violence, sexual harassment at workplace, pornography, prostitution— should become priority and every stakeholder should contribute seriously to prevent this menace of sexual violence.

LEGAL PROVISIONS

The initial major changes in law were in eighties of last century post the Mathura Rape case. Post 2012 and 2013, we have lot of legal changes in terms of sexual offences, the definitions being rewritten, procedures

Performa 1: Medicolegal examination report of sexual violence.

1. Name of the Hospital ....OPD No. ....Inpatient No. ....
2. Name .... D/o or S/o (where known)..
3. Address...
4. Age (as reported)... Date of Birth (if known)..
5. Sex (M/F/Others)..
6. Date and Time of arrival in the hospital ....
7. Date and Time of commencement of examination..
8. Brought by..(Name & signatures)
9. MLC No. ....Police Station..
10. Whether conscious, oriented in time and place and person...
11. Any physical/intellectual/psychosocial disability...
(Interpreters or special educators will be needed where the survivor has special needs such as hearing/speech disability, language barriers, intellectual or psychosocial disability.)
12. Informed Consent/refusal

I..D/o or S/o...
hereby give my consent for:

a. medical examination for treatment	Yes ()	No ()
b. this medicolegal examination	Yes ()	No ()
c. sample collection for clinical & forensic examination	Yes ()	No ()

I also understand that as per law the hospital is required to inform police, and this has been explained to me.

I want the information to be revealed to the police	Yes ()	No ()

I have understood the purpose and the procedure of the examination including the risk and benefit, explained to me by the examining doctor. My right to refuse the examination at any stage and the consequence of such refusal, including that my medical treatment will not be affected by my refusal, has also been explained and may be recorded. Contents of the above have been explained to me in .... language with the help of a special educator/ interpreter/support person (circle as appropriate).. ....

If special educator/interpreter/support person has helped, then his/her name and signature...................................

Name & signature of survivor or parent/Guardian/person in whom the child reposes trust in case of child (<12 yrs)

....

....

With Date, Time & Place

Name & signature/thumb impression of Witness

....

....

With Date, Time and Place

13. Marks of identification (Any scar/mole)
1. ....
2. ....

Left Thumb impression

14. Relevant medical/surgical history

Onset of menarche (in case of girls) Yes ( ) No ( ) Age of onset...............

Menstrual history–Cycle length and duration...............Last menstrual period...............

Menstruation at the time of incident—Yes/ No, Menstruation at the time of examination—Yes/ No

Was the survivor pregnant at time of incident—Yes/No, If yes duration of pregnancy .... weeks

Contraception use: Yes/No............ e If yes—method used: ....

Vaccination status—Tetanus (vaccinated/not vaccinated), Hepatitis B (vaccinated/not vaccinated)

15A. History of sexual violence

(i) Date of incident/s being reported (ii) Time of incident(s) (iii) Location(s)

(iv) Estimated duration: 1–7 days............ 1 week to 2 months............ 2–6 months............ >6 months............Episode: One............ Multiple ....Chronic (>6 months)............ Unknown............

(v)Number of Assailant(s) and name(s)...............
(vi) Sex of assailant(s)............... Approx. Age of assailant (s)...............If known to the survivor—relationship with the survivor............... ....

(vii) Description of incident in the words of the narrator:
Narrator of the incident: Survivor/informant (specify name and relation to survivor)
....

If this space is insufficient use extra page

15B. Type of physical violence used if any (Describe):

Hit with (Hand, fist, blunt object, sharp object)
Biting
Pinching
Violent shaking
Dragging
Any other:

Burned with
Kicking
Pulling Hair
Banging head

15C.

i. Emotional abuse or violence if any (insulting, cursing, belittling, terrorizing)...............
ii. Use of restraints if any ....
iii. Used or threatened the use of weapon(s) or objects if any...............
iv. Verbal threats (for example, threats of killing or hurting survivor or any other person in whom the survivor is interested; use of photographs for blackmailing, etc.) if any: ....
v. Luring (sweets, chocolates, money, job) if any: ....
vi. Any other:...............

15D.

i. Any H/O drug/alcohol intoxication:
ii. Whether sleeping or unconscious at the time of the incident: ....

15E. If survivor has left any marks of injury on assailant(s), enter details: ....

15F. Details regarding sexual violence:
Was penetration by penis, fingers or object or other body parts (Write Y = Yes, N = No, DNK = Don't know)

Mention and describe body part/s and/or object/s used for penetration.

	Penetration			***Emission of semen***		
Orifice of victim	By Penis	By body part of self or assailant or third party (finger, tongue or any other)	By Object	Yes	No	Don't know
Genitalia (Vagina and/or urethra)						
Anus						
Mouth						

Oral sex performed by assailant on survivor	Y	N	DNK
Forced masturbation of self by survivor	Y	N	DNK
Masturbation of assailant by survivor	Y	N	DNK
Forced manipulation of genitals of assailant	Y	N	DNK
Did ejaculation occur outside body orifice (vagina/anus/ mouth/urethra)? If yes, describe where on the body	Y	N	DNK
Kissing, licking or sucking any part of survivor's body	Y	N	If Yes, describe
Touching/Fondling	Y	N	If Yes, describe
Condom used*	Y	N	DNK
If yes status of condom	Y	N	DNK
Lubricant used*	Y	N	DNK
If yes, describe kind of lubricant used			
If object used, describe object:			
Any other forms of sexual violence			

*Explain what condom and lubricant are to the survivor:

Post incident has the survivor	***Yes/No/Do not know***	***Remarks***
• Changed clothes • Changed undergarments • Cleaned/washed clothes • Cleaned/washed undergarments • Bathed • Douched • Passed urine • Passed stools • Rinsing of mouth/Brushing/ Vomiting • (Circle any or all as appropriate)		

Time since incident: ....
H/o vaginal/anal/oral bleeding/discharge prior to the incident of sexual violence ....
H/ovaginal/anal/oralbleeding/dischargesincetheincidentofsexualviolence..
H/o painful urination/painful defecation/fissures/abdominal pain/pain in genitals or any other part since the incident of sexual violence

16. General Physical Examination
    i. Is this the first examination ....
    ii. Pulse .... BP...
    iii. Temp .... Resp. Rate ....
    iv. Pupils ....
    v. Any observation in terms of general physical wellbeing of the survivor ....

17. Examination for injuries on the body if any
The pattern of injuries sustained during an incident of sexual violence may show considerable variation. This may range from complete absence of injuries (more frequently) to grievous injuries (very rare).
(Look for bruises, physical torture injuries, nail abrasions, teeth bite marks, cuts, lacerations, fracture, tenderness, any other injury, boils, lesions, discharge specially on the scalp, face, neck, shoulders, breast, wrists, forearms, medial aspect of upper arms, thighs and buttocks) Note the Injury type, site, size, shape, color, swelling signs of healing simple/grievous, dimensions)

Scalp examination for areas of tenderness (if hair pulled out/dragged by hair)	
Facial bone injury: Orbital blackening, tenderness	
Petechial hemorrhage in eyes and other places	
Lips and Buccal Mucosa/Gums	
Behind the ears	
Eardrum	
Neck, Shoulders and Breast	
Upper Limb	
Inner aspect of upper arms	
Inner aspect of thighs	
Lower Limb Buttocks	
Other, please specify	

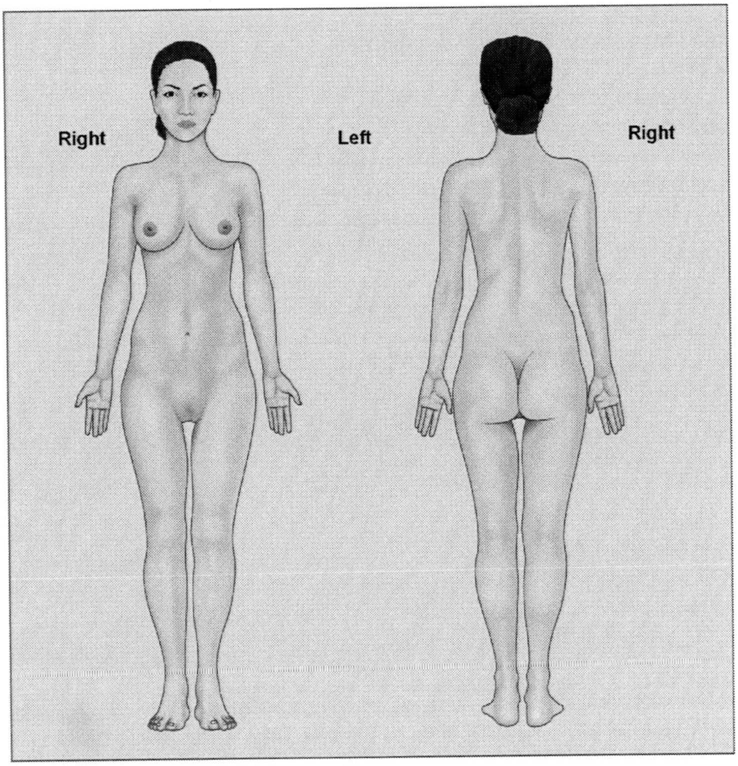

18. Local examination of genital parts/other orifices*:
   A. *External Genitalia: Record findings and state NA where not applicable.*

Body parts to be examined	***Findings***
Urethral meatus and vestibule	
Labia majora	
Labia minora	
Fourchette and Introitus	
Hymen Perineum	
External Urethral Meatus	
Penis	
Scrotum	
Testes	
Clitoro-penis	
Labio-scrotum	
Any Other	

*Per vaginum/Per speculum examination should not be done unless required for detection of injuries or for medical treatment.

   B. P/S findings if performed ....
   P/V findings if performed ....
   Record reasons if P/V of P/S examination performed ....

C. Anus and rectum (encircle the relevant)
Bleeding/tear/discharge/edema/tenderness

D. Oral Cavity (encircle the relevant)
Bleeding/discharge/ tear/edema/tenderness

19. Systemic examination:
Central Nervous System: ....
Cardiovascular System: ....
Respiratory System: ....
Chest: ....
Abdomen: ....

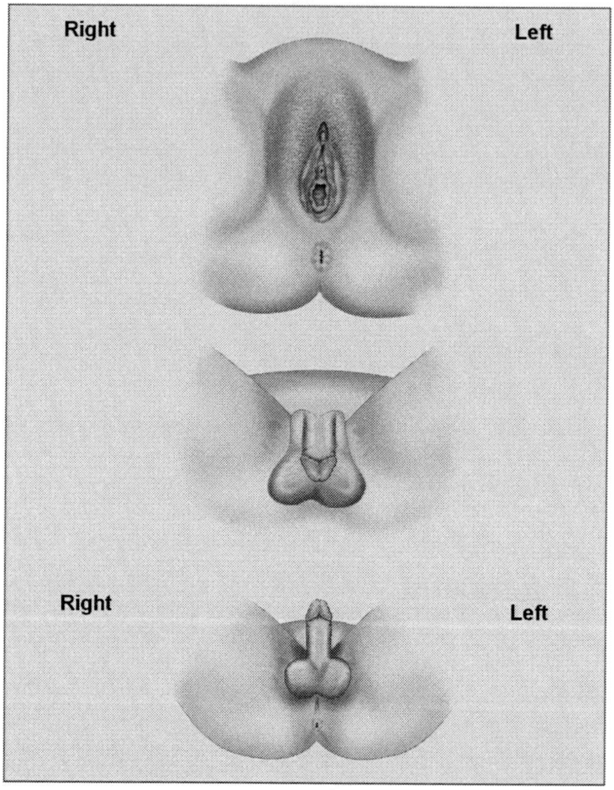

20. Sample collection/investigations for hospital laboratory/clinical laboratory:
    1. Blood for HIV, VDRL, HbsAg
    2. Urine test for pregnancy
    3. Ultrasound for pregnancy/internal injury
    4. X-ray for injury
21. Samples collection for central/state forensic science laboratory:
    1. Debris collection paper
    2. Clothing evidence where available (to be packed in separate paper bags after air drying)

List and details of clothing worn by the survivor at time of incident of sexual violence

3. Body evidence samples as appropriate (duly labeled and packed separately):

	Collected/Not collected	***Reason for not collecting***
Swabs from stains on the body (blood, semen, foreign material, others)		
Scalp hair (10–15 strands)		
Head hair combing		
Nail scrapings (both hands separately)		
Nail clippings (both hands separately)		
Oral swab		
Blood for grouping, testing		

4. Genital and anal evidence (Each sample to be packed, sealed, and labelled separately—to be placed in a bag)

*Swab sticks for collecting samples should be moistened with distilled water provided.

	Collected/not collected	***Reason for not collecting***
Matted pubic hair		
Pubic hair combing (mention if shaved)		
Cutting of pubic hair (mention if shaved)		
Two vulval swabs (for semen examination and DNA testing)		
Two vaginal swabs (for semen examination and DNA testing)		
Two Anal swabs (for semen examination and DNA testing)		
Vaginal smear (air-dried) for semen examination		
Vaginal washing		
Urethral swab		
Swab from glans of		

*Samples to be preserved as directed till handed over to police along with duly attested sample seal.

22. Provisional medical opinion:
I have examined (name of survivor)..............M/F/Other..................aged......................... reporting (type of sexual violence and circumstances) ...., XYZ days/hours after the incident, after having (bathed/douched, etc.)...................... My findings are as follows:
- Samples collected (for FSL), awaiting reports
- Samples collected (for hospital laboratory)
- Clinical findings
- Additional observations (if any)

23. Treatment prescribed:

Treatment	*Yes*	*No*	*Type and comments*
STI prevention treatment			
Emergency contraception			
Wound treatment			
Tetanus prophylaxis			
Hepatitis B vaccination			
Post-exposure prophylaxis for HIV			
Counseling			
Other			

24. Date and time of completion of examination: ....
This report contains .... number of sheets and .... number of envelopes.

Signature of Examining Doctor

Name of Examining Doctor

Place: ....

Seal

25. Final Opinion (After receiving Lab reports):
Findings in support of the above opinion, taking into account the history, clinical examination findings and laboratory reports of .... bearing identification marks described above, ... hours/days after the incident of sexual violence, I am of the opinion that:

Signature of Examining Doctor

Name of Examining Doctor

Place: ....

Seal

COPY OF THE ENTIRE MEDICAL REPORT MUST BE GIVEN TO THE SURVIVOR/VICTIM FREE OF COST IMMEDIATELY.

of investigation, medical examination, adjudication all have significantly changed. Below is write-up of sections of law which are of concern to victims/survivors, accused of sexual violence, doctors and other stakeholders dealing with these cases of sexual violence. Some of the sections of *Bharatiya Nayaya Sanhita (BNS)*—previously *Indian Penal Code (IPC)*, Protection of Children from Sexual Offences Act, Amendment Act 2019 (POCSO), *Bharatiya Nagarik Suraksha Sanhita (BNSS)*—previously *Criminal Procedure Code (CrPC)* and *Bharatiya Sakshya Adhiniyam*—previously *Indian Evidence Act (IEA)* are briefly written here.[2,8-10]

Sec 63 BNS (Previously 375 IPC)

Rape

A man is said to commit "rape" if he.................. (a) penetrates his penis, to any extent, into the vagina, mouth, urethra or anus of a woman or makes her to do so with him or any other person; or (b) inserts, to any extent, any object or a part of the body, not being the penis, into the vagina, the urethra or anus of a woman or makes her to do so with him or any other person; or (c) manipulates any part of the body of a woman so as to cause penetration into the vagina, urethra, anus or any part of body of such woman or makes her to do so with him or any other person; or (d) applies his mouth to the vagina, anus, urethra of a woman or makes her to do so with him or any other person, under the circumstances falling under any of the following seven descriptions:[1]

1. Against her will.
2. Without her consent.
3. With her consent, when her consent has been obtained by putting her or any person in whom she is interested, in fear of death or of hurt.
4. With her consent, when the man knows that he is not her husband and that her consent is given because she believes that he is another man to whom she is or believes herself to be lawfully married.
5. With her consent when, at the time of giving such consent, by reason of unsoundness of mind or intoxication or the administration by him personally or through another of any stupefying or unwholesome substance, she is unable to understand the nature and consequences of that to which she gives consent.
6. With or without her consent, when she is under eighteen years of age.
7. When she is unable to communicate consent.

Explanations:

1. For the purposes of this section, "vagina" shall also include labia majora.
2. Consent means an unequivocal voluntary agreement when the woman by words, gestures or any form of verbal or non-verbal communication, communicates willingness to participate in the specific sexual Act;
3. Provided that a woman who does not physically resist to the Act of penetration shall not by the reason only of that fact, be regarded as consenting to the sexual activity.

Exceptions:

1. A medical procedure or intervention shall not constitute rape.
2. Sexual intercourse or sexual acts by a man with his own wife, the wife not being under eighteen* years of age, is not rape. (**earlier provision of fifteen years is stuck down by the Supreme Court in 2017 in the case of Independent Thought vs. Union of India*) According to Section 64 BNS *previously* Sec 376 IPC, minimum punishment is 10 years of imprisonment to life imprisonment; if victim is less than 16 years of age, then minimum punishment is 20 years to life imprisonment and fine to cover medical expenses paid to victim *[Sec 65(1) BNS]*; if survivor is less than 12 years of age, then minimum punishment is 20 years to life imprisonment or Death penalty and fine to cover medical expenses paid to victim *[Sec 65(2) BNS]*.

Sec 397 BNSS (Previously 357C CrPC)

Treatment of Victims

All hospitals, public or private, whether run by the Central Government, the State Government, local bodies or any other person, shall immediately, provide the first-aid or medical treatment, free of cost, to the victims of any offence covered U/S 124.1 BNS (*previously* 326A IPC), *Sec 64 BNS* (*previously* 376 IPC), *Sec 66 BNS* (*previously* 376A IPC, *Sec 65.2 BNS* (*previously* 376 AB IPC), *Sec 67 BNS* (*previously* 376B IPC), *Sec 68 BNS* (*previously* 376C), *Sec 70.1 BNS* (*previously*

376D IPC), *Sec 70.2 BNS* (*previously* 376DA IPC), *Sec 70.2 BNS* (*previously* 376DB IPC) or *Sec 71 BNS* (*previously* Sec 376E IPC), and shall immediately inform the police of such incident.

Sec 200 BNS (Previously 166B IPC)

Punishment for Nontreatment of Victim

Whoever, being In-charge of a hospital, public or private, whether run by the Central Government, the State Government, local bodies or any other person, contravenes the provisions of *Sec 397 BNSS* (previously 357C CrPC) shall be punished with imprisonment for a term which may extend to one year or with fine or with both.

Sec 3 POCSO Act 2012 (Amendment) Act, 2019

Penetrative Sexual Assault

A person is said to commit "penetrative sexual assault" if—

a. he penetrates his penis, to any extent, into the vagina, mouth, urethra or anus of a child or makes the child to do so with him or any other person; or
b. he inserts, to any extent, any object or a part of the body, not being the penis, into the vagina, the urethra or anus of the child or makes the child to do so with him or any other person; or
c. he manipulates any part of the body of the child so as to cause penetration into the vagina, urethra, anus or any part of the body of the child or makes the child to-do so with him or any other person; or
d. he applies his mouth to the penis, vagina, anus, urethra of the child or makes the child to do so to such person or any other person.

As per *Sec 4 POCSO Act*, the punishment is 10 years imprisonment and fine to cover medical expenses paid to victim. If the child is less than 16 years, then the punishment is 20 years imprisonment to life imprisonment and fine to cover medical expenses paid to victim.

Sec 5 POCSO Act 2012 (Amendment) Act, 2019

Aggravated Penetrative Sexual Assault

Whoever being a Police officer, Public servant, member of Armed forces, management of Jail, remand home, protection home, observation home, custody home, Care and protection home, Hospital, educational/religious institute commits penetrative sexual assault on a child or commits Gang penetrative sexual assault, commits penetrative sexual assault using deadly weapons or causes grievous hurt, or during communal riots or natural calamity, or commits penetrative sexual assault on a pregnant child or on a child less than 12 years of age, or is suffering from HIV or physical or mental disability, or repeats with same child, commits penetrative sexual assault by stripping naked in public the child or makes the female child pregnant would have caused *aggravated penetrative sexual assault.*

As per *Sec 6 POCSO Act*, the punishment is 20 years imprisonment to life imprisonment and fine to cover medical expenses paid to victim.

Sec 7 POCSO Act 2012 (Amendment) Act, 2019

Sexual Assault

Whoever, with sexual intent touches the vagina, penis, anus or breast of the child or makes the child touch the vagina, penis, anus or breast of such person or any other person or does any other act with sexual intent which involves physical contact without penetration is said to commit sexual assault.

As per Sec 8 POCSO Act, the punishment is 3–5 years of imprisonment and fine.

Sec 9 POCSO Act 2012 (Amendment) Act, 2019

Aggravated Sexual Assault

Whoever being a police officer, public servant, member of armed forces, management of Jail, remand home, protection home, observation home, custody home, care and protection home, hospital, educational/religious institute commits sexual assault on a child or commits gang sexual assault, commits sexual assault using deadly weapons or causes grievous hurt, or during communal riots or natural calamity, or commits sexual assault on a pregnant child or on a child less than 12 years of age, or is suffering from HIV or physical or mental disability, or repeats with same child, commits sexual assault by stripping naked in public the child or makes the female child pregnant would have caused aggravated sexual assault.

(v) whoever persuades, induces, entices or coerces a child to get administered or administer or direct anyone to administer, help in getting administered any drug or hormone or any chemical substance, to a child with the intent that such child attains early sexual maturity *(New clause under POCSO Amendment Act, 2019).*

As per Sec 10 POCSO Act, the punishment is 5–7 years of imprisonment and fine.

For section 14 of the Principal Act, the following section shall be substituted, namely: "14. (1) Whoever uses a child or children for pornographic purposes shall be punished with imprisonment for a term which shall not be less than five years and shall also be liable to fine, and in the event of second or subsequent conviction with imprisonment for a term which shall not be less than seven years and also be liable to fine; (2) Whoever using a child or children for pornographic purposes under sub-section (1), commits an offence referred to in section 3 or section 5 or section 7 or section 9 by directly participating in such pornographic acts, shall be punished for the said offences also under section 4, section 6, section 8 and section 10, respectively, in addition to the punishment provided in sub-section (1)."

For section 15 of the Principal Act, the following section shall be substituted, namely: "15. (1) Any person, who stores or possesses pornographic material in any form involving a child, but fails to delete or destroy or report the same to the designated authority, as may be prescribed, with an intention to share or transmit child pornography, shall be liable to fine not less than five thousand rupees, and in the event of second or subsequent offence, with fine which shall not be less than ten thousand rupees; (2) Any person, who stores or possesses pornographic material in any form involving a child for transmitting or propagating or displaying or distributing in any manner at any time except for the purpose of reporting, as may be prescribed, or for use as evidence in court, shall be punished with imprisonment of either description which may extend to three years, or with fine, or with both; (3) Any person, who stores or possesses pornographic material in any form involving a child for commercial purpose shall be punished on the first conviction with imprisonment of either description which shall not be less than three years which may extend to five years, or with fine, or with both, and in the event of second or subsequent conviction, with imprisonment of either description which shall not be less than five years which may extend to seven years and shall also be liable to fine."

Sec 19 POCSO Act 2012 (Amendment) Act, 2019

Reporting of Offences

1. Notwithstanding anything contained in the CrPC, any person (including the child), who has apprehension that an offence under this Act is likely to be committed or has knowledge that such an offence has been committed, he shall provide such information to—(a) the Special Juvenile Police Unit, or (b) the local police.
2. Every report given under sub-section (1) shall be—(a) ascribed an entry number and recorded in writing; (b) be read over to the informant; (c) shall be entered in a book to be kept by the Police Unit.
3. Where the report under sub-section (1) is given by a child, the same shall be recorded under sub-section (2) in a simple language so that the child understands contents being recorded.
4. In case contents are being recorded in the language not understood by the child or wherever it is deemed necessary, a translator or an interpreter, having such qualifications, experience and on payment of such fees as may be prescribed, shall be provided to the child if he fails to understand the same.
5. Where the Special Juvenile Police Unit or local police is satisfied that the child against whom an offence has been committed is in need of care and protection, then, it shall, after recording the reasons in writing, make immediate arrangement to give him such care and protection (including admitting the child into shelter home or to the nearest hospital) within twenty-four hours of the report, as may be prescribed.
6. The Special Juvenile Police Unit or local police shall, without unnecessary delay but within a period of twenty-four hours, report the matter to the Child Welfare Committee and the Special Court or where no Special Court has been designated, to the Court of Session, including need of the child for care and protection and steps taken in this regard.
7. No person shall incur any liability, whether civil or criminal, for giving the information in good faith for the purpose of sub-section (1),

Sec 21 POCSO Act 2012 (Amendment) Act, 2019

Punishment for Failure to Report or Record a Case

1. Any person, who fails to report the commission of an offence under sub-section (1) of section 19 or section 20 or who fails to record such offence under sub-section (2) of section 19 shall be punished with imprisonment of either description which may extend to six months or with fine or with both.
2. Any person, being in-charge of any company or an institution (by whatever name called) who fails to report the commission of an offence under sub-section (1) of section 19 in respect of a subordinate under his control, shall be punished with imprisonment for a term which may extend to one year and with fine.
3. The revisions of sub-section (1) shall not apply to a child under this Act.

Sec 184 BNSS (Previously 164 A CrPC)

Medical Examination of the Victim of Rape

1. Where, during the stage when an offence of committing rape or attempt to commit rape is under investigation, it is proposed

to get the person of the woman with whom rape is alleged or attempted to have been committed or attempted, examined by a medical expert, such examination shall be conducted by a registered medical practitioner employed in a hospital run by the Government or a local authority and in the absence of such a practitioner, by any other registered medical practitioner, with the consent of such woman or of a person competent to give such consent on her behalf and such woman shall be sent to such registered medical practitioner within twenty-four hours from the time of receiving the information relating to the commission of such offence.

2. The registered medical practitioner, to whom such woman is sent shall, without delay, examine her person and prepare a report of his examination giving the following particulars, namely—
   i. the name and address of the woman and of the person by whom she was brought;
   ii. the age of the woman;
   iii. the description of material taken from the person of the woman for DNA profiling;
   iv. marks of injury, if any, on the person of the woman;
   v. general mental condition of the woman; and
   vi. other material particulars in reasonable detail.
3. The report shall state precisely the reasons for each conclusion arrived at.
4. The report shall specifically record that the consent of the woman or of the person competent, to give such consent on her behalf to such examination had been obtained.
5. The exact time of commencement and completion of the examination shall also be noted in the report.
6. The registered medical practitioner shall, *within a period of seven days* forward the report to the investigating officer who shall forward it to the Magistrate referred to in *Section (193)* as part of the documents referred to in clause (a) of *Sub-Section (6)* of that section.
7. Nothing in this section shall be construed as rendering lawful any examination without the consent of the woman or of any person competent to give such consent on her behalf.

Sec 27 POCSO Act 2012 (Amendment) Act, 2019

Medical Examination of a Child

(1) The medical examination of a child in respect of whom any offence has been committed under this Act, shall, notwithstanding that a First Information Report (FIR) or complaint has not been registered for the offences under this Act, be conducted in accordance with *Section S 184 BNSS* (previously 164A CrPC); (2) In case the victim is a girl child, the medical examination shall be conducted by a woman doctor; (3) The medical examination shall be conducted in the presence of the parent of the child or any other person in whom the child reposes trust or confidence; (4) Where, in case the parent of the child or other person referred to in subsection (3) cannot be present, for any reason, during the medical examination of the child. The medical examination shall be conducted in the presence of a woman nominated by the head of the medical institution.

Rule 6 POCSO Rules 2020

Medical Aid and Care

1. Where an officer of the SJPU, or the local police receives information under section 19 of the Act that an offence under the Act has been committed, and is satisfied

that the child against whom an offence has been committed is in need of urgent medical care and protection, such officer, or as the case may be, the local police shall, within 24 hours of receiving such information, arrange to take such child to the nearest hospital or medical care facility center for emergency medical care: Provided that where an offence has been committed under Sections 3, 5, 7 or 9 of the Act, the victim shall be referred to emergency medical care.

2. Emergency medical care shall be rendered in such a manner as to protect the privacy of the child, and in the presence of the parent or guardian or any other person in whom the child has trust and confidence.
3. No medical practitioner, hospital or other medical facility center rendering emergency medical care to a child shall demand any legal or magisterial requisition or other documentation as a pre-requisite to rendering such care.
4. The registered medical practitioner rendering medical care shall attend to the needs of the child, including: (a) treatment for cuts, bruises, and other injuries including genital injuries, if any; (b) treatment for exposure to sexually transmitted diseases (STDs) including prophylaxis for identified STDs; (c) treatment for exposure to human immunodeficiency virus (HIV), including prophylaxis for HIV after necessary consultation with infectious disease experts; (d) possible pregnancy and emergency contraceptives should be discussed with the pubertal child and her parent or any other person in whom the child has trust and confidence; and, (e) wherever necessary, a referral or consultation for mental or psychological health needs, or other counselling, or drug de-addiction services and programs should be made.
5. The registered medical practitioner shall submit the report on the condition of the child within 24 hours to the SJPU or Local Police.
6. Any forensic evidence collected in the course of rendering emergency medical care must be collected in accordance with Section 27 of the Act.
7. If the child is found to be pregnant, then the registered medical practitioner shall counsel the child, and her parents or guardians, or support person, regarding the various lawful options available to the child as per the Medical Termination of Pregnancy Act 1971 *(now Amendment Act, 2021)* and the Juvenile Justice (Care and Protection of Children) Act 2015.
8. If the child is found to have been administered any drugs or other intoxicating substances, access to drug deaddiction program shall be ensured.
9. If the child is a *divyang* (person with disability), suitable measure and care shall be taken as per the provisions of the Rights of Persons with Disabilities Act, 2016.

Sec 39 (1) BSA (Sec 45 IEA)

Opinion of Experts

When the Court has to form an opinion upon a point of foreign law or of science or art, or as to identity of handwritingor finger impressions, the opinions upon that point of persons especially skilled in such foreign law, science or art,or in questions as to identity of handwriting or finger impressions are relevant facts. Such persons are called experts.

CASE LAWS

Lillu@ Rajesh and Anr vs. State of Haryana

In this case, the Supreme Court of India has banned the use of two-finger test. The two-finger test and its interpretation violate the right of rape survivors to privacy, physical and mental integrity and dignity.[11]

The two-finger test was a procedural interpretation, if when two fingers can be passed into a woman's vaginal introitus with ease, then she is used to sexual intercourse; and when one finger cannot be passed even with difficulty into woman's vaginal introitus, then she is not used to sexual intercourse. This two-finger test has moved from one textbook to another without any cross-checking for any scientific research evidence and is totally a subjective-biased evidence as two finger sizes are not uniform. It perpetuates-biased approach on the chastity of a woman. The Ministry of Health and Family Welfare, Government of India does not approve of such procedure and has removed it in its proforma.[3]

Independent Thought vs. Union of India

In this case, the Supreme Court of India held all sexual activity with a child less than 18 years whether married or not will be a criminal offence. It stuck down the inconsistency between the POCSO Act and the IPC. The Court held as per section 42A POCSO Act, whenever there is an inconsistency of the provisions of POCSO Act and any other law, then POCSO Act will have an overriding effect with regard to inconsistency. POCSO Act being a special law and dealing with children will override the general law. Hence the exception 2 of Section 375 IPC exempting wife above 15 years from using the provisions of POCSO Act is stuck down and now the section 375 IPC, exception 2 reads as—"Sexual intercourse or sexual acts by a man with his own wife, the wife not being 18 years, is not rape", and this judgment will have prospective effect.[12]

This judgment has far-reaching effects with child marriages still prevalent in India and in such situations, it calls for mandatory reporting of all sexual activity between husband and the minor wife as a POCSO Act offence, wherein there may be no complaint from minor wife or her parents and they may even oppose the doctor and hospital reporting the offence under mandatory reporting to the police.

SUPREME COURT JUDGMENT ON ABORTIONS CONDUCTED BEYOND THE PROVISIONS OF MTP ACT IN SEXUAL VIOLENCE CASES

There were several instances across the country of child mothers who were in advanced stages of pregnancy due to sexual violence on them. The Supreme Court held in a 10-year-old child who was carrying a 32-week gestational age fetus that abortion cannot be permitted. This decision was taken after the medical board ruled that abortion if conducted would be detrimental to child mother, as she was in advanced stage of pregnancy. The Supreme Court also directed all States to form Medical Boards in each district so that they can advise the High Courts to take decisions in cases of pregnancy beyond twenty weeks of gestational age.[13,14]

As a result of this Supreme Court judgment, in a situation of pregnancy of women and girls due to sexual violence, beyond the twenty weeks of gestation, where MTP cannot be done as per provisions of MTP Act, 1971, they can approach the jurisdictional High Court. This is possible with several pro-bon lawyers working on this cause in each High Court. Then the High Court would give an emergency hearing and refer the matter to the medical board. And on the advice of the medical board the High Court would take a final decision whether to terminate or continue the pregnancy. The medical board has to take decision considering scientific evidence, ethical considerations, legal issues on case-to-case basis.

Key Learning Points

Here are the essential issues in the must-know area of a doctor dealing with both children and adult victims of sexual violence.[3,5-7,15]

- Every case of rape/sexual assault is a medical emergency.
- Child sexual abuse has lifelong consequences on the physical and mental health of the child. The impact of the abuse will depend on the duration and frequency of the exposure to abuse, the age of the child and the support network available.
- No medical facility, public or private, can deny emergency medical care and medical examination to a victim of suspected rape/sexual assault (Section 357C CrPC *now 397 BNSS*).
- Treatment has to be provided free of cost by the government as well as private medical facilities.
- Not providing free emergency medical care or medical examination to a victim who has been or is suspected of having been sexually violated can result in imprisonment for one year or fine or both for the doctor (Section 166B IPC *now 200 BNS*).
- Not reporting a case of sexual assault or suspected sexual assault of a child can result in imprisonment of six months, or fine or both for the doctor (Section 19 POCSO Act). The report has to be made to the nearest police station or Special Juvenile Police Unit.
- Medical examination of a child with sexual assault must be conducted in the presence of the parent or guardian of the child or some other person in whom the child has trust and confidence. If there is no such person available, the head of the medical institution must nominate a woman to be present during the examination (Section 27 POCSO Act).
- Medical examination of a victim with sexual assault must be conducted, in the case of a female child, by a female doctor.
- FIR or permission from a magistrate, police or any other authority cannot be demanded by any medical facility or center for providing emergency medical care to a victim who has been or who may have been sexually violated (Sec 357C CrPC *now 397 BNSS*, Sec 27 POCSO Act).
- In a case of rape/sexual assault, informed consent must be taken from the child above 12 years of age, or, where the child is below 12 years of age, the child's parent/guardian, before medically examining the child. In case consent is not given, informed refusal must be documented by the doctor.
- Lack of medical evidence does not mean no sexual offence was committed. Evidence may have been lost due to healing of older injuries, use of condom by the offender, and post-assault activities such as washing, douching, urination, and defecation.
- Doctors must protect children from rape/sexual assault and its consequences. They should teach parents about safe, unsafe, and uncomfortable touch and how to keep their children safe.
- Doctors must teach children how to protect themselves from rape/sexual assault.
- Doctors must provide appropriate care and treatment to the survivor of rape/sexual assault.
- Doctors should give social, psychological and legal guidance to the rape/sexual assault survivor and the family.
- In a case of rape/sexual assault doctors should help the process of justice delivery by conducting accurate and complete forensic medical examination and be willing to testify in court.
- Forensic examination needs to be conducted within 96 hours and requires evidence collection such as blood, semen, sperm, hair, etc. linking to perpetrator.
- With timely medical care and mental health support, a victim of sexual violence can resume a normal and healthy life.
- Doctors should prominently display the Childline number (1098) in their clinics and hospitals. Any case of known or suspected child abuse or neglect can be reported to this number.
- It is the duty of the doctor to prevent the occurrence of child sexual abuse by teaching parents how to talk to their children about safe, unsafe and uncomfortable touch, and teaching children about personal safety.

NATIONAL GUIDELINES

The excerpts of the Guidelines and Protocols from Ministry of Health and Family Welfare, Government of India for responding to victims/survivors of sexual violence for comprehensive care are as follows:[3]

(*Source:* Adopted from Guidelines and Protocols from Ministry of Health and Family Welfare, Government of India for Responding to Victims/Survivors of Sexual Violence[3])

1. *Informed consent:* Doctors shall inform the person being examined about the nature and purpose of examination and in case of child to the child's parent/guardian/person in whom the child reposes trust. This information should include:
   a. The medicolegal examination is to assist the investigation, arrest and prosecution of those who committed sexual offences. This may involve an examination of the mouth, breasts, vagina, anus, and rectum.
   b. To assist investigation, forensic evidence may be collected with the consent of the survivor. This may include removing and isolating clothing, scalp hair, foreign substances from the body, saliva, pubic hair, samples taken from the vagina, anus, rectum, mouth and collecting a blood sample.
   c. The survivor or in the case of child, the parent/guardian/person in whom the child reposes trust, has the right to refuse either a medicolegal examination or collection of evidence or both, but that refusal will not be used to deny treatment to survivor after sexual violence.
   d. As per the law, the hospital/examining doctor is required to inform the police about the sexual offence. However, if the survivor does not wish to participate in the police investigation, it will not result in denial of treatment for sexual violence. Informed refusal will be documented in such cases.
2. *Per vaginum examination,* commonly referred to by lay persons as 'two-finger test,' must not be conducted for establishing an incident of sexual violence and no comment on the size of vaginal introitus, elasticity of the vagina or hymen or about past sexual experience or habituation to sexual intercourse should be made as it has no bearing on a case of sexual violence. No comment on shape, size, and/or elasticity of the anal opening or about previous sexual experience or habituation to anal intercourse should be made.
3. *Injury documentation:* Examine the body parts for sexual violence related findings (such as injuries, bleeding, swelling, tenderness, discharge). This includes both micro-mucosal injuries which may heal within short period to that of severe injuries which would take longer to heal.
   - Injuries must be recorded with details—size, site, shape, color.
   - If a past history of sexual violence is reported, then record relevant findings. Sexual violence is largely perpetrated against females, but it can also be perpetrated against males, transgender and intersex persons.
4. The nature of forensic evidence collected will be determined by three main factors—nature of sexual violence, time elapsed between incident of sexual violence and examination and whether survivor has bathed or washed herself.
5. *Opinion:* The issue of whether an incident of rape/sexual assault occurred is a legal issue and not a medical diagnosis. Consequently, doctors should not, on the basis of the medical examination

conclude whether rape/sexual assault had occurred or not. Only findings in relation to medical findings should be recorded in the medical report.

- Drafting of provisional opinion should be done immediately after examination of the survivor on the basis of history and findings of detailed clinical examination of the survivor.
- It should be always kept in mind that normal examination findings neither refute nor confirm sexual violence. Hence circumstantial/other evidence may please be taken into consideration.
- *Absence of injuries may be due to:*
  - Inability of survivor to offer resistance to the assailant because of intoxication or threats
  - Delay in reporting for examination

CONCERNS

Mandatory Reporting

The intent of legislature in making the doctors/hospitals in Rape cases; and all persons in sexual assault cases to mandatorily report sexual violence cases to police have led to lot of problems.[16] This hinders the compulsory treatment provided by law. If somebody requires treatment, then because of mandatory reporting provisions they will have to agree for criminal investigation irrespective of whether they are willing to participate in criminal investigation at that material point of time. They will not have any choice (in participating in criminal investigation) if they need treatment. These mandatory reporting laws are not unique only to India. Many other countries also have, but in some of such countries (Example: USA), they have a choice whether to report to criminal investigation system or social support system. The benefits which they are entitled as victim of sexual violence are not altered in victim choosing either criminal investigation system or social support system.

Antenatal Sare (ANC) in Teenage Pregnancy

Child marriage is still in practice in India and there are several teenage pregnancies reporting to hospital as high-risk pregnancies. Antenatal care is given priority by the central government making 9th of every calendar month as a day for antenatal care. Now with all sexual activity under 18 years of age being considered as not permissible and criminal, with marriage status being no exception all such teenage pregnancies less than 18 years of married wives also become a mandatory reporting condition for doctors/hospitals.[12] Thus, if such pregnancies are considered as an offence under POCSO Act, then the husband has to be punished. And as a result, if they wish not to approach doctor/hospital, then the antenatal care gets affected and may result in increased morbidity and mortality of such high-risk pregnancy.

MTP

As per the Medical Termination of Pregnancy Act, 1971 *now Amendment Act, 2021,* doctor could terminate pregnancy under *24 weeks* of gestation if such pregnancy was due to sexual violence/rape. There is no requirement of even a police complaint/first information report. But now with mandatory reporting laws of Rape/Sexual assault, doctor even before medically terminating pregnancy of a victim of sexual violence, should mandatorily report to police. Due to these reasons, the victim may choose some crude methods for abortion risking her life just to avoid mandatory reporting. This mandatory reporting provision also contradicts the provisions of MTP Act and MTP Regulations in terms of violation of privacy and confidentiality issues.[16]

Marital Rape

The forced sexual relations with wife-aged less than 18 years are an offence under POCSO Act. But those forced sexual relations with wife above 18 years of age are not covered under the Rape definition. In addition, with changed definition of Rape, the forced sexual relations with wife either by penis into anus or urethra or oral cavity; or with penetration by objects or body parts (fingering) into vagina or anus or urethra are also not covered as a criminal offence of Rape. The wife has to not only suffer physical consequences of injuries but also mental harm due to such forced sexual relations against her wish and consent. The only solace is that such situations being redressable as domestic violence under PWDVA (Protection of Women against Domestic Violence Act, 2005). PWDVA is a civil law, and the wife could get restraint orders against husband.

MEDICOLEGAL QUESTIONS AND ANSWERS (FAQs)

(*Source:* Adopted from the book published by UNFPA and Government of Maharashtra on Answers to Frequently Asked Questions by Medical Professionals during medical examination of Survivors and Accused of Sexual Violence.[17])

- *Can you medically examine a Survivor/ Victim without a police requisition?*
  Yes. The Supreme Court had observed in State of Karnataka V Manjanna (in the year 2000) that the medical examination of Sexual violence victim should be done immediately, and no hospital/doctor should delay examination for want of police requisition. Now Section 27 POCSO Act (Protection of Children from Sexual offences Act) (in the year 2012) and Rule 6 of POCSO Rules (in the year 2020) specify not to insist for police requisition or Magistrate order before conducting medical examination. Section 357 C CrPC (Criminal Procedure Code) (in the year 2013) also states that the hospital first conducts the examination. All these legal changes thus ensure the right of sexual violence victim to voluntary report to the hospital instead of to the Police/ Court after sexual violence and also that the medical examination of Sexual violence victim is a Medico-legal emergency.
- *Is it mandatory to inform police?*
  Yes. Section 19 POCSO Act and Section 357 C CrPC *(now Sec 397 BNSS)* both instruct the doctor/hospital to mandatorily inform the police when they are examining a case of Sexual Violence. Section 21 POCSO Act and Section 166 B IPC (Indian Penal Code) *now S. 200 BNS* prescribe punishment for not following the directions of Section 19 POCSO Act and Section 357C CrPC *now Sec 397 BNSS.*
- *Are there any problems in mandatory reporting?*
  Yes. On one end, we have Section 164A CrPC *(Sec 184 BNSS)* (specific law for medical examination of the victim of rape) which insists that no part of examination is lawful without the consent of woman. But today if a woman claims she needs time to make up her mind to inform police or to initiate police investigation and asks the doctor to refrain from informing police—the doctor is in a dilemma, whether to follow the mandatory law or the ethical requirement/legal requirement of Informed consent. Section 357 C CrPC *now Sec 397 BNSS* and Rule 6 POCSO Rules specify that treatment is a must

and no hospital/doctor to deny this. But unfortunately, the 'right to treatment' and 'mandatory reporting' even when the woman has not agreed/ consented for the same are enshrined in the same section of the law. It took several decades of struggle to recognize legally the right to treatment of the victim/survivor of sexual violence. But with these mandatory reporting laws women seeking treatment and care are going to be jeopardized.

The MTP Act 1971 *now Amendment Act, 2021* (Medical Termination of Pregnancy Act) recognizes the right of the woman to MTP when her pregnancy is as a result of sexual violence. It also guarantees privacy and confidentiality of her information. But with the mandatory reporting laws of sexual violence now all these rights of the woman are being denied/affected because now such pregnancies as a result of sexual violence have to be mandatorily reported to police (even if the lady does not want that).

- *Is it mandatory to go to government hospital for sexual violence examination?*
  No, Section 357 C CrPC *now Sec 397 BNSS* now mandates all hospitals irrespective of being Government, public sector or private sector the responsibility of immediately providing first aid or medical treatment free of cost; thus, removing the major barrier which existed earlier of insisting Government hospitals only.
- *Is it necessary for a female doctor only to examine sexual violence victims?*
  Over the past decades, several High Courts liberally interpreted section 53 (2) CrPC *[now Sec 51 (2) BNSS]* and proposed that when we are insisting a female doctor to examine a female accused why cannot we extend the same privilege when the female is a victim and thus insisted sexual violence victims to be only examined by female doctors wherever available. But this change had its own problems. With only few female doctors working that too in rural hospitals, several sexual violence victims had to wait for their turn to get examined by the female doctors who were often busy with their duties to provide obstetric/maternity services. This delay in the examination led to loss of crucial medical evidence. The 2005 Criminal law amendment in section 164 A CrPC put an end to this insistence of female doctor, by stating any doctor with whom the female victim consented can carry out this examination. But the problem again resurfaced with the present Sec 27 POCSO Act insisting a female doctor only to examine a girl child (less than 18 years).
- *Is treatment part of Doctor's role?*
  There is a major shift from the past model of mere evidence collection in such cases to the present model of insisting on treatment by doctors. Rule 6 of POCSO Rules specify that treatment should include care for Injuries, STIs, HIV, Pregnancy testing, Emergency contraception, psychological counseling, drug deaddiction program, disability assessment and care. Section 357 C CrPC *now Sec 397 BNSS* insists that such treatment should be free of cost and noncompliance of such treatment can drag the doctor to one-year imprisonment and/or fine. Ideally speaking every doctor/ hospital should provide comprehensive care which also includes rehabilitation and follow-up care.
- *Are past sexual practices still documented in sexual violence examination?*
  Unfortunately, yes. Though the section 146 IEA *(now Sec 149 BSA)* and section 53A IEA (Indian Evidence Act) *(now Sec 48 BSA)* prohibits the debate on previous

sexual experience/past sexual practices in the witness box. But such insensitive things are being documented in medical practices/protocols in the form of documenting two-finger test, old hymenal injuries, past abortions, past contraceptive practices. Such documentation should stop immediately (except rarely only in cases of chronic sexual abuse and if consensual sexual intercourse is within one week of the medical examination may require such documentation).

- *Is it necessary to do age estimation?*
  The opinion is divided, when medically you cannot accurately opine the real age and can only possibly give an age range, why are the investigating authorities insisting on medical age estimation from doctors, even when they have clear documentary proof of age. But section 164 A CrPC *(now Sec 184 BNSS)* and section 15 (5A) of ITPA (Immoral Traffic Prevention Act 1956) insist on medical age estimation from doctors. Recently, the Supreme Court is of the opinion in Ashwani Kumar Saxena vs. State of MP that—'only in cases where those documents or certificates are found to be fabricated or manipulated, the court, the Juvenile Justice Board or the Committee need to go for medical report for age determination', thus again opening up the debate should there be medical age estimation when clear documentary proof of age exists. Now section 94 of JJ Act *(Juvenile Justice Act, 2015)* clearly spells out that medical examination for age estimation is to be carried out only if the Special Court or Juvenile Justice board is of the opinion that there is no availability of School records and Revenue records (birth certificate) for proving age.
- *Is it relevant to document when was the examination done?*
  Yes, it is very important because delay in examination and post-assault activities affect the outcome of medical examination. Mere non-detection in medical examination does not mean that sexual violence/crime did not occur. Each hour delay in the medical examination affects the medical evidence being detected. Many mucosal injuries heal within hours. Post-assault activities in the form of urination, defecation, washing, bathing, douching affect the medical evidence that is going to be detected. Thus, this examination should be treated as medicolegal emergency and priority be given by doctors/hospitals.
- *Who can be present while the doctor conducts a medical examination?*
  All these days, when a male doctor was conducting the examination of a female, we were insisting on the presence of disinterested, sound, major female person as a witness. Now section 27 POCSO Act insists that whenever you examine a child there should be a parent or any person whom she/he trusts to be present throughout the examination. If such persons are not available, then it is the duty of the hospital to provide one.
- *Are there any uniform guidelines and protocols for dealing with such cases?*
  Yes, today we have the Ministry of Health and Family Welfare, Government of India Guidelines and Protocols—Medicolegal care for survivors/victims of sexual violence. These guidelines address all issues including medical examination, psychosocial care, treatment, issues when dealing with children, disabled, transgender and intersex persons, persons with alternate sexual orientation, sex workers, people facing caste, class or religion-based discrimination. They also

have removed the insensitive practices in medical examination like two-finger tests, over emphasis on hymen, built of the woman, past contraceptive practices, past consensual sexual acts, past abortions, etc.

- *Is it necessary for the doctor to inform/report to the Child Welfare Committee (CWC) while dealing with a child of sexual assault?*
  Whenever the sexually assaulted child requires immediate care and protection, the doctor has to inform/report to the CWC. Issues like when there is no safe place for the child to stay; the perpetrator is in the same household of the child; there is risk of safety of the child; there is nobody available to consent for seeking health care to the child and act in the best interests of the child—the doctor can use the services of CWC. The doctors could also contact CWC members through the help of the police.
- *Can a doctor administer anesthesia to every victim/survivor of Rape/Sexual assault so as to enable medical examination?*
  The doctor cannot administer anesthesia to every victim/survivor of Rape/Sexual assault. Anesthesia can be administered only in those cases to enable medical examination which are done in the best interest of the victim/survivor (Like in cases where there is bleeding injuries, and the child victim/survivor is uncooperative).
- *Can a doctor administer HIV prophylaxis to every victim/survivor of Rape/Sexual assault?*
  The doctor has to assess whether there is high risk of possible HIV transmission as a result of this sexual violence, before deciding whether to administer HIV prophylaxis to a victim/survivor of Rape/Sexual assault.
- *Should a doctor do urine pregnancy test to every child victim/survivor of Rape/Sexual assault?*
  Based on the age of the child, if she has already attained menarche, then decision to do urine pregnancy test has to be taken depending on the phase of menstrual cycle she is in (like whether in menstrual bleeding or proliferative phase or secretory phase). If it is a case of prepubertal girl around the age of menarche, it is better to do urine pregnancy test so as to not miss any possible pregnancy in her first menstrual cycle itself.
- *What is the minimum age of a female for giving valid consent for sexual intercourse?*
  The minimum age of a female for giving valid consent for sexual intercourse is 18 years as per section 375 IPC (now Sec 63 BNS).
- *What is the minimum age of victim/survivor for giving valid consent for medical examination?*
  The minimum age of victim/survivor for giving valid consent for medical examination is 12 years as per Sections 89 and 90 IPC *(now Sec 27 and 28 BNS).*
- *What is the minimum age of victim/survivor for giving valid consent for MTP?*
  The minimum age of victim/survivor for giving valid consent for MTP is 18 years as per section 87 IPC (now Sec 25 BNS).
- *How/from who do you obtain informed consent for medical examination in case of a child who is 10 years of age and there are no natural guardians (parents) or local guardians?*
  Informed consent can be obtained from a panel of senior doctors in administrative positions in the hospital who will act in the best interest of the child.

- *How/from who do you obtain Informed consent for MTP in case of a child who is 14 years of age and there are no natural guardians (parents) or local guardians and the gestational age is 18 weeks?*
  Informed consent can be obtained from a panel of senior doctors in administrative positions in the hospital who will act in the best interest of the child *OR* from the Child Welfare Committee (CWC). *But as per Section 5 of the MTP Act of 1971 amendment act 2021, if the continuation of the pregnancy is a threat to the life of the mother, then it can be terminated by any doctor, in any hospital, at any duration of gestational age.*
- *How/from who do you obtain informed consent for MTP in case of a child who is 16 years of age and there are no natural guardians (parents) or local guardians and the gestational age is 21 weeks?*
  Informed consent has to be obtained from the jurisdictional Court for MTP as the gestational age is beyond *24 weeks [Beyond the provisions of permissible limit (20 weeks of gestational age) of MTP Act of 1971 amendment act 2021].*
- *In case of an emergency lifesaving procedure which has to be performed by a doctor on a victim/survivor of sexual violence, who will consent or how is consent obtained?*
  As per section 92 IPC, it is not an offence even if without consent, if any act is done in good faith for the benefit of the person. Thus, in an emergency lifesaving procedure which has to be performed by a doctor on a victim/survivor of sexual violence, then there is no need of any person's consent. The doctor could directly conduct the emergency lifesaving procedure.
- *In case of a mentally diseased victim/survivor who would consent for medical examination?*
  In case of medical examination of a mentally diseased victim/survivor, then informed consent is obtained from the parents or local guardian acting in the best interest of the mentally diseased victim/survivor. If the parents or local guardian are not available, then informed consent is obtained from a panel of senior doctors in administrative positions in the hospital who will act in the best interest of the victim/survivor. In the case of a child, informed consent could be obtained from the Child Welfare Committee. Otherwise even informed consent could be obtained from Jurisdictional Courts also if it is not an emergency.
- *In case of a mentally subnormal victim/survivor who would consent for medical examination?*
  In case of medical examination of a mentally subnormal victim/survivor, then informed consent is obtained from the parents or local guardian acting in the best interest of the mentally subnormal victim/survivor. If the parents or local guardian are not available, then informed consent is obtained from a panel of senior doctors in administrative positions in the hospital who will act in the best interest of the victim/survivor. In the case of a child, informed consent could be obtained from the Child Welfare Committee. Otherwise even informed consent could be obtained from Jurisdictional Courts also if it is not an emergency.
- *In case of a deaf/mute/dumb-victim/survivor who would consent for medical examination?*
  In the case of medical examination of a deaf/mute/dumb-victim/survivor, then

informed consent is obtained from the parents or local guardian acting in the best interest of the deaf/mute/dumb-victim/ survivor. If the parents or local guardian are not available, then informed consent is obtained from a panel of senior doctors in administrative positions in the hospital who will act in the best interest of the victim/ survivor. In the case of a child, informed consent could be obtained from the Child Welfare Committee. Otherwise even informed consent could be obtained from Jurisdictional Courts also if it is not an emergency.

- *In case of an intoxicated or drugged victim/ survivor who would consent for medical examination?*
  In the case of medical examination of an intoxicated or drugged victim/ survivor, then informed consent is obtained from the parents or local guardian acting in the best interest of the intoxicated or drugged victim/ survivor. If the parents or local guardian are not available, then informed consent is obtained from a panel of senior doctors in administrative positions in the hospital who will act in the best interest of the victim/survivor. In the case of a child, informed consent could be obtained from the Child Welfare Committee.
- *Is it necessary to obtain a court order for medical examination of a victim/survivor of sexual violence who does not consent for the same?*
  No. Court or person could force a medical examination on a victim/ survivor, when the victim/survivor of sexual violence does not consent for the same.
- *Is it necessary for presence of injuries in all sexual violence cases?*
  No, the research evidence speaks contrary. The WHO evidence states that in only 33% of cases of sexual violence there are injuries; that means out of 3 cases of sexual violence you do not find injuries in 2 cases. This absence of injuries could be due to various reasons—the victim being unconscious either due to trauma or being drugged/intoxicated, overpowered, silenced with fear. Even the use of lubricants in sexual violence decreases injuries. Now the Explanation 2 to section 375 IPC *(63 BNS)* states that if someone does not resist the sexual violence that alone cannot be construed as offering consent to the Act. Thus, now the law also does not insist the woman for offering resistance (*that means presence of resistance injuries is not required to prove a case of sexual violence).*
- *What is the relevance of special tests/ investigations?*
  With the research evidence divided on the use of colposcopy to detect microinjuries, Toluidine dye test having its own limitations in detecting microinjuries of only sexual violence, false-positive results with use of Wood's lamp examinationfor detecting semen, insisting for use of these special tests/investigations should be done with caution.
- *What is the relevance of DNA examination in sexual violence cases?*
  Yes, DNA is crucial comparable evidence in sexual violence cases if collected and profiled properly. But unfortunately, in Indian scenario, the accused is not caught/arrested at all or immediately not caught/arrested. Thus, this comparable evidence cannot be put to use at all. The other problem is with both Section 164A CrPC *(now Sec 184 BNSS)* and Section 53A CrPC *(now Sec 52 BNSS)* insisting for collection of DNA evidence in all cases of sexual violence, nobody has thought of the workload it puts on our understaffed

Forensic Science Laboratories (FSL). Other problems with India are that we do not have DNA database of population or at least criminals; nor do we have more government Forensic Science Laboratories neither at least private laboratories to test DNA. The other issue is that of the standards/quality of our FSLs as many of them are not accredited laboratories. The law insisting on such quality control—DNA Technology (Use and Application) Regulation Bill, 2019 is pending in the Parliament.

- *Should you do a medical examination and collect evidence if woman is menstruating?* There are always chances of losing trace evidence in cases of heavy menstrual blood flow occurring at the time of assault, as well as at the time of medical examination. In situations of menstruation at the time of medical examination, then a repeat medical examination is warranted. But it is always wise to collect whatever evidence is available at the time of medical examination even if the woman is menstruating. (*It would be wrong to delay the medical examination just because the woman is menstruating as it affects not only evidence collection, but also would delay the commencement of treatment of STIs/Injuries, psychological counseling, etc.)*
- *Is it necessary to collect all evidence in all cases—even when there is delayed reporting after the alleged sexual violence?* The type(s) of evidence to be collected in each case depends on both the nature of sexual violence (*penetrative or nonpenetrative; penile or nonpenile; orifice penetrated—vagina/anus/mouth/urethra; ejaculation occurred or not; post-assault activities like bathing, douching, washing, urination, defecation*) and the actual time of medical examination post-sexual violence (*keeping in mind that there are many a times delay in reaching for medical examination due to various social issues/barriers*). Clothes which were worn at the time of assault are to be collected even in delayed medical examinations (*if they are still worn*). Swabs/Slides for evidence of motile spermatozoa till 12–24 hours post-assault; Swabs/Slides for evidence of spermatozoa till 24–48 hours post-assault; Swabs for evidence of Semen/Blood stain/Lubricant till 4–5 days post- assault; Loose hair and any other trace evidence (buttons, paint, etc.), whenever present along with nail clippings to be collected during the time of medical examination.
- *What should the doctor/hospital do in case there is a delay on the part of police in collecting the sealed evidentiary materials/packets?* The doctor can always pack, seal and label all the evidentiary materials/packets and dispatch them along with the report to the police for onward transfer to laboratories (FSL and/or hospital laboratory) for testing and opinion(s). If in the case, there is any delay on the part of the police in collecting the same, then a reminder letter/phone call can be made to speed up the process. If they still fail to collect, then a letter/phone call can be made to the superior police officers, explaining about the urgent need of collection of evidentiary materials/packets from the doctor/hospital for onward transfer to laboratories (FSL and/or hospital laboratory) for testing and opinion(s) *(In 2008, the Delhi High Court was of the opinion that the evidentiary materials/packets should be stored in the hospital itself till such time that the police prepare*

necessary documents for onward transfer to FSL. This order was made keeping in mind the storage facilities in the hospital are far superior in comparison to that of a police station) (Delhi Commission for women vs. Delhi Police, In the High Court of Delhi, WP (CRL) 696/2008).

- *How long the products of conception could/should be kept in the hospital?*
  Products of conception are collected for doing DNA profiling and to ascertain whether it matches with that of the accused. Ideally speaking it has to be sent to the DNA laboratory immediately. If this is not possible, then the products of conception should be stored in a container and maintaining the cold chain/cold storage (at 4°C) should be sent to the DNA laboratory as early as possible. This depends also on the standard operating procedures (SOPs) of each of the Forensic Science Laboratory doing the DNA profiling.
- *In case of a full-term delivery, then what samples of the fetus should be collected to send for DNA analysis?*
  Some of the DNA laboratories prefer the whole fetus to be sent to them if it can be sent immediately. If there is a delay, some prefer femur sample instead to be sent to them as early as possible. Some laboratories prefer blood samples. It is better to refer to the standard operating procedures (SOPs) of each of the Forensic Science Laboratory doing the DNA profiling so as to decide what sample/how much sample/transit or transportation time/preservative to be used, etc. for DNA analysis.
- *Can the doctor give opinion on whether Rape or Sexual assault occurred?*
  Rape and Sexual assault are legal terms and as doctors are only doing medical examination, they cannot opine whether Rape or Sexual assault occurred or not.
- *Should a doctor give provisional opinion in every case examined?*
  Yes, whenever the doctor has got the positive examination findings (presence of injuries/STIs) and also when wet smear examination is positive for spermatozoa—the doctor should give provisional opinion immediately after the medical examination incorporating these. Otherwise, the Investigating officer gets stranded being unable to frame charges against the accused and/or to arrest the accused. But in every case of medical examination, there may not be an affirmative provisional opinion. This would largely depend on—the delay in reporting for medical examination post-assault, post-assault activities, type of sexual violence, facilities available at the time of medical examination, etc.
- *When can a doctor issue final opinion?*
  If a doctor had reserved the opinion for want of laboratory investigative reports, then the doctor could issue the final opinion immediately after the receipt of these laboratory investigative reports both/either from the hospital laboratory and/or FSL.
- *Is it necessary that the final opinion be affirmative in every case?*
  In every case of medical examination, there may not be an affirmative final opinion. This would largely depend on—the delay in reporting for medical examination post assault, post assault activities, type of sexual violence, facilities available at the time of medical examination and laboratory investigations, etc.
- *What points constitute medical opinion?*
  Medical opinion consists of the following:
  - Any evidence of sexual violence (penetrative by penis and/or body part and/or object or non-penetrative);

   - Any evidence to ascertain mental incapacity to give consent due to the effect of the disease/ethyl alcohol/narcotic drug/psychotropic substance;
   - Any evidence for medical age determination which would be crucial in deciding incapacity to give consent and/or increase in the punishment;
   - Any evidence to identify assailants through medical examination in the form of collection of DNA material through collection of hair, semen, blood, nails clippings, etc.
- *What are the limitations of medical opinion?*
  Limitations of medical opinion are as follows:
   - Post-assault activities in the form of bathing/douching/washing and urination/defecation; delay in reporting for medical examination; Healing of injuries and STIs;
   - Use of condom which was not recovered; Non corroboration of treatment received.
- *Is it difficult/not possible to issue Provisional Opinion?*
  The doctor can provide provisional opinion about the presence of spermatozoa if any, injuries if any, and then age of injuries. But as a defensive practice the doctor only opines—'reserved pending for want of FSL/laboratory reports', thus fixing the Investigating officer in a spot of bother, unable to proceed further in the investigation of the case and worst of all the accused gets the benefit of doubt and may even get a bail as an outcome of defensive practices of doctors.
- *How should the final opinion be furnished?*
  Section 164A CrPC insists the doctor provide a reasoned opinion. Thus, the negative evidence—for example, absence of semen whether it is due to use of condom or the woman was menstruating or due to washing of genitals/bathing or due to delay in medical examination, etc. has to be explained. It is always better if the doctor provides/finalizes the final opinion well before getting into the witness box.
- *What is the relevance of medical opinion and current Law?*
  Earlier courts were giving lot of credit to the medical evidence for proving a charge of Rape/Sexual assault (*when the law of rape was looking for penetrative penovaginal sexual intercourse).* Now that the law of Rape/ Sexual assault is changed from recognizing even non-penetrative acts and also penetrative acts into anus/ oral/urethra/vagina by either penis or objects or body parts (fingering). Thus, there could be several situations of Rape/ Sexual assault with no medical evidence at all. This has to be clearly understood by Doctors, Police, Lawyers, Courts and all other stakeholders in providing justice to the sexual violence victims.
- *Are there any templates for issuing reasoned medical opinions?*
  Yes, the doctors could refer to the templates given in the guidelines and protocols, medicolegal care for survivors/ victims of sexual violence—manual issued by Ministry of Health and Family Welfare before issuing reasoned medical opinions after medical examinations.
- *How to ascertain/opine about sexual violence when both physical/genital injuries are absent and also FSL reports are negative for presence of semen/alcohol/ drug/lubricant?*
  In such cases, if the history is positive for sexual violence but medical examination

does not find any injuries nor FSL could detect any presence of semen/alcohol/drug/lubricant—then the medical opinion could be that *the possibility of sexual violence could not be ruled out by medical examination and laboratory investigations.* This could be due to healing of injuries or absence of injuries; post-assault activities like bathing/douching/washing/urination/defecation; use of condom which is not recovered; type of sexual violence—penetrative by objects/body parts or non-penetrative assault; delay in medical examination, etc. In such cases, the investigating officer has to look for other corroborative evidence(s) and beyond medical evidence.

- *Can medical opinion be given only on the basis of history when nothing is evident from the clinical findings (medical examination) and also by laboratory investigations?*
  Yes, medical opinion in such cases can be given only on the basis of history like, for example, *'the possibility of sexual violence could not be ruled out by medical examination and laboratory investigations.'* This (history suggestive of sexual violence, but the clinical findings being negative as well as laboratory investigations being negative) could be due to healing of injuries or absence of injuries; post-assault activities like bathing/douching/washing/urination/defecation; use of condom which is not recovered; type of sexual violence—penetrative by objects/body parts or non-penetrative assault; delay in medical examination, etc.
- *How should the doctor respond to the police requisition asking to 'rule out rape' after medical examination of the person?*
  As per law, the police could ask any question to the doctor based on their investigation in the said case. But the doctor has to respond only based on what is possible to be inferred from the medical examination of that person. Rape is a legal term. Thus, the doctor is not possible to 'rule out rape' by medical examination. Hence in such cases the doctor after medical examination concludes opining only with those positive or negative findings of the medical examination.
- *How should the doctor respond to the police requisition asking to find out whether the person is 'habituated to sex' after medical examination of the person?*
  As per section 146 IEA *(now Sec 149 BSA)* and section 53A IEA *(now Sec 48 BSA)*, it is illegal to ask questions related to past sexual acts to the survivor/victim. That means past consensual sexual acts are immaterial when the current act of sexual violence is being adjudicated. Hence, the doctor also is not needed to opine to the question of the police requisition asking to find out whether the person is 'habituated to sex'.
  (Below are the questions commonly faced in the witness box by the doctor while deposing evidence in the cases of medical examination of Sexual Violence cases)
- *Did you inform police before doing MTP?*
  Yes, as this pregnancy was a result of Rape/Sexual assault; as per the provisions of mandatory reporting (Section 357C CrPC *(now Sec 397 BNSS)*/Section 19 POCSO) I have informed police before doing MTP. *OR* As the age of this pregnant woman is less than 18 years and is unmarried/married, I have informed police before doing MTP as the minimum legal age for consenting for sexual intercourse by a woman is 18 years.
- *Before doing MTP, why did you not wait till police arrival?*

No, as per provisions of mandatory reporting, I had to only inform the police, which I have done through MLC intimation and also again reminded the police the day when I was doing MTP *OR* As per law, I have already informed police and subsequently I could not wait till the arrival of police, as it was a case of threatened abortion and it would have ended in complications. And as per law (Section 357C CrPC, *now Sec 397 BNSS*), I have to compulsorily treat the person; otherwise, I am liable for punishment under section 166 B IPC *now Sec 200 BNS*.

- *Whether rape occurred or not?*
  Rape is a legal term and as a doctor by doing medical examination, I cannot opine whether Rape occurred or not.
- *Whether the victim is habituated to sexual intercourse or not?*
  As per law [section 146 IEA *(now Sec 149 BSA)* and section 53A *(now Sec 48 BSA)* IEA], it is not required to know whether the victim is habituated to sexual intercourse or not. And also, as per the Guidelines and protocols, Medicolegal care for survivors/victims of Sexual Violence—manual issued by Ministry of Health and Family Welfare, I am not supposed to comment on whether the victim is habituated to sexual intercourse or not.
- *Why is semen absent in this case? OR When there is no semen, how do you say it is a case of rape/sexual assault?*
  It is not necessary that in every case of Rape/Sexual assault, we could find Semen. If it is non-penile penetration (Objects or body parts) or if its penile penetration but no ejaculation or if its penile penetration but ejaculated outside the body or its penile penetration but a condom was used and was not recovered—in all these situations, semen may be absent in case of Rape/Sexual assault.
- *Why are spermatozoa absent in this case?*
  It is not necessary that in every case of Rape/Sexual assault, we could find spermatozoa. If it is non-penile penetration (Objects or body parts) or if its penile penetration but no ejaculation or if its penile penetration but ejaculated outside the body or its penile penetration but a condom was used and was not recovered *OR* the accused person was azoospermic *OR* had the disease of vas deferens *OR* there is such inordinate delay between the sexual violence and the medical examination that even if spermatozoa were present at the time of sexual violence—now they all are disintegrated and are beyond recognition.
- *Was there a female assistant during medical examination?*
  This may be relevant whenever a male doctor is examining a female victim/survivor. Accordingly, it can be answered Yes or No depending on whether a male doctor or female doctor does the medical examination of female victim/survivor. *Whenever a male doctor is medically examining a female, then there should be a disinterested adult female witnessing the medical examination (chaperone).*
- *Can the Judges/Lawyers/Police ask the doctors to comment on the status of the hymen? Is it relevant? Why?*
  The old injuries or scars of the hymen may be immaterial in the adjudication of the current forceful sexual act/sexual violence. This is because the hymen could be torn in a non-sexual act and need not be torn in a sexual act. However, fresh injuries on the hymen are always helpful in interpreting use of force (genital force). But in those cases of chronic/repetitive non-consensual sexual acts/sexual violence even the documentation of old

hymenal injuries/scars is necessary. Depending on the case the Judges/ Lawyers/Police can ask the doctors to comment on the status of the hymen.

CONCLUSION

In this section, we understood the magnitude of the problem of sexual violence, steps in medicolegal management of victims of sexual violence, preventive steps, legal provisions, important judgments from Supreme Court and National Guidelines from Government of India. The key learning points summarize the take home messages and the concerns section red flags the issues which need more concerted attention.

REFERENCES

1. Rai D. Sexual violence pandemic in India: Rape cases doubled in last 17 years, India Today, December 13, 2019. Available online at https://www.indiatoday.in/diu/story/sexual-violence-pandemic-india-rape-cases-doubled-seventeen-years-1628143-2019-12-13. accessed on 12/7/2020.
2. Criminal Law (Amendment) Act 2013: Sexual offences, available online at https://www.lawctopus.com/academike/criminal-law-amendment/, accessed on 12/7/2020.
3. Ministry of Health and Family Welfare, Government of India, Guidelines and Protocols Medicolegal care for Survivors/ Victims of Sexual violence, available online at https://main.mohfw.gov.in/sites/default/files/953522324.pdf, accessed on 12/7/2020.
4. One Stop Centre Scheme, Ministry of Women and Child Development, Implementation Guidelines for State Governments/UT administrations, December 2017, available at https://wcd.nic.in/sites/default/files/OSC_G.pdf, accessed on 12/7/2020.
5. Narayanareddy J. Procedure of examination and certification in rape /Sexual Assault case. In Pillay VV (Ed) NACPFMT's Practical Medicolegal Manual for Forensic and Clinical students and Practitioners, Vol 1. Paras Medical Publisher. 2019. Pp. 200-53.
6. Narayanareddy J, Medical Evidence in examination of rape/sexual assault survivor. In Biswas G (Ed). Recent Advances in Forensic Medicine and Toxicology, Good Practice Guidelines and Current Medicolegal issues. Jaypee Brothers Medical Publishers. 2018;2:18-40.
7. Jagadeesh N. Legal changes towards justice for sexual assault victims. Indian Journal of Medical Ethics. [S.l.], v.7, n.2, p. 108, Nov. 2016. ISSN 0975-5691. Available online at https://ijme.in/articles/legal-changes-towards-justice-for-sexual-assault-victims/ accesed on 12/7/2020.
8. The Protection of Children from Sexual Offences Act 2012, available online at https://wcd.nic.in/sites/default/files/POCSO%20Act%2C%202012.pdf, accessed on 12/7/2020.
9. The Protection of Children from Sexual Offences Rules 2020, available online at http://egazette.nic.in/WriteReadData/2020/218601.pdf, accessed on 12/7/2020.
10. The Indian Evidence Act, 1872 available online at https://www.indiacode.nic.in/handle/123456789/2188?sam_handle=123456789/1362, accessed on 12/7/2020.
11. Lillu @ Rajesh and Anr V State of Haryana, Supreme Court, 11 April, 2013, available online at https://indiankanoon.org/doc/78844212/, accessed on 13/7/2020.
12. Independent Thought vs. Union of India, Supreme Court, 11 October, 2017, available online at https://indiankanoon.org/doc/87705010/, accessed on 13/7/2020.
13. Chandigarh 10-year-old's rape case: Verdict against uncles today, Hindustan Times, Chandigarh, 31st October, 2017, available online at https://www.hindustantimes.com/chandigarh/chandigarh-10-year-old-s-rape-case-verdict-against-uncles-today/story-sHQ9SWLyzscKFBBs4NIMPI.html, accessed on 13/7/2020.
14. Indian Court rejects abortion for 10-year-old rape victim, BBC News, India 28 July, 2017, available online at https://www.bbc.com/

news/world-asia-india-40753409, accessed on 13/7/2020.

15. Stop Child Sexual Abuse, IMA White paper on Child sexual abuse, available online at https://www.ima-india.org/ima/left-side-bar.php?pid=232, accessed on 13/7/2020.
16. Jagadeesh N, Bhate-Deosthali P, Rege S, Ethical concerns related to mandatory reporting of sexual violence. Indian Journal of Medical Ethics, [S.l.], v. 2, n. 2 (NS), p. 116, Nov. 2016. ISSN 0975-5691. Available online at https://ijme.in/articles/ethical-concerns-related-to-mandatory-reporting-of-sexual-violence/ , accessed on 13/7/2020.
17. Jagadeesh N. Answers to Frequently Asked Questions by Medical Professionals during Medical Examination of Survivors and Accused of Sexual Violence, 2017, Government of Maharashtra and United Nations Population Fund.

SECTION 5

Medicolegal Issues in Family Planning Services

CHAPTER 12

Medicolegal Aspects of Female Contraception and Sterilization

Ranabir Pal, Amrita Ghosh

No woman can call herself free who does not control her own body.

—Margaret Sanger

INTRODUCTION

The concept of reproductive health was introduced at the International Conference on Population and Development in 1994. Reproductive rights (WHO) rest on the recognition of the basic rights of all couples and individuals to decide freely and responsibly the number, spacing and timing of their children and to have the information and means to do so, and the right to attain the highest standard of sexual and reproductive health. They also include the right of all to make decisions concerning reproduction free of discrimination, coercion and violence. Ensuring access to contraception is a fundamental part of upholding human rights as well as contributing to improved health outcomes, with direct benefit for individuals, families, communities and wider society. Various international treaties and policy tools have gradually codified sexual and reproductive health rights. These recognize sexual and reproductive health within a rights-based framework and require the state to safeguard, promote, and fulfil these rights. Since the International Conference on Human Rights Declaration in 1968 and the International Conference on Population and Development in 1994, reproductive rights have been steadily recognized as human rights. The International Covenant on Economic, Social, and Cultural Rights (ICESCR) of 1996 and the Convention on the Elimination of all Forms of Discrimination Against Women (CEDAW) of 1979 both emphasize the importance of focusing on reproductive rights in attaining women's fundamental rights. As a signatory to these covenants and conventions, India is responsible for ensuring that these objectives are met in its policies and laws.

Milestones in Reproductive Health

1952	First country to launch the National Family Planning program (Clinic-based approach)
1992	Child survival and safe motherhood (CSSM)
2000	National Population Policy to promote voluntary and informed choice and continuation of 'target-free' approach in family planning service delivery
2005	NRHM—to provide accessible, affordable and quality healthcare delivery system
2005	Conditional cash transfer scheme like Janani Suraksha Yojana (to promote institutional delivery)
2012	Family planning 2020 was launched to intensify family welfare measures
2013	NHM—National Health Mission included RNMCH-A and control of communicable and non-communicable diseases
2021	The Union Cabinet has cleared the proposal to increase the minimum age for marriage of women from 18 to 21 years

When it comes to reproductive health and rights (RHR), national laws and regulations show a varied picture of compliance as well as significant gaps. Women's reproductive health rights are impacted directly or indirectly by laws that allow for medical termination of pregnancy (abortion), protection against sex selection, maternity benefits, and protection from domestic abuse, including sexual violence by an intimate partner. The insufficiency of this legislation has been criticized on several occasions. A proposal has been made to broaden the focus beyond maternal health to cover different life stages. The National Health Mission (NHM) (2012–2017) embraced the Reproductive Maternal Neonatal Child and Adolescent Health (RMNCH+A) program, as well as the *Rashtriya Kishor Swasthya Karyakram* (RKSK) downstream, in order to realistically visualize the ground realities and assessments of the public healthcare system in order to provide convergence for synergistic effects.[1]

Contraceptive Behavior: NFHS-5 in Comparison to NFHS-4

Recently published NFHS-5 from MoHFW GOI report shows a breakthrough, i.e., the replacement level of total fertility rate (TFR) is 2.1, at which a population exactly replaces itself from one generation to the next has been achieved in most of the states/UTs. India has achieved below this to 2.0 NFHS-5 while only 3 states, *viz.* Manipur (2.2), Meghalaya (2.9) and Bihar (3.0) have TFR above replacement levels till now. Contraceptive prevalence rate (CPR) is the proportion of women of reproductive age who are using (or whose partner is using) a contraceptive method at a given point in time. CPR increased in most States/UTs, and highest prevalence rate found in Himachal Pradesh and West Bengal (74%). Unmet needs of family planning point, the gap between women's reproductive intentions and their contraceptive behavior to become pregnant by their own plans of family welfare which follows a declining trend over the last few years. The CPR has come down to less than 10% in all States except Meghalaya and Mizoram.

Table 1 shows the comparison between NFHS-4 and NFHS-5.[2]

METHODS OF CONTRACEPTION

There are a variety of contraception methods that can be used either temporarily for spacing or permanently for sterilization. Beneficiaries can choose from a variety of contraception options based on their needs and preferences. Surgical sterilization is a well-known and common technique of contraception. It provides highly effective pregnancy prevention; it has a very low risk of problems when performed according to approved medical standards; and it eliminates the need for long-term contraceptive supplies because it is a one-time treatment. Because modern sterilization techniques are safe and straightforward, male and female sterilizations can be performed as outpatient procedures. Because this method of contraception is permanent, it is critical to make an informed decision and get proper counseling.

There are a variety of contraception methods that can be used either temporarily for spacing or permanently for sterilization. Beneficiaries can choose from a variety of contraception options based on their needs and preferences.

Because there is no "optimal" form of birth control for every woman, the following complicated process is commonly referred to as the "Cafeteria Approach." The birth control method that is right for one and one's partner is determined by a variety of factors, including whether she wants to get pregnant

TABLE 1: Comparison between NFHS-4 and NFHS-5.

Indicators	*NFHS-5 (2019–2020)*			*NFHS-4 (2015–2016)*
	Urban	***Rural***	***Total***	***Total***
Marriage and Fertility				
Women use 20–24 years married before age 18 years (%)	14.7	27.0	23.3	26.8
Men age 25–29 years married before age 21 years (%)	11.3	21.1	17.1	20.3
Total fertility rate (children per women)	1.6	2.1	2.0	2.2
Women age 15–19 years who were already mother or pregnant at the time of survey (%)	3.8	7.9	6.8	7.9
Adolescent fertility rate for women age 15–19 years	27	49	43	51
Current use of family planning method (currently married women age 15–49 years)				
Any method	69.3	65.6	66.7	53.5
Any modern method (%)	58.5	55.5	56.5	47.8
Female sterilization (%)	36.3	38.7	37.9	36.0
Male sterilization (%)	0.2	0.3	0.3	0.3
IUD/PPIUD (%)	2.7	1.8	2.1	1.5
Pill (%)	4.4	5.4	5.1	4.1
Condom (%)	13.6	7.6	9.5	5.6
Injections (%)	0.4	0.6	0.6	0.2
Unmet needs for family planning (currently married women age 15–49 years)				
Total unmet need (%)	8.4	9.9	9.4	12.9
Unmet need for spacing (%)	3.6		4.0	5.7

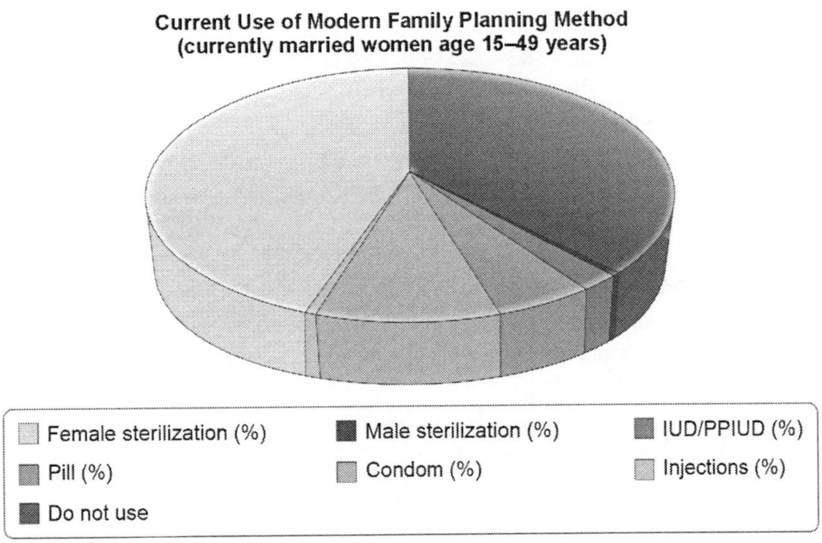

soon, within a few years, or never; possible advantages and disadvantages; how often they have sex; number of sex partners; overall health of the users, including the presence and absence of co-morbidities; and how comfortable and confident she is with using the method (for example, can she remember to take a pill every day? Will she insist on her spouse using a condom every time?)

"Even the most successful birth control techniques can fail if the use is inconsistent, erroneous, and of poor-quality logistics," it is necessary to clarify to the beneficiaries. Methods for avoiding pregnancy, from most effective to least effective: Female and male sterilization (female tubal ligation or occlusion, male vasectomy)—Birth control that prevents pregnancy for the rest of life through surgery or a medical procedure.

- *Long-acting reversible contraceptives or "LARC" methods (intrauterine devices, hormonal implants):* The user does not have to remember to use birth control every day or month because the health-care provider inserts it once. Depending on the procedure, LARCs can endure anywhere from 3 to 10 years.
- *Short-acting hormonal methods (pill, mini pills, patch, shot, vaginal ring):* Remember to take at least once a day or once a month. Every three months, the user must get a shot from a healthcare provider.
- *Barrier methods (condoms, diaphragms, sponge, cervical cap):* Birth control user use each time user have sex.
- *Natural rhythm methods*: Instead of utilizing birth control, users should avoid sex and/or use birth control only on days when they are most fertile (most likely to get pregnant). A fertility monitor or an ovulation home test kit can assist users in determining the most fertile days.[3]

Medical Eligibility (Tables 2 and 3)

Medical eligibility criteria are useful tools for clinicians to use when prescribing the most appropriate and safe contraceptive treatment for each woman. Although different criteria may be useful for some complex conditions, prescribers should remember that these criteria are only guidelines, and clinical judgment should always take precedence.

TABLE 2: Definitions and interpretation of the WHO-MEC 2015 categories.[5]

	Definition of category	*Interpretation of the category in practice*
Category 1 (Accept)	A condition for which there is no restriction on the use of the contraceptive method	Use method in any circumstances
Category 2 (Caution)	A condition where the advantages of using the method generally outweigh the theoretical or proven risks	Generally, use the method
Category 3 (Delay)	A condition where the theoretical or proven risks usually outweigh the advantages of using the method	Use of method is not usually recommended unless other more appropriate methods are not available or not acceptable
Category 4 (Special)	A condition which represents an unacceptable health risk if the contraceptive method is used	Method not to be used

TABLE 3: Conditions included in Caution, Delay and Special categories.

Caution	*Delay*	*Special*
Previous abdominal or pelvic surgery	Severe iron deficiency anemia (Hemoglobin <7 gm/dL)	Conditions that increase chances of heart disease or stroke, i.e., older age, smoking, high BP or diabetes
Obesity	Current pregnancy	Blood pressure >160/100
Controlled BP (140–159/90–99 mm Hg)	8–42 days postpartum	Complicated heart disease
Uncomplicated heart disease	Pregnancy with severe pre-eclampsia or eclampsia	Coagulation disorders
History of ischemic heart disease	Postpartum or postabortion complications (Infection, hemorrhage and trauma)	Chronic lung diseases (Asthma or emphysema)
Stroke	Current DVT/PE	Endometriosis
History of cerebrovascular accident	Major surgery with prolonged immobilization	Pelvic tuberculosis
History of deep vein thrombosis or pulmonary embolism	Abdominal skin infections	Fixed uterus due to previous surgery or infection
Epilepsy	Current ischemic heart disease	Abdominal wall or umbilical hernia
Depressive disorders	Lung disease like pneumonia	Postpartum or postabortion uterine rupture or perforation
Current breast cancer	Systemic infection	Diabetes of 20 years standing with organ damage
Uterine fibroids	Unexplained vaginal bleeding	Hyperthyroidism
PID without subsequent pregnancy	Large collection of blood in uterus	Severe cirrhosis of liver
Uncomplicated diabetes	Malignant trophoblastic disease	AIDS
Hypothyroidism	Cancers of the genital tract	
Mild cirrhosis	Current PID	
Liver tumors	Current purulent cervicitis, Chlamydia, Gonorrhea	
Kidney disease	Current gallbladder disease	
Thalassemia and sickle cell disease	Uncontrolled diabetes	
HIV		

General eligibility criteria:[4]

- The clients must have been married.
- Female clients should be below the age of 45 years and above 22 years.
- The couple should have at least one child whose age is above one year unless the sterilization is medically indicated.
- Clients or their spouses must not have undergone sterilization in the past (not applicable in the cases of failure of previous sterilization).
- Clients must be in a normal state of mind so as to understand the full implications of sterilization.
- A psychiatrist must certify mentally ill individuals, and a legal guardian or spouse must provide consent.

The conditions included in Caution, Delay and Special categories are shown in **Table 3.**[6]

Eligibility Criteria from WHO[7]

	COC P CVR	CIC	POP	DMPA NET-EN	LNG ETG	Cu-IUD	LNG-IUD	Barr		
								Co	S	D
CARDIOVASCULAR RISK FACTORS OR DISEASES										
SMOKING										
Age ≥ 35 years										
< 15 cigarettes/day	3	2	1	1	1	1	1	1	1	1
≥ 15 cigarettes/day	4	3	1	1	1	1	1	1	1	1
MULTIPLE RISK FACTORS FOR ARTERIAL CARDIOVASCULAR DISEASE										
e.g. older age, smoking, diabetes, hypertension and known dyslipidaemias	3/4	3/4	2	3	2	1	2	1	1	1
HYPERTENSION										
History of hypertension, where blood pressure CANNOT be evaluated (incl. hypertension in pregnancy)	3	3	2	2	2	1	2	1	1	1
Adequately controlled hypertension, where blood pressure CAN be evaluated	3	3	1	2	1	1	1	1	1	1
Elevated blood pressure levels (properly taken measurements)										
SYS 140-159 or DIA 90-99 mm Hg	3	3	1	2	1	1	1	1	1	1
SYS ≥ 160 or DIA ≥ 100 mm Hg	4	4	2	3	2	1	2	1	1	1
Vascular disease	4	4	2	3	2	1	2	1	1	1
DEEP VEIN THROMBOSIS (DVT) / PULMONARY EMBOLISM (PE)										
History of DVT/PE	4	4	2	2	2	1	2	1	1	1
Acute DVT/PE	4	4	3	3	3	1	3	1	1	1
DVT/PE and established on anticoagulant therapy	4	4	2	2	2	1	2	1	1	1
Major surgery with prolonged immobilisation	4	4	2	2	2	1	2	1	1	1
KNOWN THROMBOGENIC MUTATIONS										
e.g. Factor V Leiden, prothrombin mutation, protein S, protein C, and antithrombin deficiencies	4	4	2	2	2	1	2	1	1	1

Contd...

Contd...

ISCHAEMIC HEART DISEASE										
Current and history	4	4	I: 2, C: 3	3	I: 2, C: 3	1	I: 2, C: 3	1	1	1
STROKE										
History of cerebrovascular accident	4	4	I: 2, C: 3	3	I: 2, C: 3	1	2	1	1	1
VALVULAR HEART DISEASE										
Complicated valvular heart disease (pulmonary hypertension, risk of atrial fibrillation, history of subacute bacterial endocarditis)	4	4	1	1	1	2	2	1	1	2
RHEUMATIC DISEASES										
SYSTEMIC LUPUS ERYTHEMATOSUS										
Positive or unknown antiphospholipid antibodies	4	4	3	I: 3, C: 3	3	I: 1, C: 1	3	1	1	1
Severe thrombocytopenia	2	2	2	I: 3, C: 2	2	I: 3, C: 2	2	1	1	1
NEUROLOGIC CONDITIONS										
MIGRAINE WITHOUT AURA										
Age < 35 years	I: 2, C: 3	I: 2, C: 3	I: 1, C: 2	2	2	1	2	1	1	1
Age ≥ 35 years	I: 3, C: 4	I: 3, C: 4	I: 1, C: 2	2	2	1	2	1	1	1
MIGRAINE WITH AURA										
Any age	4	4	I: 2, C: 3	I: 2, C: 3	I: 2, C: 3	1	I: 2, C: 3	1	1	1
BREAST CANCER										
Current	4	4	4	4	4	1	4	1	1	1
Past and no evidence of current disease for 5 years	3	3	3	3	3	1	3	1	1	1
OTHER REPRODUCTIVE TRACT INFECTIONS OR DISORDERS										
Unexplained vaginal bleeding (suspicion for serious condition) – before evaluation	2	2	2	3	3	I: 4, C: 2	I: 4, C: 2	1	1	1
Immediate post-septic abortion	1	1	1	1	1	4	4	1	1	1
Gestational trophoblastic disease										
Decreasing or undetectable β-hCG levels	1	1	1	1	1	3	3	1	1	1
Persistently elevated β-hCG levels or malignant disease	1	1	1	1	1	4	4	1	1	1
Cervical cancer (awaiting treatment)	2	2	1	2	2	I: 4, C: 2	I: 4, C: 2	1	2	1
Endometrial cancer	1	1	1	1	1	I: 4, C: 2	I: 4, C: 2	1	1	1
Ovarian cancer	1	1	1	1	1	I: 3, C: 2	I: 3, C: 2	1	1	1
Uterine fibroids with distortion of the uterine cavity	1	1	1	1	1	4	4	1	1	1
Anatomical abnormalities – Distorted uterine cavity incompatible with IUD insertion	-	-	-	-	-	4	4	1	1	NA
Current pelvic inflammatory disease	1	1	1	1	1	I: 4, C: 2	I: 4, C: 2	1	1	1

Contd...

Contd...

HIV/AIDS and OTHER INFECTIONS										
High risk of HIV	1	1	1	1	1	2	2	1	4	4
Asymptomatic or mild HIV clinical disease (WHO stage 1 or 2)	1	1	1	1	1	2	2	1	3	3
Severe or advanced HIV clinical disease (WHO stage 3 or 4)	1	1	1	1	1	I: 3, C: 2	I: 3, C: 2	1	3	3
History of toxic shock syndrome	-	-	-	-	-	-, -	-, -	1	1	3
Pelvic tuberculosis	1	1	1	1	1	I: 4, C: 3	I: 4, C: 3	1	1	1
Current purulent cervicitis or chlamydial infection or gonorrhoea	1	1	1	1	1	I: 4, C: 2	I: 4, C: 2	1	1	1
ENDOCRINE CONDITIONS										
DIABETES										
With nephropathy/retinopathy/neuropathy	3/4	3/4	2	3	2	1	2	1	1	1
Other vascular disease or diabetes of > 20 years' duration	3/4	3/4	2	3	2	1	2	1	1	1
GASTROINTESTINAL CONDITIONS										
SYMPTOMATIC GALL BLADDER DISEASE										
Medically treated	3	2	2	2	2	1	2	1	1	1
Current	3	2	2	2	2	1	2	1	1	1
HISTORY OF CHOLESTASIS										
Past-COC related	3	2	2	2	2	1	2	1	1	1
VIRAL HEPATITIS										
Acute or flare	I: 3/4, C: 2	I: 3, C: 2	1	1	1	1	1	1	1	1
CIRRHOSIS										
Severe (decompensated)	4	3	3	3	3	1	3	1	1	1
LIVER TUMOURS										
Benign hepatocellular adenoma	4	3	3	3	3	1	3	1	1	1
Malignant (hepatoma)	4	3/4	3	3	3	1	3	1	1	1

Barr: barrier methods; C: continuation; CIC: combined injectable contraceptive; Co: condom; COC: combined oral contraceptive; Cu-IUD: copper-bearing intrauterine device; CVR: combined contraceptive vaginal ring; D: diaphragm (with spermicide), cervical cap; DIA: diastolic; DMPA: depot medroxyprogesterone acetate (injectable); DVT: deep venous thrombosis; I: initiation; LNG/ETG: levonorgestrel and etonorgestrel (implants); LNG-IUD: levonorgestrel-releasing intrauterine device; NA: not applicable; NET-EN: noresthisterone enanthate injectable contraceptive; P: combined contraceptive patch; PE: pulmonary embolism; POC: progestogen-only contraceptive; POP: progestogen-only pill; S: spermicide; SYS: systolic.[7]

COUNSELING

Counseling is the process of assisting clients in making educated and voluntary fertility decisions. Before the client signs the consent form, the following actions must be taken:

1. They must be informed of all family planning options available to them, as well as the fact that this procedure is, for all intents and purposes, permanent.
2. Clients must willingly make an educated decision on sterilization.
3. They need to be counseled in their own language.
4. Clients must be made aware of what will happen before, during, and after the procedure, as well as any potential complications or adverse effects.
5. The following features of the sterilization procedure may be explained to the client:

a. It is a long-term method of preventing future pregnancies.
b. It is a surgical treatment with the risk of complications, including failure, necessitating additional management.
c. It has no effect on sexual pleasure, performance, or ability.
d. It will have no effect on the client's strength or capacity to complete daily tasks.
e. Sterilization does not protect against RTIs, STIs, HIV/AIDS, or other sexually transmitted infections.
f. Clients must be informed that this operation can be reversed, but that doing so requires extensive surgery and that success cannot be assured.

6. Clients should be encouraged to ask questions in order to clear up any doubts they may have.
7. Clients must be informed that they can refuse the operation at any time without jeopardizing their access to other reproductive health services.

PRE-PROCEDURE INSTRUCTIONS

Prior to surgery, the client's medical history, menstruation and obstetrics history, physical examination, and any necessary laboratory investigations should be completed to determine the client's eligibility for surgery.[8]

a. Carcinoma of the breast (known or suspected) or personal history of breast cancer
b. Carcinoma of the endometrium or other known or suspected estrogen-dependent neoplasia
c. Cerebral vascular or coronary artery disease (current or history of)
d. Cholestatic jaundice of pregnancy or jaundice with previous oral contraceptive pill use
e. Combination of smoking and age older than 35 years
f. Diabetes mellitus with complications
g. Headaches with focal neurologic symptoms
h. Hepatic adenomas or carcinoma
i. Hepatocellular disease (acute or chronic) with abnormal liver function
j. Hypersensitivity to any component in oral contraceptive pills
k. Major surgery with prolonged immobilization
l. Pregnancy (known or suspected)
m. Severe hypertension
n. Stroke
o. Systemic lupus erythematosus with antiphospholipid antibodies
p. Undiagnosed abnormal genital bleeding
q. Valvular heart disease with complications

Consent/Role of Spouse in Consent

- Consent for a sterilization procedure should not be gained under duress or while the client is sedated.
- Before the surgery, the client must sign a sterilization permission document.
- Sterilization does not require the consent of the husband. The Consent Form should be written in both English and the local dialect.
- The consent of the husband is not required, although it is preferable, in order to avoid a violation of the recent Supreme Court rule (The Supreme Court's ruling was for any surgery that could harm a spouse's reproductive capacity).

Failure of Sterilization Procedure and Litigation

- The failure of an operation that results in pregnancy could be due to a technical flaw in the surgery or spontaneous recanalization.
- During the pregnancy, the patient should be offered MTP or be medically assisted. She should be given the opportunity to have the procedure again. Tubectomy predisposes to ectopic pregnancy, which must be ruled out.

COMPLICATIONS

Medicolegal problems can arise due to following reasons:

- Unqualified persons—inadequate training
- Unrecognized place Improper consent
- Wrong selection of patient

Intraoperative complications:

a. Nausea and vomiting
b. Vasovagal attack
c. Respiratory depression or arrest
d. Cardiac arrest
e. Uterine perforation
f. Bleeding from the mesosalpinx
g. Injury to the urinary bladder
h. Injury to intra-abdominal viscera—small or large bowel and blood vessels
i. Convulsions and toxic reactions to local anesthesia

Postoperative complications:

a. Wound sepsis
b. Hematoma in the abdominal wall
c. Intestinal obstruction, paralytic ileus and peritonitis
d. Tetanus
e. Incisional hernia

As with any surgical treatment, regular protocols and care should be followed. A complete discharge narrative with all pertinent facts and stern directions on what to do if she misses her period should be supplied. Postoperative instructions must be given in the local language, both in writing and orally. Special wound-care instructions must be followed. If there is a missed period/suspected pregnancy within two weeks of the missed period, the client must be invited to return to the clinic.

Documentation/Certificate of Sterilization

Certificate of sterilization should be issued after the second follow-up after ruling out any pregnancy.[9]

Smt. Anita Devi vs. State of Raj & Ors. on 13 December, 2011[10]

The cause of action in this petition is alleged to be based on a failed sterilization procedure that the petitioner underwent on January 27, 2009. According to the petitioner, she conceived and gave birth to an unwanted child as a result of the unsuccessful sterilization, and she is therefore entitled to compensation of ₹5,00,000 for raising the child. Alternatively, the petitioner is entitled to compensation under the Family Planning Insurance Scheme designed by the Government of India (Ministry of Health and Family Welfare) via circular dated 06.07.2006 for failed sterilization.

The issue of payment of compensation following a failed sterilization and the birth of an unwanted child is fully covered by the Hon'ble Supreme Court's decision in the case of State of Punjab vs. Shiv Ram & Ors. [(2005) 7 SCC 1], in which the Hon'ble Supreme Court held that such compensation could not be granted.

However, it appears that the petitioner has not made a proper representation/claim before the competent authority as provided

सही उम्र में शादी
सोच कर बच्चे

ज़िम्मेदारी निभाओ
प्लान बनाओ

Sterilization Certificate

Hospital Registration No. (IPD/OPD) ______________

1. This is to certify that Smt/ Shri.. S/O; W/O Shri .... working as .... residing at .... has undergone Minilap Tubectomy – (Interval/Post-Partum/Post Abortion/Concurrent with other procedures)//Laparoscopic Tubal Occulsion (Interval/Post Abortion/Concurrent with other surgeries)/Vasectomy Conventional/ NSV) in this facility/hospital ....(Name of facility/Hospital) on .... by Dr...

For Female Sterilization:

2. She has resumed her menstrual Cycle (LMP_____) or she has not resumed her menses within the month of sterilization but pregnancy test is negative.

For Male Sterilization:

3. His semen examination undertaken on (Date)________________ revealed no sperm (azoospermia)

**Strike out whichever is not applicable*

She/ He is therefore certified to be sterile

Signature of Medical Officer I/c

Name..................................

Date ....

Seal ....

Note: Client should acknowledge 'received' on the duplicate copy before receiving the original copy. The duplicate to be maintained as a record in the facility as per state norms.

Department of Health & Family Welfare, U.T., Chandigarh.

for in the Family Planning Insurance Scheme as framed by the Government of India (Ministry of Health and Family Welfare) for a failed sterilization under its circular dated 06.07.2006.

MEDICOLEGAL ASPECTS OF FEMALE CONTRACEPTION AND STERILIZATION

In India, the Medical Termination of Pregnancy Act of 1971 (MTP) forbids indiscriminate abortion, as amended in 2002. Sex selection is prohibited in India under the Pre-Natal Diagnostic Techniques (Regulation and Prevention of Misuse) Act, 1994. (PNDT). In 2003, the law was amended to include the Pre-Conception and Pre-Natal Diagnostic Techniques (Prohibition of Sex Selection) Act (The PCPNDT Act). The purpose of this change was to increase coverage of the unborn in the womb's safety in relation to emerging technologies used in sex selection, followed by abortion as a prophylactic measure owing to widespread rejection of the female gender as a future family member. Only a few situations are exempt from the MTP Act's abortion prohibition. The PCPNDT Act, on the other hand, forbids the sex selection of an unborn living child for the purpose of terminating the pregnancy, with a focus on the female gender.

MTP Act[11]

In India, causing an abortion is illegal, even if done by the pregnant woman herself, unless it is done with the ostensible intention of saving a life, in which case it is punishable by up to three years in prison, a fine, or both. This Act allows any registered medical practitioner to perform an abortion under the following conditions: (a) the pregnancy must not have lasted more than 12 weeks; (b) the pregnancy poses a significant risk to the woman's life or physical or mental health; and (c) the pregnancy poses a significant risk to the child's physical or mental abnormalities and severe handicapping after birth. This Act enables abortion (a) in cases of rape resulting in grave psychosocial injury to the pregnant woman, and (b) in cases of alleged failure of the couple's conventional contraceptives to limit family size, if certain conditions are met. Two medical practitioners must agree on the medical necessity of an abortion in pregnancies of 12 weeks to less than 20 weeks; in pregnancies of 12 weeks to less than 20 weeks, one medical practitioner's opinion is sufficient for abortion. Abortions must be performed at public healthcare institutions regardless of the length of pregnancy.

The Medical Termination of Pregnancy (Amendment) Act, 2021[12]

Salient Features of Amendments

- Increasing the upper gestation limit from 20 to 24 weeks for particular groups of women, as described in the MTP Rules, which would include rape survivors, incest victims, and other vulnerable women (such as differently abled women, children), among others.
- Only one provider's opinion will be necessary up to 20 weeks of pregnancy, and two physicians' opinions will be required for terminations between 20 and 24 weeks of pregnancy.
- In cases of significant prenatal anomalies diagnosed by the Medical Board, the upper gestation restriction will not apply. The Medical Board's composition, functions, and other elements will be prescribed later under the Act's Rules.

- The name and other personal information of a woman whose pregnancy has been terminated shall not be disclosed to anyone unless authorized by law.
- The grounds for contraceptive failure have been widened to include women and their partners.

The Medical Termination of Pregnancy (Amendment) Bill of 2021—aims to increase women's access to safe and legal abortions for therapeutic, eugenic, humanitarian, or societal reasons. The amendments include the substitution of certain subsections and the insertion of certain new clauses under certain sections of the existing Medical Termination of Pregnancy Act, 1971, with the goal of raising the upper gestation limit for termination of pregnancy under certain conditions and strengthening access to comprehensive abortion care, under strict conditions, without jeopardizing service and quality-of-safe abortion.

The Pre-conception and Pre-natal Diagnostic Techniques (Prohibition of Sex Selection) Amendment Act 2002[13]

In reaction to the misuse of the MTP Act, the Pre-natal Diagnostic Techniques (Regulation and Prevention of Misuse) Act of 1994 (PNDT) was enacted in 1994. This act was changed in 2002 in order to close loopholes in the original Act. Citizens and healthcare practitioners are subject to the following restrictions under the Act: Regulate prenatal diagnostic procedures for the detection of genetic abnormalities (such as amniocentesis, ultrasonography, and others) and restrict their use to registered facilities and qualified professionals only. Any sort of sex selection before or after conception should be prohibited. Prevent sex selection techniques from being used for sex selection before or after conception.

- Any process for determining a person's sex should not be marketed.
- The sale of ultrasound machines to unregistered individuals is prohibited under this Act.
- Offenses are cognizable, non-bailable, and non-compoundable, and they carry a five-year jail sentence and a monetary penalty.[13]

Assisted Reproductive Technology (ART) Regulation Bill, 2020[14]

We are on the verge of declining fertility as a result of India's socio-demographic transformation, which includes more working women, a prevalent preference for late marriage, divorce, and single parenthood. According to the World Health Organization, up to 19 million Indian couples are infertile at any given time, with 25% of adults trying to start a family.

There was no separate legislation governing ART in India a few years ago. The proposed Assisted Reproductive Technology Bill was first introduced in 2008 and modified in 2017. The Union Cabinet has approved the Assisted Reproductive Technology (ART) Regulation Bill, 2020, which will regulate all medical treatments used to assist infertile couples and ensure that ARTs in India are legal and ethical with primary characteristics as follows:

a. Use of safe and ethical ART to maintain anonymity and respect children's rights.
b. Pre-genetic Implantation Testing is essential to rule out the chance of defective chromosomes before they are delivered to the uterus, thus lowering the risk of genetic disorder.
c. A National Board to draught a code of ethics and minimum standards for

laboratory and diagnostic equipment as well as ART clinic practices.

d. An ART Bank is a facility that supplies sperm/semen, oocyte donors, and surrogate mothers to people who want to have a family.
e. The National Board's plans and policies for clinics and banks must be followed by state and union territory regulatory boards and agencies.
f. A national registry and registration authority to keep the database of the National Board up to date.
g. The Bill proposes draconian penalties for such illegal activities as sex selection, selling human embryos or gametes, and running an agency/racket/organization, including a fine of ₹10 lakh in the first occurrence and a sentence of up to 12 years in the second instance.

National Family Planning Program[15]

India, the world's second most populated country, was the first to implement a nationwide family planning program in 1952 in order to reduce fertility and slow growth. The transformation and molting from a narrow objective of population stabilization to broader vistas of reproductive health promotion, women empowerment, life-cycle approach, and male engagement during the last seven decades has opened the way for a holistic futuristic vision of welfare. Since 1997, the Family Welfare Program has been integrated with the Reproductive and Child Health (RCH) Program, which covers client choice, service quality, gender concerns, and underserved groups, including teenagers. The 'London Summit on Family Planning' (2012) focused on global family planning, with the goal of reaching an additional 120 million females in the world's poorest countries by 2020 with family planning services and knowledge channels. Following in their footsteps, the Indian government launched a new method to focus family planning efforts on the Reproductive, Maternal, Newborn, and Child Health and Adolescents (RMNCH+A) program, which covers the entire reproductive, maternal, newborn, and child health spectrum. Beyond population stabilization, this paradigm changes in family welfare concept recognized the long-term goal of a "target-free strategy." Customized empathetic quality control in family planning approaches, institutionalization of fixed day services, rejuvenating 'Postpartum' and 'Post-abortion' contraceptive services, participatory approaches from males, community-oriented schemes through ASHAs, streamlining commodity security, and Public-Private Partnerships (PPPs) were used to accelerate translational research and client-centric interventions. In public policy advocacy, capacity building, and a targeted Behavior Change Communication campaign, evaluation and assessments, quality improvement, feasibility studies, software development, development of resource materials including E-learning modules, social marketing, social franchising, and the provision of skilled human resource, the government has embraced multidisciplinary approaches. India's four-pronged family welfare approach includes: (a) A greater emphasis on spacing services, (b) The adoption of family planning based on perceived need, (c) Emphasis on male participation, (d) Approach based on rights. '*Mission Parivar Vikas*' was launched in 2016 to improve the quality of family planning healthcare services in high fertility districts in seven states: Bihar, Jharkhand, Madhya Pradesh, Chhattisgarh, Uttar Pradesh, Assam, and Rajasthan, with a focus on temporary methods to reduce the national fertility rate to 2.1 by 2025. Through '*Hum Do*,' the National Family Planning Program seeks to give informed guidance and tailor-made contraceptive services to needy couples.

CONCLUSION

In general terms, reproductive rights are the domains of every individual to decide freely and responsibly the number, spacing and timing of their children. It also includes the right to information and means to do so right to the highest standard of reproductive health, right to make decisions concerning reproduction free of discrimination, coercion and violence.

In 1952, India was the first country in the world to initiate National Family Planning Program which achieved many successes over decades. '*Mission Parivar Vikas*' was launched in 2016 to improve the quality of family planning healthcare services in high fertility districts in seven states: Bihar, Jharkhand, Madhya Pradesh, Chhattisgarh, Uttar Pradesh, Assam, and Rajasthan, with a focus on temporary methods to reduce the national fertility rate to 2.1 by 2025. NFHS-5 report, recently published by MoHFW GOI, showed the TFR of India as 2.0, which is below replacement level (2.1), but still 3 states viz. Manipur (2.2), Meghalaya (2.9) and Bihar (3.0) had TFR above replacement level. So, we have to go a long way to improve health literacy, women empowerment, and social movement to minimize the number of adolescent marriage and adolescence pregnancy, increase of the contraceptive prevalence to sustain the goal that we have achieved after seven decades of motivation, hard work and vast use of national resources with active community participation.

Moreover, contraceptive prevalence rate for India is as high as 67.8% (highest for West Bengal 74%). CPR includes percentage of women of reproductive age (15–49 years), either married or in union using any method of contraception, i.e., modern or traditional (use of modern method—61.7%).

Further, policy makers at all levels should think of revision (s) of laws related to female contraception and sterilization to upheld rights of women. Moreover, healthcare providers should be aware of legal and administrative aspects all the ethical and legal issues to help implement women's health. Implement lifecycle approach and improve healthy lifestyle for adolescents of both genders.

Key Learning Points/Carry Home Messages

- Women empowerment, i.e., promoting women's sense of self-worth, their ability to determine their own health choices, and their right to influence social changes for themselves and for others will play the crucial role in achieving CPR 100% and keep the national fertility rate below replacement level. Unmet need of India is below 10% which also need to keep to the minimum.
- Information education communication with emphasis on health education and especially reproductive health (sex education) is the need of hour, should be implemented at all levels from childhood to highest levels to improve the acceptance of responsibilities regarding family welfare.
- Right to reproductive health requires contraceptive services be available, accessible, acceptable and of good quality, and provided without discrimination as per proclamation of Universal Health Care in line with Health for All by the WHO.
- *The Medical Termination of Pregnancy (Amendment) Act, 2021:* This amendment increased the upper gestation limit from 20 to 24 weeks for particular groups of women, as described in the MTP Rules, which would include rape survivors, incest victims, and other vulnerable women (such as differently abled women, neuropsychiatric cases, children), among others.

The Pre-conception and Pre-natal Diagnostic Techniques (Prohibition of Sex Selection) Amendment Act 2002: In reaction to the misuse of the MTP Act, the Pre-natal Diagnostic Techniques (Regulation and Prevention of Misuse) Act of 1994 (PNDT) was enacted in 1994. This act was changed in 2002 in order to close loopholes of the original version. Citizens and healthcare practitioners are subject to the following restrictions under the Act: Regulate prenatal diagnostic procedures for the detection of genetic abnormalities (such as amniocentesis, ultrasonography, and others) and restrict their use to registered facilities and qualified professionals only. Overall literacy needs to be improved for the achievement of optimum level of female contraceptive behavior.

REFERENCES

1. Status of Human Rights in the Context of Sexual Health and Reproductive Health Rights in India, April 2018. SAMA Resource Group for Women and Health. Available from: https://nhrc.nic.in/sites/default/files/sexual_health_reproductive_health_rights_SAMA_PLD_2018_01012019_1.pdf.
2. National Family Health Survey-5 2019–2021. India Fact sheet. Available from: http://rchiips.org/nfhs/NFHS-5_FCTS/India.pdf.
3. 9 types of contraception you can use to prevent pregnancy. Available from: https://www.health.qld.gov.au/news-events/news/types-contraception-women-condoms-pill-iud-ring-implant-injection-diaphram.
4. Female Sterilization ICOG FOGSI Recommendations for Good Clinical Practice. Available from: Female_Sterilization_FOGSI_Good clinical Practice.pdf.
5. Medical eligibility criteria for contraceptive use Fifth edition, 3 February 2015 | Guideline Available from: https://www.who.int/publications/i/item/9789241549158.
6. Reference Manual for Female Sterilization, Family Planning Division Ministry of Health and Family Welfare Government of India, 2014 Available from: http://cghealth.nic.in/dhs/NEW%20OFFERINGSFP%20GUIDELINES/Ref%20Manual%20for%20Female%20Sterilization%202014.pdf [Accessed on 15/12/2021].
7. Serfaty D. Update on the contraceptive contraindications. J Gynecol Obstet Hum Reprod. 2019;48(5):297-307. doi: 10.1016/j.jogoh.2019.02.006.
8. ICOG FOGSI Recommendations for Good Clinical Practice, Available from: https://www.fogsi.org/wp-content/uploads/fogsi-focus/Female_Sterilization.pdf.
9. Sterilization Certificate. Department of Health & Family Welfare, UT Chandigarh. Available from: http://www.nrhmchd.gov.in/sites/default/files/Sterilization_Certificate.pdf.
10. Rajasthan High Court Smt Anita Devi vs. State of Raj & Ors. on 13th Dec, 2011 Available from: https://indiankanoon.org/doc/84457926.
11. MTPAct1971.Availablefrom:http://ncwapps.nic.in/acts/THEMEDICALTERMINATIONOFPREGNANCYACT1971.pdf.
12. Ministry of Health and Family Welfare Rajya Sabha passes. The Medical Termination of Pregnancy (Amendment) Bill, 2021 Posted On: 17 MAR 2021 12:12 PM by PIB Delhi Available from: https://pib.gov.in/PressReleasePage.aspx?PRID=1705381.
13. The Pre-conception and Pre-natal Diagnostic Techniques (Prohibition of Sex Selection) Amendment Act 2002. Gazette of India. Extraordinary Part II, Section 1, No.15. Dated January 20, 2003.
14. The Assisted Reproductive Technology (Regulation) Bill, 2020 [Ministry: Health and Family Welfare] Available from:https://prsindia.org/billtrack/the-assisted-reproductive-technology-regulation-bill-2020Mm
15. National Programme for Family Planning Available from: https://www.nhp.gov.in/national-programme-for-family-planning_pg.

CHAPTER 13

Medicolegal Aspects of Surrogacy and Assisted Reproductive Technology in India

Roya Rozati, RS Sharma, Charulata Chatterjee

INTRODUCTION

Upon reviewing the ancient Indian Vedic literature, which dates back thousands of years, and considering the findings from modern science in fields such as molecular biology, genetics, and DNA research, it becomes evident that motherhood is a deeply ingrained, instinctual physiological process.[1-3]

The maternal instinct is a core drive shared by all living beings, both animals and humans. According to ancient Indian philosophy, the biological essence of life is to transmit genetic traits to future generations. In this view, all living creatures exist in a transitional state, playing a role in safeguarding the survival and continuity of their genes.[4]

The primary objective of any species is propagation, meaning that the birth of offspring is shaped by factors that enhance their chances of survival. For instance, birds travel vast distances to find environments that can support their young. In the Canadian Inuit community, located 300 miles north of the Arctic Circle, seasonal patterns were documented until the 1970s, reflecting the importance of timing for survival.[5] However, due to modernization and the decline of traditional ways of life, seasonality has not been reported in recent years.

In India, infertility is often associated with social stigma, and its emotional and psychological impact is most intensely felt by the couples who face it. Although infertility does not lead to death, it can be profoundly distressing, as individuals grapple with the inability to fulfil the biological role of parenthood, despite having no personal fault in the matter.

Indian society is characterized by a strong family structure, a deep desire for children, and a cultural emphasis on having sons to carry on the family lineage, or "Vansh." However, with significant advancements in medical science, infertility can now be treated through modern techniques such as assisted reproductive technology (ART), including procedures like in vitro fertilization (IVF) and intracytoplasmic sperm injection (ICSI), among others.

GUIDELINE OF SURROGACY

Surrogacy is a procedure whereby a woman decides to have a pregnancy for intended couple by ART—assisted reproductive techniques. After the baby is born, surrogate gives custody and guardianship to the intended parent or parents **(Fig. 1)**.

Surrogacy is an assisted reproductive technique that is becoming more popular due to the growing demand for parenthood among infertile couples who are unable to have children through other means.

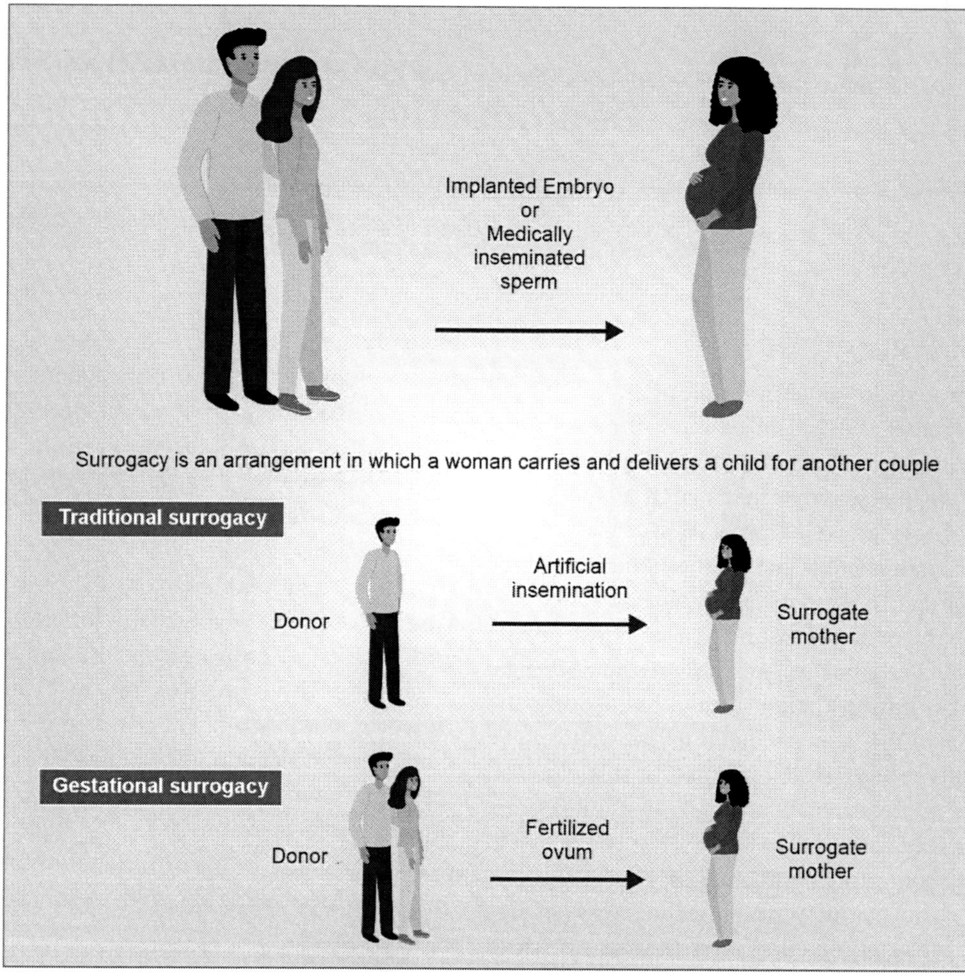

Fig. 1: Surrogacy and its types.
Courtesy: Syed Khaled Shahbaaz

LEGISLATION RELATED TO ASSISTED REPRODUCTIVE TECHNOLOGY AND SURROGACY: OVERVIEW [6-8]

- In response to the increasing number of surrogacy cases, India introduced the assisted reproductive technology (ART) Bill in 2010. The Government of India decided to enact a law to address potential future challenges related to surrogacy, aiming to regulate both surrogacy and ART in the country. An expert committee was formed, which submitted a draft of the proposed bill to the government, and it was subsequently approved.
- The Assisted Reproductive Technology (Regulation) Act, 2021[6] received the assent of the President and was published in the Gazette of India on 18th December 2021. This Act has been enacted for:
  - the regulation and supervision of the assisted reproductive technology clinics and the assisted reproductive technology banks.

- prevention of misuse.
- safe and ethical practice of assisted reproductive technology services for addressing the issues of reproductive health where assisted reproductive technology is required for becoming a parent or for freezing gametes, embryos, embryonic tissues for further use due to infertility, disease or social or medical concerns and for regulation and supervision of research and development and for matters connected therewith or incidental thereto.

- The Surrogacy (Regulation) Act 2021[7] (SRA) was approved by the Parliament with intention to establish and regulate the surrogacy procedure. The Act came into force on 25th January 2022, after the issuance of the notification in the Official Gazette by the Union Government.
- Surrogacy (Regulation) Act, 2021 and Assisted Reproductive Technology (Regulation) Act, 2021 to come into force with effect from January 25, 2022.
- In exercise of the powers conferred by section 50 of the Surrogacy (Regulation) Act, 2021 (47 of 2021), the Central Government made the following rules, namely, the Surrogacy (Regulation) Rules, 2022.[8]

SALIENT FEATURES FOR SURROGACY (REGULATION) RULES 2022[8]

(1) Legal Aspect

The Bill bans commercial surrogacy while permitting altruistic surrogacy. Altruistic surrogacy involves no financial compensation for the surrogate mother, beyond covering medical expenses and insurance during the pregnancy. In contrast, commercial surrogacy refers to surrogacy or related procedures performed for a financial reward or benefit that exceeds the basic medical expenses and insurance coverage.

(2) Couple Defined

The act defines a 'couple' as two individuals a legally married man and woman living together in a recognized sexual relationship under Indian law. The Act further clarified and restricted surrogacy laws in India, allowing only Indian married couples, unmarried women, and divorced or widowed women to opt for surrogacy while excluding same-sex couples and foreigners.

Couples of Indian origins, where the wife is between 23 and 50 years old and the husband is between 26 and 55 years old, are eligible for surrogacy. The intended couple or single woman must not have any surviving children (biological, adopted, or surrogate), except in cases where the child has a physical or mental disability, life-threatening condition, or fatal illness.

(3) Surrogate Mother

Surrogacy Act clearly specifies that surrogate should be a married woman having a child of her own and between the age of 25–35 years on the day of implantation.

(4) Cost

The intended couple will bear the medical expenses and insurance coverage for the surrogate mother.

(5) Insurance Coverage

The intending woman or couple must obtain general health insurance coverage for the surrogate mother from an insurance company or agent recognized by the Insurance Regulatory and Development Authority (IRDA), as established under the

Insurance Regulatory and Development Authority Act (41 of 1999). The coverage must be for a period of 36 months and be sufficient to cover all expenses related to pregnancy complications, as well as any postpartum delivery complications [under Surrogacy (Regulation) Rules, 2022].

(6) Number of Attempts of Surrogacy Procedure

A surrogate mother can undergo a surrogacy procedure a maximum of three times.

(7) Consent of a Surrogate Mother

The consent of a surrogate mother shall be as specified in Form 2 in the Act titled as Consent of the Surrogate Mother and Agreement for Surrogacy.

(8) Number of Embryos to be Transferred in the Uterus of the Surrogate Mother

The gynecologist shall transfer one embryo into the uterus of a surrogate mother during a treatment cycle. Provided that only in special circumstances up to three embryos may be transferred.

(9) Conditions under Which the Surrogate Mother may be Allowed for Abortion

The surrogate mother may be allowed for abortion during the process of surrogacy in accordance with the Medical Termination of Pregnancy Act, 1971 (34 of 1971).

(10) The Form, Procedure, and Fee for Registering a Surrogacy Clinic

(1) A surrogacy clinic conducting procedures related to surrogacy, as outlined in the Act, must submit an application for registration to the appropriate authority using Form 3.

(2) Each application for registration must be accompanied by a non-refundable fee of two lakh rupees for the surrogacy clinic. However, if the application is rejected by the appropriate authority, no fee will be required for re-submission of the same clinic's application. Additionally, government-run institutions are exempt from paying the application fee.

(11) Period, Manner and Form for Certificate of Registration

(1) The appropriate authority shall, after conducting the necessary inquiry and ensuring that the applicant has met all the requirements, issue a certificate of registration in Form 4 to the applicant.

(2) The registered surrogacy clinic shall prominently display a copy of its certificate of registration at a visible location within its business premises.

(12) Appeal

(1) The surrogacy clinic, intending woman, or couple may appeal against an order of rejection, suspension, or cancellation of registration under Section 13, or the rejection of certificates under Section 14, within 30 days of receiving the relevant communication from the appropriate authority.

(2) The form of appeal shall be as specified in Form 5.

(13) The Procedure for Seizing Documents, Records, Objects, etc., and the Preparation and Delivery of the Seizure List

(1) Every surrogacy clinic shall permit the National Board, National Registry, State Board, Appropriate Authority, or any other authorized person to inspect its premises, equipment, and records.

(2) An inspection of an already registered clinic may be conducted without prior notice during the clinic's working hours.

(3) The authorities mentioned in subsection (1) shall ensure that the entry and search procedures do not jeopardize the gametes or embryos stored in the facility.

(14) Medical Conditions Requiring Gestational Surrogacy

A woman may opt for surrogacy if:

(a) she has no uterus or missing uterus or abnormal uterus (like hypoplastic uterus or intrauterine adhesions or thin endometrium or small unicornuate uterus, T-shaped uterus) or if the uterus is surgically removed due to any medical conditions such as gynecological cancer;

(b) intended parent or woman who has repeatedly failed to conceive after multiple in vitro fertilization or intracytoplasmic sperm injection attempts (Recurrent implantation failure);

(c) multiple pregnancy losses resulting from an unexplained medical reason, unexplained graft rejection due to exaggerated immune response;

(d) any illness that makes it impossible for woman to carry a pregnancy to viability or pregnancy that is life threatening.

(15) ART Banks

(1) ART banks are specialized facilities that procure, store, and supply sperm and oocytes for use in assisted reproduction procedures. They act as a resource for ART clinics and patients seeking donor gametes.

Complete details of surrogates and donors will be stored at government-certified ART banks. The State Board will issue certificates to these ART banks. This independent body will have the authority to register, oversee, and monitor the operations of the ART banks.

(16) Sex Determination

Sex determination of the baby and 'selective childbirth' through surrogacy is illegal.

(17) Offences and Penalties

(1) Any medical geneticist, gynecologist, registered medical practitioner or any person shall not:

(a) abandon, disown or exploit or cause to be abandoned, disowned or exploited in any form the child or children born through assisted reproductive technology;

(b) sell human embryos or gametes, run an agency, a racket or an organization for selling, purchasing or trading in human embryos or gametes;

(c) import or help in getting imported in whatsoever manner, the human embryos or human gametes;

(d) exploit the commissioning couple, woman or the gamete donor in any form;

(e) transfer human embryo into a male person or an animal;

(f) sell any human embryo or gamete for the purpose of research; or

(g) use any intermediates to obtain gamete donors or purchase gamete donors.

(2) Whoever contravenes the provisions of clauses (a) to (g) of sub-section (1), shall be punishable with a fine which shall not be less than five lakh rupees but may extend to 10 lakh rupees for the first contravention and for subsequent contravention, shall be punishable with imprisonment for a term which shall not be less than three years but may extend to eight years and with fine which shall not be less than 10 lakh rupees but may extend to 20 lakh rupees.

(18) Restrictions on the Sale of Human Gametes, Zygotes, and Embryos

The sale, transfer, or use of gametes, zygotes, embryos, or any related information, either directly or indirectly, to any party within or outside India, shall be prohibited. However, the transfer of one's own gametes and embryos for personal use is permitted, provided it is done with the approval of the National Board.

SURROGACY (REGULATION) AMENDMENT RULES, 2024[9]

- The Central Government made amended the Surrogacy (Regulation) Rules, 2022, namely, the Surrogacy (Regulation) Amendment Rules, 2024.
- As per the amendment in the Surrogacy (Regulation) Rules, 2022, Form 2 (*Consent of the Surrogate Mother and Agreement for Surrogacy*) has been updated.
- The previous paragraph 1(d)* of Form 2 has been removed and replaced with a new provision as follows:
  "1(d)(i) couple undergoing surrogacy must have both gametes from the intending couple. However, in case when the District Medical Board certifies that either husband or wife constituting the intending couple suffers from medical condition necessitating use of donor gamete then surrogacy using donor gamete is allowed subject to the condition that the child to be born through surrogacy must have at least one gamete from the intending couple;
  (ii) single woman (widow or divorcee) undergoing surrogacy must use self-eggs and donor sperms to avail surrogacy procedure".

**The previous paragraph 1(d) which is no more in force and has been removed and replaced was as follows:*

1. *That I understand that the methods of treatment may include:*

(d) *the fertilization of a donor oocyte by the sperm of the husband*

ART GUIDELINES

Since its inception, advancements in assisted reproductive technology (ART) have helped thousands of individuals worldwide achieve pregnancy. ART plays a crucial role in enabling people to build their families and alleviating the psychological distress associated with infertility. However, the practice of ART is not without controversy, and significant ethical concerns persist in both research and clinical settings.

Level 1 ART Clinic

An ART (Assisted Reproductive Technology) Level 1 clinic is a facility that performs basic infertility treatments like intrauterine insemination (IUI). These clinics also conduct preliminary investigations to diagnose the cause of infertility.

At least one gynecologist must be present at all times and the clinic must register with the authorities.

Staff and Equipment Requirement

Minimum staff: One gynecologist with degree of medical postgraduate in gynecology and obstetrics.

Microscope, Centrifuge, and Refrigerator are the minimum requirement to apply for the registration.

Level 2 ART Clinic

Registered Level 2 can undertake procedures and techniques that attempt to obtain a pregnancy such as surgical retrieval of gametes, embryo transfer, storage of gametes, etc.

Staff and Minimum Equipment Requirement

Minimum staff required for level 2 clinic is one gynecologist, one anesthetist, one embryologist and one counselor.

The additional staff at the level of Director and Andrologist may be employed but not mandatory.

Equipment: (a) Microscope; (b) Incubator (minimum 2 in number); (c) Laminar airflow; (d) Sperm counting chambers; (e) Centrifuge; (f) Refrigerator; (g) Equipment for cryopreservation; (h) Ovum Aspiration Pump; (i) USG machine with transvaginal probe and needle guard; (j) Test tube warmer; and (k) Anesthesia resuscitation trolley.

These are minimum requirements to get registered, failure to have any of these equipment. Appropriate authority may reject the application.

Qualification

Gynecologist: Postgraduate in Obs/Gyne with at least 50 OPU along with 3 years of experience in Infertility or MD or FNB with at least 3 years of experience.

Anesthetist: Anesthetist will be a medical postgraduate in Anesthesia.

Embryologist: Full-time MCE with 3 years human ART laboratory experiences in handling human gametes and embryos; Full-time PhD (Thesis related to Clinical Embryology or ART or fertility) with additional one year of human ART laboratory experience in handling human gametes and embryos; MBBS or BVSc should have MCE (full time) with 2 years ART laboratory experience in handling human gametes and embryos; MSc in Biotech or Life Sciences minimum of one year of onsite, Full-time clinical embryology certified training in addition to four years' experience in handling human gametes and embryos in a registered ART level 2 clinic.

Counselor: A person who is a graduate in Psychology or Clinical Psychology or Nursing or Life Sciences.

Director: The director should have a postgraduate degree in Medical or Life Sciences or Management Sciences. This post is not a mandatory requirement.

Andrologist: The Andrologist shall be MCh/DNB in urology or MS (General Surgery) or FNB/MCh/DM in reproductive medicine with minimum 2 years of experience and having hands-on experience of minimum 15 surgical sperm retrieval (namely PESA/TESA/TESE/MESA/MICROTESE procedures). This post is not a mandatory requirement.

Location of the IVF Laboratory

Though not specified in the ART Act ideally the location of an IVF laboratory is critical to ensuring high-quality standards. The lab must be free from pathogens and provide a safe, non-toxic, and stable environment. Thus, selecting the site requires careful consideration. The laboratory's setting plays a key role in maintaining consistent success rates, and it should be positioned away from polluted areas, such as industrial zones or areas with heavy traffic. IVF labs should also be situated far from gas stations and parking lots. Furthermore, locations prone to pollutants should be avoided to minimize any adverse effects on embryo culture.

Necessities for an ART Clinic

The success of any assisted reproductive technology (ART) program depends heavily on the quality of its IVF laboratory. The primary role of an ART laboratory is to create an optimal environment for the development of embryos and handling of gametes.

When setting up an ART laboratory, three key factors must be considered:

The location of the laboratory, the expertise of the embryologists and the protocols and quality control measures, including the laboratory design.

Additionally, the layout of the ART laboratory, the consumables, and the equipment used in the IVF process are crucial components in establishing a well-functioning IVF laboratory for any fertility clinic.

ETHICAL GUIDELINES

Ethical guidelines deliver a predominant background for the department of ART in both research and clinical practice. These ethical guidelines similarly support the right to fair and reasonable access to health care, including ART. These ethical guidelines have been established primarily for Human Research Ethics Committees (HRECs), ART Clinicians, Embryologists, Clinic Nurses, Administrators, Counselors and Researchers. Recognizing the guiding principles should inform the researchers and clinicians to develop the procedures at their facilities. The Ethical guidelines protection all events associated with ART as they happen in clinical practice and research.

IVF Laboratory Design

Before establishing an IVF facility, the laboratory design must be carefully planned based on the expected workload. The design of the laboratory is crucial to meet both structural and environmental requirements.

Structural design aspects include specifications for the laboratory layout, such as flooring, ceiling height, lighting, and wall finishes.

When painting laboratory walls, it is highly recommended to use non-toxic, odorless, non-volatile, and glossy paint. The ceiling should be solid, while the flooring should be slip-resistant, preferably vinyl, to facilitate easy cleaning. Cupboards and tabletops should have a washable, matte finish and be constructed from heat-resistant materials. Furniture should be of standard working height and ergonomically designed to reduce staff fatigue.

The lighting system should be dimmable, and there should be sufficient electrical outlets. The power supply should be stable, with an alarm system to alert staff about any interruptions or issues with major equipment such as micromanipulators, incubators, freezing machines, refrigerators, etc.[10] Additionally, the laboratory should be equipped with a wall-mounted data logger to continuously monitor and display ambient temperature and humidity levels.

Environmental design focuses on ensuring that the quality of the ambient air is suitable for all procedures. This involves selecting appropriate materials and implementing engineering measures to minimize contamination from air-handling systems and the laboratory structure, which could impact air composition.[11]

The IVF laboratory should be located adjacent to the operating theater or procedure room, as recommended by the American Society for Reproductive Medicine.[12] Additionally, consulting with clean-room experts is highly advised to eliminate chemical air contaminants (CACs) and volatile organic compounds (VOCs) within the laboratory environment.

Green IVF not only limits the use of fertility drugs but also reduces use of disposables in the IVF laboratory. However, to achieve *Net Zero* emissions in IVF laboratories, it is essential that to take the action from today to reduce energy consumption, waste, and water use.

The vision for sustainable IVF extends beyond current practices. To redefine the field, one must explore innovative approaches that challenge conventional norms. For example, flexible lab design that allows add on without breaking the existence structure. Use of biodegradable material instead of plastic.

A well-designed ART laboratory should consist of four main sections:

1. *Andrology section:* This area is dedicated to semen analysis, sperm preparation, and sperm function test.
2. *Embryology section:* This section handles oocyte retrieval, embryo culture, and embryo-transfer procedures. Surgical sperm collection can also be done here.
3. *Cryopreservation section:* The focus here is on the vitrification or freezing of oocytes, sperm, embryos, as well as testicular and ovarian tissues in liquid nitrogen.
4. *Micromanipulation section:* This section is responsible for procedures such as assisted hatching, intracytoplasmic sperm injection (ICSI), as well as embryo, blastocyst, and polar body biopsy.

Air Quality

Air quality in an in vitro fertilization (IVF) lab is important for embryo development and IVF success. Air quality control in IVF labs involves using high-efficiency filtration systems, maintaining optimal humidity levels, and controlling volatile organic compounds (VOCs).

Air Filtration

HEPA filters: High-efficiency particulate air (HEPA) filters remove airborne particles.[13]

Positive air pressure: Positive air pressure moves air through the filters to remove particulates.

HVAC systems: Heating, ventilation, and air-conditioning (HVAC) systems should be properly installed, maintained, and cleaned.

Humidity

Optimal humidity levels: Maintaining humidity levels between 50–70% helps prevent condensation and bacterial growth.

VOCs

VOC levels: It is recommended to keep VOC levels below 400–800 ppb. VOCs can be found in cleaning agents, plastic ware, and more.[11]

VOC filtration: VOCs can be filtered using activated carbon filters.

Particle counts: Particle counts are used to assess cleanroom classification.

Equipment for an IVF Lab

Incubators

An IVF incubator will serve as an artificial uterus for the embryos to grow and develop until such time that it is mature enough to be transferred or preserved for future use.

The CO_2 incubator plays a crucial role in maintaining the optimal temperature, controlling humidity levels, and regulating essential gases such as oxygen and carbon dioxide. In addition to these functions, the incubator also safeguards valuable cultures from microbial contamination, ensuring a sterile environment for cell growth and development.

In addition to maintaining the appropriate gas concentrations and temperature, pH plays a critical role in the embryos' development. To support optimal growth, the culture media should be maintained within a pH range of 7.2–7.4. The water (H_2O) in the cells can form a carbonic acid buffer by reacting with CO_2. This combination produces bicarbonate and carbonic acid, which helps maintain the pH within the neutral range. In other words, adding the right amount of CO_2 is crucial for keeping the pH stable and promoting healthy embryo growth. An environment that is too acidic or too basic can hinder cell growth and disrupt the cells' metabolism, leading to adverse effects.

Functional aspects of the incubator, such as gas capability and sensor type, as well as temperature control and size/patient capacity need to be considered. Beside that embryos development improves if cultured at low level of oxygen. Big box CO_2 incubators had other limitations as achieving CO_2 level after door opening is longer time taking.[14] Hence advances are made as Bench-top incubator with low oxygen level.[15]

Advanced bench top IVF incubators are smaller, more efficient, and have more stable conditions than traditional incubators. This allows for better embryo development and higher success rates.

Features of Advanced IVF Incubators

Compact size: Advanced incubators are smaller and can hold fewer samples or have individual chambers for each sample.

Time-lapse imaging: Advanced incubators can take continuous images of embryos to monitor their development without removing them from the incubator.

Stable conditions: Advanced incubators maintain the right temperature, pH, and gas levels to mimic the environment of a female uterus.

Inline gas filters: Inline filters can reduce particle counts and VOCs in the gas supply.

Laminar Flow

Laminar flow creates a sterile environment for handling eggs, sperm, and embryos. This equipment is designed to prevent contamination and increase the chances of successful fertilization.

Laminar flow uses a vertical airflow system to move fluid particles in a smooth path, parallel to each other. It uses a filtration system to provide clean air and has a positively pressurized interior to prevent contamination from entering the work zone.

Micromanipulator

A micromanipulator is a device used in in vitro fertilization (IVF) labs to manipulate gametes and embryos under a microscope. It is a tool that allows for precise and delicate manipulation of cells and embryos.

The micromanipulator is used in conjunction with an inverted microscope and a joystick.

They can also be used to perform ICSI and biopsy procedures.

Centrifuge

A centrifuge is necessary for preparing sperm for IVF insemination or intracytoplasmic sperm injection (ICSI).

The laboratory should be cleaned with quaternary ammonium compound or distilled water. Any media preparation should be done with ultra-pure tissue grade water.[16]

Cryopreservation

Slow freezing is performed using a freezing machine that gradually lowers the temperature over a period of 2–2½ hours. This method is ideal for freezing cleavage stage embryos, blastocysts, and ovarian tissue. While these machines are costly and require regular maintenance, recent advancements in vitrification may eventually reduce the need for such advanced freezing machines, as vitrification protocols become more widely adopted.[17] For the cryopreservation of embryos, ovarian tissue, and gametes, liquid nitrogen tanks are essential.

The most critical step in setting up a new laboratory is purchasing the appropriate equipment. It is recommended to invest in well-established, reputable models that have been in use for a long time in recognized centers. When selecting equipment, key factors such as reliability, quality, safety, and the completion of electrical leakage tests by biomedical engineers should be prioritized. The equipment must also come with reliable breakdown services and maintenance support. After the equipment is purchased, regular maintenance and servicing are essential to ensure optimal functioning. Suppliers should provide backup equipment in case of malfunctions, and all equipment should be equipped with a backup power supply, as well as a trigger alarm or call-back service to address potential power interruptions.

Quality Control and Quality Assurance

Once the new laboratory is completed, several important steps must be taken before it becomes operational. The laboratory should undergo a thorough cleaning, and all equipment should be wiped down before being moved in. The ventilation rate should be increased, and air pressures should be elevated to help purge any irritants or volatile organic compounds (VOCs) released by new materials, furniture, and construction. New clean-room facilities, such as ART laboratories, require a significant curing period.[13] The length of this period depends on factors such as the materials used in construction and the cleaning processes applied. During this "burn-in" period, the laboratory should remain free from human activity and traffic to ensure the environment is properly conditioned before use.

All consumables used in ART procedures should be sourced from reputable brands known to be safe for the culture of embryos and gametes, with a proven track record in established centers. Certain plastic items, such as test tubes, embryo transfer catheters, graduated pipettes, petri dishes, and four-well culture dishes, are designed for single use only. Similarly, some glassware, including ICSI holders and injection needles, should be single-use. Oocyte aspiration needles and embryo transfer catheters must also be used only once. Tissue culture-grade, powder-free gloves should be worn in all IVF clinics, with each batch clearly marked with a batch number and expiration date. To maintain consistency and quality, it is crucial to avoid using different suppliers for ART procedures, as standardization across supplies is essential.

In the past, culture media were prepared within IVF laboratories, a process requiring strict quality control and significant effort. However, high-quality commercially prepared culture media are now widely available and increasingly used in laboratories globally. It is crucial to use media that are well-established in literature as suitable for culturing embryos and human oocytes. Additionally, the media selected should be easily accessible. Only media that are properly registered should be used in IVF procedures. Each batch of media must be certified for osmolarity, pH, sperm survival, and endotoxin levels. All media containers must display the date of manufacture, batch number, and lot number. If the media is manufactured internationally, proper packaging and temperature control during shipping should be ensured. Media from different companies should not be mixed, and manufacturer instructions must be strictly followed when using the medium.

Each ART laboratory should maintain a comprehensive manual that outlines all procedures performed within the facility. Laboratory protocols must be documented as standard operating procedures (SOPs). All activities conducted in the ART laboratory should be thoroughly documented, providing enough detail on the techniques used.[18] Each SOP must be signed and dated, and all SOPs should be readily accessible to staff to ensure strict adherence. Any deviation from SOPs must be treated seriously and not overlooked. During procedures, at least two individuals should be present to handle patient specimens. Patient identifiers, such as names and identity numbers, should be used, and the batch numbers of culture media and all consumables should be recorded for each patient.

A manual double witness system[19] or an electronic witness system should be implemented at each step of the procedure to ensure accuracy and accountability. A quality control sheet should be designed to align with the specific workflows of the laboratory and should be diligently maintained. A comprehensive quality program should be established, covering daily, weekly, monthly, quarterly, half-yearly, and yearly intervals, to ensure consistent monitoring of laboratory practices. Regular internal and external audits should be conducted to assess adherence to standards and identify areas for improvement. Additionally, obtaining quality accreditation certificates will be instrumental in maintaining high standards and continuous quality assurance in the ART laboratory.

ASSISTED REPRODUCTIVE TECHNOLOGY (ART) PROCEDURES

Assisted reproductive technology (ART) procedures prioritize patient protection as a primary concern. Equally important is the care and handling of embryos and gametes, which form a new entity of life. It is essential for all ART clinics to strictly adhere to scientific and ethical practices. Patients undergoing ART treatments must be fully informed about all the procedures involved. They should have a clear understanding of the significance of each ART procedure, ensuring that they are well-informed and able to make decisions with confidence.

ART clinics must notify the State Board or National Advisory Board on an ongoing basis if they are implementing any novel procedures for ART treatments. This ensures transparency and compliance with regulations. Various procedures are employed in ART clinics, each designed to address specific fertility issues, and it is important for clinics to stay updated on the latest advancements and practices in the field to provide the best care for patients.

ART procedures include:

1. Artificial insemination with husband's semen (AIH)
2. Artificial insemination with donor semen (AID)
3. IVF-associated techniques
4. In vitro fertilization and embryo transfer (IVF-ET)

5. Intracytoplasmic sperm injection (ICSI) with ejaculated, epididymal or testicular spermatozoa
6. Oocyte donation (OD) or embryo donation (ED)
7. Cryopreservation
8. Biopsy
9. Surgical sperm collection
10. Any add on procedures

CONCLUSION

The Assisted Reproductive Technology (Regulation) Act, 2021 was enacted to safeguard the rights of infertile couples and surrogate mothers seeking ART services. The Act also aims to ensure that ART clinics and banks are properly regulated and licensed.

ART is generally considered a safe procedure, with single embryo implantation being a strategy to maximize success rates. However, it is essential for couples to provide informed consent, fully understanding both the risks and benefits involved in the procedure.

Maintaining and achieving high success rates in ART requires a commitment to quality, which can only be achieved through effective teamwork. The coordinated efforts of all professionals involved, from clinicians to laboratory staff, are vital for optimizing outcomes and ensuring the best possible care for patients.

REFERENCES

1. Hrdy SB. Mother nature: maternal instincts and how they shape the human species? New York: Ballantine Books; 2000.
2. Szabo L. Researchers link maternal instincts, Tots' Smiles, Virginia. USA Today, 2008 Jul; Sect 7.
3. Tierney H. Women's Studies Encyclopedia, 3rd edn. Westport (CT): Greenwood Publishing Group; 2008. 3 vols.
4. Gupta PD, Lino A, Swarankar ML. Mothering a cause: practical knowledge of reproduction and motherhood. Bikaner: Capricorn Publishing House, 2010.
5. Condon RG. Birth seasonality, photoperiod, and social change in the Central Canadian Arctic. Human ecology. 1991;19:287-321.
6. The Assisted Reproductive Technology (Regulation) Act, 2021. [Internet]. [cited 2024 Feb 10]. Available from:https://thc.nic.in/Central%20Governmental%20Acts/Assisted%20Reproductive%20Technology%20(Regulation)%20Act,2021.pdf.
7. The Surrogacy (Regulation) Act, 2021. [cited 2024 Feb 10]. Available from: https://thc.nic.in/Central%20Governmental%20Acts/Assisted%20Reproductive%20Technology%20(Regulation)%20Act,2021.pdf.
8. The Surrogacy (Regulation) Rules, 2022. [cited 2024 Feb 11]. Available from: https://thc.nic.in/Central%20Governmental%20Rules/Surrogacy%20(Regulation)%20Rules,%202022.pdf.
9. The Surrogacy (Regulation) Amendment Rules, 2024 [cited 2024 Feb 18]. Available from: https://egazette.gov.in/WriteReadData/2024/252270.pdf.
10. Gianaroli L, Plachot M, van Kooij R, Al-Hasani S, Dawson K, DeVos A, Magli MC, Mandelbaum J, Selva J, van Inzen W. ESHRE guidelines for good practice in IVF laboratories. Human Reproduction. 2000;15(10):2241-6.
11. Cohen J, Gilligan A, Willadsen S. Culture and quality control of embryos. Hum Reprod. 1998;13(Suppl 3):137-44.
12. The American Society for Reproductive Medicine. Revised Guidelines for Human Embryology and Andrology Laboratories. Fertil Steril. 2008;90: S45-59.
13. Boone WR, Johnson JE, Locke AJ, Crane MM 4th, Price TM. Control of air quality in an assisted reproductive technology laboratory. Fertil Steril. 1999;71:150-4.
14. Abramczuk JW, Lopata A. Incubator performance in the clinical in vitro fertilization program: importance of temperature conditions for the fertilization and cleavage of human oocytes. Fertil Steril. 1986;46:132-4.

15. Meintjes M, Chantlis SJ, Douglas JD, Rodriguez AJ, Guerami AR, Bookout DM, Barnett BD, Madden JD. A controlled randomized trial evaluating the effect of lowered incubator oxygen tension on live births in a predominantly blastocyst transfer program. Hum Reprod. 2009;24(2): 300-7.
16. Wiemer KE, Anderson A, Stewart B. The importance of water quality for media preparation. Hum Reprod. 1998;13(Suppl 4): 166-72.
17. Balaban B, Urman B, Ata B, Isiklar A, Larman MG, Hamilton R, Gardner DK. A randomized controlled study of human Day 3 embryo cryopreservation by slow freezing or vitrification: vitrification is associated with higher survival, metabolism and blastocyst formation. Hum Reprod. 2008;23(9):1976-82.
18. Kastrop P. Quality management in the ART laboratory. Reprod Biomed Online. 2003;7: 691-4.
19. Pool TB. Practices contributing to quality performance in the embryo laboratory and the status of laboratory regulation in the US. Hum Reprod. 1997;12:2591-3.

SECTION 6

Medicolegal Issues in Obstetrics

CHAPTER 14

Medicolegal Aspects of Cesarean Delivery

Ritu Sharma, Pinky Mishra

INTRODUCTION

Advancement of healthcare system and the strengthened National Health Mission with initiatives like JSSK (*Janani Shishu Suraksha Karyakaram*) and JSY (*Janani Suraksha Yojna*), have increased the number of institutional deliveries in India. This has improved both the maternal and perinatal outcome. Improvement in surgical and anesthesia procedures supported with blood bank facilities and antimicrobials have made cesarean section a safe mode of delivery. Early diagnosis of complications and timely management/referral; changes in the population profile like advanced maternal age, obesity, medical complications, assisted reproduction have contributed to increase in the cesarean delivery rates.

Rates of cesarean deliveries in India, as reported by National family health surveys-4 (2015–2016), has doubled from 9 to 17.2% over a decade. Amongst them, 55% of cesarean sections were decided before the onset of labor pains. Higher cesarean rates have shown association with primigravidas (24%), higher level of education (28%), higher socioeconomic status (36%), private facilities (41%) and urban settings (28%).[1] WHO advocates universal adoption of Robson's classification system for cesarean delivery so as to keep a check on overall cesarean rate.[2]

No doubt cesarean delivery has improved the fetomaternal outcome but the risks associated with cesarean, being a major surgical procedure, should not be underestimated emphasizing its judicious use. As per WHO report increasing cesarean rates beyond 10% at population level has not shown further reduction in fetomaternal mortality; to achieve a specific target rate, the women in need should not be denied cesarean delivery; and considering socioeconomic factors and associated morbidity, it is difficult to recommend ideal cesarean rate for a given population, thereby challenging its previous recommendation of ideal cesarean rate of 10–15% where only mortality was taken into account. The study also emphasized that the benefits of cesarean delivery are maximized in medically indicated cases only.[3,4]

After inclusion of medical services under the ambit of the Consumer Protection Act, *defensive obstetrics* for the fear of litigation has significantly contributed to the rise in cesarean rates. Defensive medicine is defined as doctor's deviation from standard medical practice brought about by threat of liability.[5,6] WHO also recognizes the association of '*fear of litigation*' with rise in cesarean section rates.[7] Involvement of two lives (mother and fetus) in Obstetrics, and generalized perception that there is no risk associated with labor, denying its dynamic character, has led to the practice of defensive Obstetrics. It is advisable that, in order to avoid the lawsuits, the Obstetricians should follow the principles of ethics, good communication, counseling and proper documentation.

MEDICOLEGAL ASPECTS ASSOCIATED WITH CESAREAN SECTIONS

For the sake of understanding the medicolegal aspects associated with cesarean sections, the indications for cesarean sections are discussed under the following three categories:

1. Medically indicated cesarean delivery
2. Refusal of medically indicated cesarean delivery
3. Cesarean delivery on maternal request (CDMR)

MEDICALLY INDICATED CESAREAN DELIVERY

Medically indicated cesarean sections are done for fetomaternal indications where risk-benefit ratio favors cesarean delivery over vaginal delivery. Some indications are absolute (cephalopelvic disproportion, severe degrees of placenta previa, etc.) while some are relative (meconium, previous cesarean delivery, etc.). Medically indicated cesarean delivery can be planned electively or in an emergency. Cesarean delivery, even if medically indicated is not without associated short-term and long-term complications (sepsis, hemorrhage, visceral injuries, neonatal respiratory distress; placenta accreta, risk of uterine rupture in subsequent delivery, subfertility, etc.).[2]

While performing an indicated surgery, one should always follow the medicolegal principles, viz, professional ethics, evidence-based practice as per clinical guidelines, diligent and reasonable care, respecting patient's autonomy and shared decision regarding plan of care, informed consent, and documentation.

How to Avoid Medical Negligence Lawsuit?

In order to avoid any medical negligence lawsuits, before proceeding with cesarean delivery, the surgeon must have a justifiable reply to the following medicolegal queries:

- Is the hospital equipped for conducting cesarean delivery *(infrastructure)*?
- Am I familiar with the process of *informed consent*?
- Am I well versed with medicolegal aspects of *intraoperative/postoperative complications*?

Infrastructure

Cesarean section, being a major operation, should be performed in a hospital with *well-equipped, and functional operational theater* having all necessary requirements for safe surgery (*experienced anesthesiologist and OT staff, equipment, medicines, blood arrangement, ICU facility, if required*) as well as newborn resuscitation arrangements. The facility should *have a blood bank* or at least should have access to a nearby blood bank, if need arises. It is preferable to cross-match blood/blood products for all patients undergoing cesarean delivery considering unpredictability of the requirement, but in high-risk cases like antepartum hemorrhage, severe anemia, etc. it is must. However, in certain emergency conditions (like acute fetal distress with otherwise low-risk pregnancy) obstetrician may proceed without blood provided the information has been conveyed to the patient and attendants and informed consent has been taken.[8] It is preferable that the ICU facility is available within the hospital. In case the ICU facility is not available within the premises of the hospital, then the hospital must be safe transport of patient to the nearby ICU in an ACLS ambulance.

A *multidisciplinary team* including skilled obstetrician, anesthetist, and a pediatrician along with other supporting nursing staff is a must. Performing cesarean delivery at a place, which is not adequately equipped in infrastructure and manpower amounts to negligence.

Informed Consent Procedure in Cesarean Delivery

Once LSCS has been decided, patients and her attendants should be briefed about the need for the procedure. This involves communication, informed consent and documentation. Good *communication skills* are the key element in the informed consent process. It should be done in the language she understands, avoiding medical jargons. Based on availability of evidence, the counseling for cesarean should be directive when it is the only medically reasonable option available; and non-directive when the indications are uncertain, thereby allowing the patient to make an informed decision regarding either mode of delivery with their merits and demerits.[9] Adherence to the standard guidelines and ignoring self-interest is expected from the Obstetrician-Gynecologist during the counseling.

It is recommended to provide *adequate evidence-based information to help* them make a rationale decision as too much information may make them confuse or scare them. Due to lack of clear parameters for adequate information, there is a need for designing the consent forms for various surgical procedures by experts from national organizations. The obstetrician-gynecologist should provide reasonable information which must include present maternal-fetal condition, the mode of delivery planned and its indication, alternatives available, the risk benefit ratio of each procedure, associated high-risk maternal factors (anemia, diabetes, hypertension, obesity, etc.) and their consequences, anticipated and unforeseen complications that may arise intra-operatively (visceral injuries, excessive blood loss, need for hysterectomy) or postoperatively (sepsis, wound infections), prior consent for any additional surgical procedure if need arise (like hysterectomy in case of suspected uterine rupture or adherent placenta), implications on future child bearing and adverse consequences of refusal of treatment should be well addressed. If tubal ligation is desired, consent for the same in specific format should also be included; blood transfusion consent, if anticipated, to be taken. Consent for anesthesia is always taken separately from the surgical consent by anesthetist. It needs to be emphasized that favorable outcomes cannot be guaranteed in all cases. Consent should be procedure specific as all encompassing blanket consents are not acceptable legally. If a patient is examined or any procedure on her is observed for educational purpose; or we want to publish any case report or photographs in medical journals, a prior consent is mandatory.[10-12]

Informed consent is a dynamic process where the patient voluntarily and freely (free from coercion or undue influence) accepts an intervention or procedure after understanding its nature, associated risks and benefits and merits and demerits of the available alternative options. If the patient refuses the recommended medical treatment, this will be termed as *informed refusal*. Patient should ideally write down and sign the consent herself which should be countersigned by the doctor and two witnesses with proper mentioning of date and time. Unilaterally executed consents are void. In case a patient is unable to sign, her

Format for Cesarean Section Consent

(Separate consent to be taken for anesthesia)

The consent should include the following:

1. Patient's particular
2. Details of procedure-indication, risks and benefits of the procedure
3. Alternative option of vaginal delivery with associated risks and benefits pertaining for the given situation
4. Associated high risk factors, if any and their consequences
5. Mention anticipated and unforeseen complications which if occur will be managed as per standard guidelines
6. Consequences of refusing recommended cesarean section
7. Consent for blood transfusion, if anticipated
8. Additional consent of hysterectomy, depending upon the indication of cesarean section
9. Consent for tubal ligation if demanded
10. Implications on future child bearing (in CDMR especially)
11. Emphasize that the favorable outcome cannot be guaranteed in all cases
12. Additional consent for observing the procedure or taking photographs for educational purpose

Signature/thumb impression of patient/surrogate derision maker

Name

Witness:	Name	Signature	
1.			
2.			
Doctor:	Designation	Name	Signature
Date		Time	

Fig. 1: Sample of consent form for cesarean delivery.

left thumb impression can be taken where witnessed consents become even more legally dependable.[13-15] A sample consent form is displayed in **Figure 1**.

Legally and ethically patient reserves the right to give the informed consent, provided she is decisionally capable which can be determined by her mental acquity, comprehension, age (major >18 years) and state of consciousness.[16] In case of doubt, proxy consent of her near relative or lawful guardian can be taken and the person giving consent is known as surrogate decision maker.[17] In case of absence of any relative and patient being decisionally incapable, surgeon may proceed with presumptive consent after informing hospital administration.[18]

Informed consent or refusal should be well documented. In consumer court, the complainant has to prove the negligence and in criminal court the obstetrician has to prove her/his innocence. In both the scenario well-documented records prove to be the savior. It should be remembered that if nothing was documented then nothing happened also.[17,19] The prenatal visits should be utilized to counsel the woman about the process of labor, its dynamic nature responsible for converting it into high risk abruptly without any warning and clearing her doubts, if any. This communication will help the woman in informed and shared decision making later on in case of emergency and this is known as preventive ethics approach.[9]

Intraoperative/Postoperative Complications

Negligence during a surgical procedure may be attributed by anesthetist, surgeon, or the assistant staff but the brunt is usually faced by the surgeon. Obstetrician-gynecologist may attract legal action due to acts of omission like failure to take informed consent and perform cesarean timely compromising fetomaternal outcome, improper postoperative care and follow-up advice; and acts of commission like accidentally leaving swabs/instruments in the abdomen, removing reproductive organs without consent, using infected instruments or causing some major complication which was not diagnosed well in time in preoperative or postoperative period. Only adhering to the guidelines and standard operating protocols can safeguard the obstetrician from litigation. It is important that all complications should be disclosed with the patient and attendant and mentioned in the records.[20] Since a normal low-risk cesarean can abruptly become a high risk, unnecessary cesarean section should be avoided.

It is advisable to take consent for any anticipated change in surgical plan or any additional surgery depending on individual case before starting the cesarean itself as additional consent on table, even if patient is under regional anesthesia, will not be considered valid due to the presumption that under influence of anesthesia drugs and stress of surgery, patient is not decisionally capable. Only in life-threatening situations, one can proceed with additional consent from surrogate decision maker and involving second obstetrician in decision making.[18]

Practice Points

- In case the facility lacks the pre-requisites for conducting cesarean delivery, it is advisable to refer woman to an adequately equipped facility timely.
- Consent should be procedure specific. Consent is not valid if it is blanket, not voluntary and free or taken from a decisionally incapable patient.
- Patient herself is empowered to give or refute consent (by exercising her power of autonomy). In case of decisionally incapable patient, one may proceed with proxy consent and in case of life-threatening conditions presumptive consent is permitted.
- Ideally the informed consent should be taken by the concerned obstetrician-gynecologist as the interpretation and understanding may vary otherwise. An assistant doctor is also allowed to take the consent if required.[21-23]
- In the case of procedures compromising the reproductive functions (hysterectomy, sterilization operation) apart from patient, consent of spouse is advisable though may not be legally required.[12]
- Additional consent on the table is not considered valid; hence it is advisable to take consent for any additional anticipated surgery beforehand depending on the individual case.
- Only adhering to the guidelines and standard operating protocols can safeguard the obstetrician from litigation.
- Informed consent, surgical procedure, any complication and its management—all need to be properly documented, which will be the only evidence acceptable before law.

REFUSAL OF MEDICALLY INDICATED CESAREAN DELIVERY: MEDICOLEGAL ASPECTS

The cesarean section is indicated for either fetal indications or maternal indications. The ethical issues emerge when the woman refuses medically indicated cesarean leading to adverse outcomes or endangering the life of fetus, or herself or both.[24] The Obstetrician-Gynecologist in such circumstances remains in a dilemma due the conflict arising between patient's autonomy and the fetal rights as well as the obstetrician's professional integrity and conscience. Obstetricians may be worried regarding the adverse outcome due to refusal and the resulting legal issues that may emerge.

Ethical analysis of all fetomaternal issues depends on how the maternal-fetal dyad is conceptualized—either as one patient or as two separate patients. Usually, the maternal and fetal interests are common, the problems arise when their interests diverge. In these situations, the Obstetrician-Gynecologist's primary responsibility is towards the pregnant woman.[24,25] One may say that obstetrician has beneficence and nonmalificence-based obligation towards the mother and beneficence-based motivation towards her fetus. Any fetal intervention will affect mother's bodily integrity and health and therefore her informed consent is the pre-requisite for the same. Forced compliance interfering with patient's autonomy and bodily integrity raises ethical concerns.[26,27]

Informed consent plays a pivotal role in informed and voluntary decision making in such emergency conditions. The obstetrician plays an active role via directive counseling but should refrain from coercion or threats to influence her decision as this may invite legal action. The first and foremost step to deal with such a scenario is to understand the reasons for her refusal to recommended cesarean like social and cultural issues, financial burden, fear of surgery, past traumatic experience, concerns related to future reproductive problems, language barriers and poor understanding of the seriousness of the situation. It is the prime responsibility of the Obstetrician-Gynecologist to provide her accurate and evidence-based information in understandable language and answer her all queries. Involvement of multidisciplinary team (neonatologist, anesthetist, intensivist, social worker, nursing staff as well as her family members) further aids counseling. Effective open and non-judgmental communication skills can do wonders to persuade her to reconsider the decision.

If even after extensive counseling the woman continue to refuse the medically indicated cesarean, document her informed refusal including the need for recommended treatment with its benefits and risks, the available alternative options with their risks and benefits, the reason for refusal and its consequences. The institutional ethics committee should be approached to resolve the issue. The involvement of court is discouraged as there is no such compulsion for Obstetrician-Gynecologist and it may sometimes worsen the situation further instead of improving upon due to the prognostic uncertainty, thereby threatening the patient-obstetrician relationship.[24,28]

It is emphasized that like non-pregnant woman, a pregnant woman reserves the right to refuse unwanted medical interventions, right to bodily integrity and privacy and her decision must be paramount. If the decisional capacity of mother is questionable, psychiatry consultation may be required and seeking a surrogate decision maker (husband, family member, guardian) is permitted. In dire emergency where the patient is decisionally incapable of giving consent due to her present condition, her preference is unknown and there is unavailability of surrogate decision maker, presumptive consent may be used.[8,29] Though there are no universal recommendations for managing such complex situations, obstetrician-gynecologist should follow the ethics principle-based practice points, respecting woman's autonomy being the core principle.

Practice Points

- Decisionally capable pregnant woman's autonomy to refuse medically indicated cesarean should be respected.
- The first step to deal with this scenario is to understand patient's perspective and try to counsel and educate her accordingly and ensure her understanding of relevant consequences of refusal.
- Team approach involving neonatologist, anesthetist, intensivist, social worker, nursing staff as well as her family members will be helpful in resolving the issue.
- Use of coercion to influence the woman's decision is neither ethically permissible nor medically advisable in view of prognostic uncertainty, i.e., inability to guarantee that the intervention will definitely benefit the fetus and will not harm the mother.
- Document her informed refusal in medical records with her signatures countersigned by two witnesses and doctor.
- The institutional ethics committee should be approached regarding resolution of the conflict.
- In case of non-performance of life-saving surgery citing the informed refusal by the patient or the authorized representative as the reason, two doctors should document and confirm the same and the hospital administration should be informed.[10]
- ACOG discourages involving court-ordered interventions in managing such cases.
- In case of adverse outcome due to refusal of medically indicated cesarean, support in the form of resources and counseling to be provided to both the woman as well as the obstetrician-gynecologist.

CESAREAN DELIVERY ON MATERNAL REQUEST: MEDICOLEGAL ASPECTS

Cesarean delivery on maternal request (CDMR) is defined as the primary cesarean delivery performed primarily on maternal request and not in view of any valid fetomaternal indication.[30] It is estimated that in United States, CDMR contributes to 2.5% of all births, however its exact global contribution to the rising cesarean rate is unknown due to scarcity of data. The panel of experts at the National Institute of Health concluded that in absence of any valid fetomaternal indication, the paucity of data comparing planned vaginal delivery with CDMR does not provide basis for recommending either of them.[31]

When the evidence is uncertain, medical ethics and patient values need to be considered. In recent decades, medical ethics in obstetrics has been dominated by principle-based ethics approach including—autonomy, beneficence, non-malfeasance and justice to address ethical issues.[32,33]

Beneficence and Nonmaleficence-based Considerations[30,34-36]

The ethical principle of beneficence obligates the obstetrician-gynecologist to promote the benefits to the woman and that of nonmaleficence obligates not to harm the woman, thereby striking a greater balance of clinical goods over clinical harms in patient care. Beneficence and patient's autonomy may conflict with each other. The benefits of performing cesarean delivery on maternal request (reduced risk of urinary incontinence, pelvic organ prolapse, intrapartum hypoxia, birth injuries, stillbirth, etc.) have low level of evidence. Also as earlier discussed, the procedure is not without the surgical risks and risk of negative impact on future reproductive outcomes (adherent placenta, risk of uterine rupture, etc.). So, at present there is insufficient evidence to recommend CDMR over planned vaginal delivery for maternal or neonatal outcomes.

Justice-based Considerations[37,38]

Justice is the process of fair allocation of benefits and burdens expecting a fair outcome, i.e., there should be proportionate benefit to the burdened individual—the substantive justice. Justice explicates the ethical significance of the number of patients that need to be treated to produce a clinical benefit. To prevent a single morbidity resulting from vaginal delivery—one case of cerebral palsy due to intrapartum hypoxia or one fetal death from umbilical cord accidents, thousands of cesarean deliveries would be required which is neither acceptable nor justified as the substantive justice is not fulfilled.

Autonomy-based Considerations[37,38]

Autonomy is derived from a Greek word "autos + nomos" which means "self- rule"; and gives woman right to make an informed decision. Patients' autonomy should be respected.

When a patient requests a cesarean, physician has obligations to enquire about the reason behind her request and offer medically reasonable alternatives to help in making informed decisions. If CDMR is based on fear of labor pain, poor obstetrical experience, personal values and cultural context, proper counseling related to the factors responsible for past experience, availability of labor analgesia and providing emotional support can help her in reconsidering the decision.[39] While discussing CMDR, women should be asked about her future reproductive plans, explained the expected rate of unplanned pregnancies and advised to give due consideration to the risk of uterine rupture and placental abnormalities given the high rate of cesarean in subsequent pregnancies; while deciding for CDMR.[40] If the patient still insists for CDMR, document the *informed consent* ensuring that the patient is apprised and fully understands the consequences. It is then ethically permissible to acknowledge her request. ACOG recommends such cesarean deliveries to be performed after 39 weeks only if no other reason for early delivery exists.[9,30]

Professional integrity gives obstetricians the right to refuse autonomy-based decisions, especially when it could not be supported by beneficence and justice-based considerations. Striking a balance between the obstetrician's conscience and professional ethics is of utmost importance to ensure that patient's wellbeing is not compromised. The three principles—beneficence, justice and autonomy-based considerations do not support routine recommendation of CDMR.[9,30]

Practice Points

- Both ACOG and FIGO recommend vaginal delivery in the absence of fetal or maternal indications for cesarean delivery.[9,30]
- Whenever a woman requests cesarean delivery, obstetrician-gynecologist should respect her autonomy and should

not disregard her request in first instance; instead should enquire regarding the reason behind her choice and counsel her accordingly.

- Discussing about her future reproductive plans and consequences of CDMR may aid her in reconsidering the decision.
- If the patient still insists on CDMR, document the informed consent. It is ethically permissible to acknowledge her request after 39 weeks only in absence of any other indication.[9,30]
- However, if obstetrician-gynecologist, whose consciences does not allow him/her in conducting CDMR, is free to refuse to honor the patient's request exercising his/her own professional autonomy and refer the patient timely to other center without any further argument respecting patient's autonomy.[41]

REFERENCES

1. International Institute for Population Sciences (IIPS) and ICF, 2017. National Family Health Survey (NFHS-4), 2015-16: India. Mumbai: IIPS.
2. WHO Statement on Caesarean Section Rates. Geneva: World Health Organization; 2015 (WHO/RHR/15.02).
3. Betran AP, Torloni MR, Zhang J, et al. What is the optimal rate of caesarean section at population level? A systematic review of ecologic studies. Reprod Health. 2015;12(1):57.
4. Ye J, Zhang J, Mikolajczyk R, et al. Association between rates of caesarean section and maternal and neonatal mortality in the 21st century: a worldwide population-based ecological study with longitudinal data. BJOG. 2016;123:745-53.
5. Hershey N. The defensive practice of medicine: myth or reality. Milbank Mem Fund Q. 1972;50:69-98.
6. Klingman D, Localio AR, Sugarman J, et al. Measuring defensive medicine using clinical scenario surveys. J Health Polit Policy Law. 1996;21(2):185-217.
7. Zwecker P, Azoulay L, Abenhaim HA. Effect of fear of litigation on obstetric care: a nationwide analysis on obstetric practice. Am J Perinatol. 2011;28(4):277-84.
8. FOGSI GCPR. Consensus statement for cesarean section. Reviewed at the Consensus group meeting at Amby Valley, July, 2014.
9. FIGO Ethics and Professionalism Guideline: Decision Making about Vaginal and Caesarean Delivery. FIGO Statement 26 June, 2020.
10. Waisel DB. Legal aspects of anesthesia care. In: Miller RD, Eriksson LI, Fleisher LA, Wiener-Kronish JP, Young WL (Eds). Miller's Anesthesia, 7th edition. Philadelphia USA: Churchill Livingstone, Elsevier; 2010. pp. 221-33.
11. Satyanarayana Rao KH. Informed consent: an ethical obligation or legal compulsion? J Cutan Aesthet Surg. 2008;1:33-5.
12. Indian Medical Council (Professional Conduct, Etiquette and Ethics) Regulations, 2002. Published in Part-III, Section 4 of the Gazette of India, dated 6th April, 2002, Amended up to December; 2010.
13. Jonsen AR, Siegler M, Winslade WJ. Clinical ethics: a practical approach to ethical decisions in clinical medicine, 6th edition. New York (NY): McGraw-Hill; 2006.
14. Bastia BK, Kuruvilla A, Saralaya KM. Validity of consent: a review of statutes. Indian J Med Sci. 2005;59:74-8.
15. Bastia BK. Consent to treatment: practice vis-à-vis principle. Indian J Med Ethics. 2008;5:113-4.
16. Grisso T, Appelbaum PS. Assessing competence to consent to treatment: a guide for physicians and other health professionals. New York (NY): Oxford University Press; 1998.
17. Trivedi LK. Consent: Does it concern? In: Malhotra J, Patel MC, Goel RN, Malhotra N (Eds). FOGSI Focus Medicolegal Issues in Obstetrics and Gynecology practice, 1st edition. New Delhi: Jaypee Brothers Medical Publishers. 2018. pp. 45-7.

18. Kumar A, Mullick P, Prakash S, et al. Consent and the Indian Medical Practitioner. Indian J Anaesth. 2015;59:695-700.
19. Mathioudakis A, Rousalova I, Gagnat AA, et al. How to keep good clinical records? Breathe. 2016;12:371-5.
20. Sharma RK. Legal issues in surgical practice and death on operation table. In: Sharma RK (Ed). How to face medical negligence in clinical practice? Institute of Medicolegal Publication, 1st edition. Noida; 2019. pp. 57-8.
21. Moore GP, Moffet PM, Fider C, et al. What emergency physicians should know about informed consent: legal scenarios, cases, and caveats? Acad Emerg Med. 2014;21(8):922-7.
22. Sharma G, Bhatt H. Consents in Obstetrics and Gynaecology. Mumbai: B & S Medicolegal Consultancies; 2013.
23. Sharma G. Consent in medical context. In: Malhotra J, Mittal P, Rajaram S, Bharti R (Eds). FOGSI Focus Surgical Skills in Obstetrics and Gynecology. New Delhi: Jaypee Brothers Medical Publishers. 2018. pp. 6-8.
24. Refusal of Medically Recommended Treatment During Pregnancy. ACOG Committee Opinion No. 664 American College of Obstetricians and Gynecologists' Committee on Ethics. Obstet Gynecol. 2016 (reaffirmed 2019);127(6):e175-82.
25. Lyerly AD, Little MO, Faden RR. A critique of the 'fetus as patient'. Am J Bioeth. 2008;8:42-4.
26. Informed consent. ACOG Committee Opinion No. 439. American College of Obstetricians and Gynecologists. Obstet Gynecol. 2009;114:401-8.
27. Maternal-fetal intervention and fetal care centers. Committee Opinion No. 501. American College of Obstetricians and Gynecologists. Obstet Gynecol. 2011;118:405-10.
28. Deshpande NA, Oxford CM. Management of pregnant patients who refuse medically indicated cesarean delivery. Rev Obstet Gynecol. 2012;5(314):e144-50.
29. Moskop JC. Informed consent in the emergency department. Emerg Med Clin North Am. 1999;17:327–40, ix–x.
30. Cesarean Delivery on Maternal Request. ACOG Committee Opinion No. 761. Obstet Gynecol. 2019;133(1):e73-e77. doi: 10.1097/AOG.0000000000003006. PMID: 30575678.
31. NIH State-of-the-Science Conference Statement on cesarean delivery on maternal request. NIH Consens State Sci Statements. 2006;23:1-29. Available at: https://consensus.nih.gov/2006/cesarean.htm.
32. Campell AV. The virtues (and vices) of the four principles. J Med Ethics. 2003;29:292-6.
33. Beauchamp TL, Childress JF. Principles of biomedical ethics, 5th edition. New York (NY): Oxford University Press; 2001.
34. Rortveit G, Daltveit AK, Hannestad YS, et al. Urinary Incontinence after vaginal delivery or cesarean section. N Engl J Med. 2003;348:900-7.
35. Gonen R, Tamir A, Degani S. Obstetricians' opinions regarding patient choice in cesarean delivery. Obstet Gynecol. 2002;99:577- 80.
36. Groom KM, Paterson-Brown S, Fisk NM. Temporal and Geographical Variation in UK Obstetricians' Personal Preference regarding Mode of Delivery. Eur J Obstet Gynecol Reprod Biol. 2002;100:185-8.
37. Minkoff H, Powderly KR, Chervenak F, et al. Ethical dimensions of elective primary cesarean delivery. Obstet Gynecol. 2004;103(2):387-92.
38. Ethical Decision Making in Obstetrics and Gynecology. ACOG Committee Opinion No. 390. Obstet Gynecol. 2007;110(6):1479-87. doi: 10.1097/01.AOG.0000291573.09193.36.
39. Obstetric Analgesia and Anesthesia. Practice Bulletin No. 177. American College of Obstetricians and Gynecologists. Obstet Gynecol. 2017;129:e73-89.
40. Keeton K, Zikmund-Fisher BJ, Ubel PA, et al. The accuracy of predicting parity as a prerequisite for cesarean delivery on maternal request. Obstet Gynecol. 2008;112: 285-9.
41. The Limits of Conscientious Refusal in Reproductive Medicine. ACOG Committee Opinion No. 385. American College of Obstetricians and Gynecologists. Obstet Gynecol. 2007;110:1203-8.

CHAPTER 15

Medicolegal Aspects of Antenatal Care and Fetal Monitoring

Sunil K Juneja, Pawneet Kaur

INTRODUCTION

Pregnancy is one of the most cherished moments in a woman's life. A normal ongoing pregnancy may or may not have a smooth course. A pregnancy which is running smoothly may end with disastrous result. To prevent any mishap, antenatal care is being provided to all the pregnant women to have a smooth sailing to get a healthy mother and healthy baby after delivery. Antenatal care and fetal monitoring are governed by several clinical, legal, and ethical considerations. Healthcare providers have a legal obligation to provide safe and competent care to their patients. They are also required to adhere to established standards of care and maintain accurate and complete medical records. Failure to provide appropriate care or document the care provided can lead to malpractice claims against the healthcare provider or facility. This chapter serves to discuss the medico-legal aspects of antenatal care and fetal monitoring.

WHO defines antenatal care (ANC) as the care provided by skilled healthcare professionals to pregnant women aiming to ensure the best health conditions for both mother and baby during pregnancy.[1] Antenatal care is a type of preventive healthcare. It refers to a comprehensive antepartum program which involves a coordinated approach to medical care, continuous risk assessment and psychosocial support that optimally begins before pregnancy and extends throughout the postpartum and inter-pregnancy period (ACOG 2017).

ANC helps in preventing and reducing maternal and fetal morbidity and mortality. Antenatal period not only provides a platform for health promotion, screening and diagnosis but also helps in disease prevention and exercising timely and appropriate evidence-based practices.[1]

AIM OF ANTENATAL CARE

- To maintain the physiology of pregnancy as near to the normal as possible
- To identify any high-risk factor and appropriate management.
- To prevent the development of any complications and to treat if any arises.
- To decrease maternal and fetal mortality and morbidity
- To remove the stress and worries of the mother regarding the delivery process.
- To teach the mother about childcare, nutrition, sanitation and hygiene.
- To advise about family planning methods.

SALIENT FEATURES OF ANTENATAL CARE AND FETAL MONITORING

Early Detection of Pregnancy

To ensure adequate care to pregnant women, fetal growth and development and safe delivery, early detection of pregnancy is necessary. It should be undertaken as early as possible after the first missed period using urine pregnancy kits.[5]

Early Antenatal Visit and Pregnancy Registration

All pregnancies are to be registered according to WHO and Indian NHM guidelines.[1,2] First visit for seeking antenatal care must be planned in first trimester and as early as possible after the missed periods.

General Considerations for Antenatal Care

Number of Antenatal Visits:

- *Indian Guidelines*: As per Indian guidelines, minimum four antenatal check-ups should be ensured for every pregnant woman as per the schedule below:
  1st visit: Within 12 weeks, preferably as soon as pregnancy is suspected
  2nd visit: Between 14–26 weeks
  3rd visit: Between 28–36 weeks
  4th visit: Between 36 weeks and term.[2]
- *WHO Antenatal Care Model*: According to the new WHO Antenatal Care Model, the number of antenatal visits a pregnant women should have with healthcare provider, have been increased to eight. It recommends the first visit in the first 12 weeks and subsequent contacts at 20, 26, 30, 34, 36, 38, and 40 weeks in order to detect complications, improve communication, increase positive birth experience and prevent stillbirth.[4]
- *NICE 2021 guidelines:* According to NICE 2021 guidelines, for nulliparous women, 10 routine antenatal appointments are recommended. For multiparous women, seven routine antenatal appointments are recommended.[3]

History Taking and Documentation: Detailed history taking and documentation in the case sheets of pregnant lady has immense clinical as well as medicolegal significance. Obtain history in detail, which should include the following:

- Take menstrual history, ask LMP and calculate EDD, prepare a birth plan.
- Stillbirth or neonatal loss, abortions, obstructed labor, premature births, twins, or multiple pregnancies, mode of delivery, weight of the previous baby, admission for hypertension or pre-eclampsia/eclampsia in the previous pregnancy, congenital anomaly· Ask whether the baby cried immediately after birth or not, sex of baby. weight of the baby, duration of breastfeeding, immunization status of baby and anti-D given to mother or not, if baby was Rh-positive.
- Treatment for infertility
- Rh-negative in the previous pregnancy
- Birth interval
- History of consanguineous marriage
- Ask about general health and wellbeing and symptoms if any.
- *Normal symptoms during pregnancy*: Nausea and vomiting, heartburn, constipation, and increased frequency of urination.[3]
- Discuss pre-existing medical, surgical, or mental health issues and family history.
- Take history of any drug abuse, alcohol and tobacco intake, medication intake, exposure to X-rays, any fever with rash.

Examination (At every visit):

- General physical examination (look for pallor, jaundice, pedal edema)
- Record pulse rate, respiratory rate, temperature, blood pressure, weight, height, and calculate BMI.
- Look for the sign and symptoms of hypothyroidism like-feeling tired,

funable-to-tolerate cold temperatures, hoarse voice, swelling of the face, weight gain, constipation, skin and hair changes, including dry skin and loss of eyebrows, carpal tunnel syndrome (hand tingling or pain), slow heart rate, muscle cramps and irregular menstrual periods.

- *Breast examination:* Palpate for any lump or tenderness, identify inverted or flat nipples and correct accordingly.
- *Abdominal examination:*
  1. Measure and record fundal height and abdominal girth to monitor the progress of pregnancy and fetal growth
  2. Check for fetal lie and presentation
  3. Assess uterine tone
  4. Auscultate fetal heart sounds
- *Vaginal examination:* if indicated (pain abdomen, leaking per vaginum, discharge per vaginum, etc.)[2]

Laboratory investigations: According to GOI 2021, the following lab investigations are recommended to be undertaken at *first visit* for ANC assessment:

- Pregnancy detection test
- Hemoglobin test
- Complete urine analysis—urine test for albumin and sugar, pus cells and casts
- Blood sugar testing
- Testing for Malaria if the woman complains of fever with chills
- HIV (Antibodies to HIV-1 and 2)
- RDT for HBsAg
- RDT for syphilis
- Hb electrophoresis or HPLC for HbA2[2]
- *Ultrasonography:* According to WHO, an ultrasound scan is recommended before 24 weeks of gestation to estimate gestational age, detection of fetal anomalies and to reduce induction of labor for post-term pregnancies.[4]

According to NICE 2021, an ultrasound scan should be offered:

a. Between 11+2 weeks and 14+1 weeks to:
   - Determine gestational age
   - Detect multiple pregnancy
   - Screen for Down's syndrome, Edwards' syndrome and Patau's syndrome (if opted)

b. Between 18+0 weeks and 20+6 weeks to screen fetal anomalies and determine placental location

c. At 28 weeks, offer a blood test to check full blood count, blood group and antibodies and give anti-D prophylaxis to rhesus-negative women

d. Offer screening for GDM at first antenatal visit and then at 24–28 weeks of gestation.

WHO recommends counseling about healthy eating and promotion of physical activity during pregnancy.[4]

At each antenatal visit, update antenatal records including history details, test results, medicines, examination findings and follow-up plan.

Prophylaxis during pregnancy: According to GOI (2021):

- Folic Acid (500 μg) during 1st trimester—to prevent neural tube defects in fetus.[2]
- *Iron folic acid (IFA):* 60 mg of elemental Iron and 0.5 mg folic acid in second and third trimester of pregnancy for 6 months.[2]
- *Injection tetanus toxoid (TT):* 0.5 mL, 2 injections one month apart or one booster (IM in upper arm) to prevent maternal and neonatal tetanus.[2]
- *Tablet Calcium 500 mg and 250 IU Vitamin D3:* One tablet twice a day (total 1 g calcium daily) from second trimester (14 weeks) onwards throughout pregnancy.[2]
- Tablet Albendazole (Deworming) 400 mg one tablet once only after 12 weeks of

gestation for worm infestation and to prevent anemia and malnutrition.
- WHO also recommends daily oral iron and folic acid supplementation with 30–60 mg of elemental iron and 0.4 mg of folic acid.[1]

Antenatal Counseling: All pregnant mothers need to be counseled for the following:
- Birth preparedness for safe institutional delivery
- Early identification of complications—recognizing danger signs during pregnancy, labor and after delivery/abortion
- Nutritional counseling
- Importance of Breastfeeding
- Sex during pregnancy
- Prevention of domestic violence
- Post-natal family planning

Fetal Monitoring

Fetal monitoring is an essential component of pregnancy management. The primary goal of fetal monitoring is to assess the fetal well-being in utero, interpret the fetal monitoring results and early intervention to prevent stillbirth and birth defects.

1. *Fetal monitoring techniques:* There are a number of fetal surveillance tests in clinical use which include maternal fetal movement count, contraction stress test, non-stress test, biophysical profile, modified biophysical profile and umbilical artery Doppler velocimetry.[6]
2. *When to begin fetal monitoring during antenatal period?*

According to ACOG 2021,[6] conditions in which antenatal fetal monitoring should be started are:
- *At the time of diagnosis:*
  - Growth restriction with umbilical artery Doppler—normal/increased or AEDF or REDF—at diagnosis
  - Dichorionic twins with fetal growth restriction
  - Decreased fetal movement
  - Poorly controlled maternal chronic hypertension
  - Preeclampsia with/without severe features
  - Complicated SLE/sickle cell disease
  - Intrahepatic cholestasis of pregnancy
  - Placental abruption/APH
  - Isolated oligohydramnios
- *32 weeks onwards:*
  - Uncomplicated twins—monochorionic-diamniotic
  - Chronic hypertension controlled with medications
  - Gestational diabetes controlled with medications/poorly controlled/pregestational diabetes
  - Uncomplicated medical conditions like—SLE/APLA/Sickle cell disease/renal disease
  - Previous stillbirth/FGR/preeclampsia—requiring preterm delivery
  - Polyhydramnios (moderate to severe)
- *36 weeks onwards:*
  - Single umbilical artery/velamentous cord insertion
  - Uncomplicated dichorionic twins
- *Individualized:*
  - Twins-complicated monochorionic-diamniotic (TTTS)
  - Twins—monoamniotic
  - Triplets and higher order multiple gestations
  - Hemoglobinopathies
  - Late term—41 weeks

RECENT ADVANCES IN ANTENATAL CARE AND FETAL MONITORING

The WHO antenatal care model 2016 is a set of guidelines for providing health care to pregnant women, designed by the World Health Organization (WHO). This model seeks to streamline antenatal care and standardize best practices across the world.

Key Features of WHO Antenatal Care Model

1. The model recommends eight to 12 antenatal care visits, depending on a woman's individual needs and risk factors.
2. *Integrated care:* The model recommends that care providers integrate all aspects of antenatal care, including screening, diagnosis, treatment, health promotion, and counseling.
3. *Risk assessment:* The model recommends that care providers assess a woman's individual risk factors and adjust the frequency and intensity of antenatal care accordingly.
4. *Individualization:* The model emphasizes the importance of providing individualized care, based on a woman's cultural and social background and her individual needs and preferences.
5. *Continuity of care:* The model recommends that care providers ensure continuity of care throughout the antenatal period and establish a plan for postnatal care.

The WHO antenatal care model has been widely adopted and implemented in many countries around the world. The model has been shown to improve maternal and fetal outcomes, reduce perinatal mortality, and improve the quality of antenatal care overall.[1]

FDA has recently approved a fully remote, medical-grade maternal-fetal monitoring solution named INVU which is based on fetal and maternal echocardiography inputs. INVU is non-invasive, measures and displays FHR and MHR tracings via a sensor band worn by the mother which can be self-applied without the need of device repositioning by a professional. It passively collects multiple sources of physiological signals. During the reading, the mother can access personalized insights via a smartphone app, while her provider receives detailed data on maternal and fetal heart rate over time. INVU is indicated for use by low risk pregnant women who need fetal monitoring documentation at and beyond 32 weeks period of gestation.[10]

Points to Remember

1. If mother's blood group is Rh-negative, get done husband's blood group.
2. If Rh-negative mother has delivered earlier, get Rh-antibody titers (ICT).
3. If mother is not iso-immunized, give anti-D at 28 weeks.
4. Prescribe iron tablets and if patient is not taking, write on prescription that she is non-compliant.
5. Document the non-compliance on prescription slip if patient is not getting investigations done or does not follow-up for routine antenatal visits as scheduled.
6. If mother is thalassemia minor, get HPLC/HbA2 of father done and if father is also thalassemia minor, explain to the couple the risk of thalassemia major (25%) chances in the offspring and offer fetal screening test for thalassemia.
7. If any high-risk factor identified, document the clinical findings on each visit.
8. If pregnant women are VDRL or HIV reactive, get husband also tested. Treat the couple as appropriate.
9. If any invasive procedure is to be done during antenatal period, must document and get informed consent signed explaining all the possible risks and complications and give inj. Anti-D if mother is Rh negative and father positive.
10. If patient is hypothyroid, adjust the dosage of medications during pregnancy and routinely follow up with TSH. Get endocrinology or medicine consultation also.

11. If patient is with Gestational Diabetes Mellitus, involve endocrinologist in management protocol and explain all the risks to the patient.
12. Treat and document asymptomatic bacteriuria
13. In later weeks of pregnancy, tell the patient to note down the feral movements. Document Daily Fetal Movement Count on prescription (daily fetal movements perceived for 1 hour each—post-breakfast, post-lunch and post-dinner).
14. The pregnant women should be advised with documentation on prescription to report to you if there is decreased fetal movements, bleeding per vaginum, leaking per vaginum or pain abdomen.
15. If mother is more than 35 years explain the risk of down syndrome. Offer her dual test, quadruple test, NIPT and or amniocentesis as appropriate.
16. *Advise safe prenatal exercises under supervision of expert:*
    - *Pelvic floor exercise (Kegel's exercise):* Tighten the pelvic floor as if to lift the internal organs or to stop urination in mid-stream. Hold as tight as possible for a slow count of 3 (gradually work-up to count of 10) and then release. Repeat 3–4 times throughout the day, wherever possible.
    - *Wall slide squats:* Stand against the wall with feet slightly apart, slowly slide down and stay for 3–5 seconds and then slide up. Relax and repeat 5–10 times.
    - *Knee extension:* Sit in a relaxed comfortable position, slowly lift your leg and make your knee straight in line with the hip. Hold it for 15 seconds and bring it down. Repeat with alternate legs.
    - *Tailor sitting:* Sit on the floor with legs apart and heels together. You will feel a stretch in the inner side of your thighs. Hold for 5–10 seconds. Relax and repeat 5 times.
    - *Walking lunge:* Stand in a walking position, slowly go forward and down and come to the starting position. Repeat by alternating lunge with opposite legs.
    - *Step-ups:* Use a staircase or small stool. Go up, hold and come down slowly. Repeat with alternate legs.
    - *Wall press:* Stand facing a wall, with hands on the wall, slowly push your hands against the wall. Your upper body will move forward, and your shoulders will stretch backwards as if in normal push-ups. Inhale slowly and deeply as you move forward, hold with your stretch for 5–10 seconds. Relax and repeat 3–5 times.
    - *Neck rotation:* Sit in a relaxed comfortable position with your hand either on your lap over a pillow. Shoulders released. Move your neck upwards, downwards and to the side slowly and to a gentle rotation on both sides.
    - *Outer thigh lift:* Lying on your sides, slightly lift your leg to a comfortable range. Hold it for 3–5 seconds and slowly bring it down. Do 5–10 times and then turn to the other side and repeat.

DO'S AND DONT'S DURING PREGNANCY

Provide general instructions on diet, exercise, physical care, travel safety, etc. to the patients verbally as well as in the form of reading material.

Do's

- Continue usual activities
- Take sleep of 8 hours in night and 2 hours of rest in noon (preferably in left lateral position)
- Plenty of fluids
- Regular bath
- Wear loose comfortable clothes
- Take care of dental hygiene
- *Care of breast:* Retracted nipples need to be corrected in later months.
- For travelling, rail is preferred over bus. Avoid long journeys as long sitting can lead to venous stasis and thromboembolism. If travelling by car seatbelt should be below the abdomen. Air traveling may not be safe if patient is having placenta previa, preeclampsia, anemias and sickle cell anemia.

- Always prefer to have institutional delivery.

Dont's

- Avoid hard and strenuous work
- Coitus should be avoided during the first trimester and during the last 6 weeks.
- Travelling should be avoided, especially in the first trimester and during last 6 weeks. Air travelling is avoided after 32 weeks.
- Stop alcohol, active and passive smoking and any other drug abuse.
- No self-medication
- Do not wear high heels.

LEGAL PROVISIONS AND RELEVANT CASES RELATED TO ANTENATAL CARE AND FETAL MONITORING

Practices like documentation of findings, record keeping, patient counseling, timely intervention, informed and shared decision making not only prevents undue mistakes but also helps to defend the doctors in the court of law in case of a medicolegal complaint.

CASE 1: State of HP & Ors. vs. Dinesh Chauhan & Ors. on 29 March 2018[7]

Facts of the Case

On July 25, 1996, a primigravida presented to the Civil Hospital Solan with complaint of bleeding and was admitted in the evening by. The doctor was on duty, but the obstetrician did not attend her at that time and did not respond to the calls made by patient's relatives and performed the examination and ultrasound the next day when the fetus was found to be dead. Patient also died after delivery and was not timely referred to higher center. Lawsuit was filed by the husband of deceased women for the damages complaining that, had the gynecologist attended to the patient promptly and properly she and her baby would not have died.[7]

Patient's Allegation

Patient's husband alleged that patient had died due to carelessness of the obstetrician because had she examined patient well in time and given proper treatment, her life could have been saved. They accused that patient had died due to breach of duty on the part of the doctor as even despite emergency, the doctor did not attend her on time.[7]

Doctor's Defense

Doctor's defense was that patient was admitted and was under the care of other on duty doctor and she was only available during 9 AM to 5 PM according to roster. Despite not on call, she came to see the patient at night around 3:30 AM when the on-duty doctor called her for help and found that patient was in labor but fetal status could not be assessed. No ultrasound facility was available at night at civil hospital. She then again checked the patient at 9 AM when the ultrasound was done, and fetus was reported to be dead and a retroplacental clot was reported. She gave patient IV infusion, medications and blood transfusion which was available at the hospital. Patient delivered the dead baby and developed postpartum hemorrhage due to which she collapsed. The doctor also called an anesthetist, physician and surgeon on call who helped in resuscitation but the patient could not be revived. All the findings were documented on the patient's file and were produced in the court.

Findings of the Court

The court mentioned that the plaintiff has led no evidence to show that in what manner defendant obstetrician has not acted with standard of care, whereas defendant obstetrician has led sufficient evidence to show that she acted in accordance with the general and approved practice. Although it was said that the patient died in the hospital, but her death cannot be attributed to any laxity or negligence on the part of the doctors, attending to her, more particularly defendant obstetrician.[7]

CASE 2: B Dilip Reddy s/o B Sunder ... vs. Rainbow Children's Hospital & ... on 19 Jan 2018)[8]

Facts of the Case

The parents of the child filed a case against the treating doctors for not detecting fetal congenital forearm limb amputation in an antenatal period. During the course of periodical check-up and examinations, prenatal scanning for four times on the advice of opposite party was performed but all were reported normal with no gross fetal anomalies, however at birth, the male child was diagnosed to have right hand deformity. A legal notice to the doctors was served demanding to pay compensation worth ₹99,67,010 for prosthesis, not taking reasonable care and skill in the diagnosis of the fetal anomaly and giving wrong reports and loss of valuable time for correcting the deformity in the right hand of the child.[8]

Patient's Allegation

Child's parents filed a complaint against doctors for not providing reasonable care during antenatal period and missed the fetal anomaly.

Doctor's Defense

Doctors pleaded that the non-detection is not due to any omission of the doctors but due to a false negative in the ultrasound reports. There had been immediate postnatal detection of abnormality and the process of initiating the counseling by experts has been adopted along with appropriate multidisciplinary guidance towards rehabilitation. There are no treatments which can be done before the birth of the child/in the fetal stage and the complainants could not have done anything differently if the scan reports had stated the amputation of the right forearm. This treatment is possible only after the birth of the child and in the present case nothing was amiss in helping the complainant couple plan the treatment of the child after birth. The defect is part of a natural process which can rarely affect fetuses and is positively not caused by ultrasound scans.

Findings of the Court

The judgment stated that it is not sure that had the opposite parties detected the deformity they can rectify the problem successfully. It is not that due to the negligence of the opposite parties during delivery of the complainant, the child has become handicapped, but it is only due to structural or functional abnormalities present at birth that cause physical or mental disability.[8]

But looking into the negligence made by the opposite parties in not detecting the congenital deformity of the baby resulting which causing the complainants to undergo agony, the complainants are entitled to compensation of ₹5,00,000.[8]

CURRENT STATUS ON MATERNAL MORTALITY[9]

UNICEF has reported a decline in the global maternal mortality ratio (MMR) by 34% from 342 deaths to 223 deaths per 100,000 live births, according to UN interagency estimates from year 2000 to 2020. India is also thriving towards achieving the sustainable development goal (SDG) of 70 maternal deaths per 100,000 live births by 2030. In India, the MMR has dropped from 384 to 103 deaths per 1,00,000 live births over a period of 20 years. The credit goes to antenatal care being provided by the healthcare personnel in cutting down the maternal mortality rate.

CONCLUSION

Antenatal care and fetal monitoring are essential components of pregnancy management. Healthcare providers must be aware of the recent advances in clinical, legal, and ethical considerations surrounding these interventions to provide safe and competent care to their patients. Accurate and complete documentation of the care provided is essential to maintain a legal record and provide a strong defense in case of false accusation and legal claims.

REFERENCES

1. WHO Recommendations on Antenatal Care for a Positive Pregnancy Experience. Geneva: World Health Organization; 2016. PMID: 28079998.
2. Training Manual on Care during Pregnancy and Childbirth for Community Health Officer at Ayushman Bharat—Health and Wellness Centres; 2021
3. Antenatal Care. National Institute for Health and Care Excellence (NICE), 19 August 2021.
4. Lattof SR, Moran AC, Kidula N, et al. Implementation of the new WHO antenatal care model for a positive pregnancy experience: a monitoring framework. BMJ Global Health. 2020;5:e002605. doi:10.1136/bmjgh-2020-002605.
5. Moller, Ann-Beth, et al. Early antenatal care visit: a systematic analysis of regional and global levels and trends of coverage from 1990 to 2013. The Lancet Global Health.2017;5(10):e977-83.
6. American College of Obstetricians and Gynecologists' Committee on Practice Bulletins—Obstetrics. "Antepartum Fetal Surveillance: ACOG Practice Bulletin, Number 229." Obstetrics and Gynecology.2021; 137(6):e116-27. doi:10.1097/AOG.0000000000004410.
7. State of HP and Others vs. Dinesh Chauhan and Others on 29 March 2018.
8. B Dilip Reddy s/o B Sunder ... vs 1. Rainbow Childrens Hospital & ... on 19 January 2018.
9. WHO, UNICEF, UNFPA, The World Bank Group and the United Nations Population Division. Trends in Maternal Mortality: 2000 to 2020. WHO, Geneva, 2023. Available from: https://www.who.int/publications/i/item/9789240068759.
10. Jain S, Acharya N. Fetal Wellbeing Monitoring: A Review Article. Cureus. 2022;14(9):e29039. doi: 10.7759/cureus.29039. PMID: 36249607; PMCID: PMC9550204.

CHAPTER 16

Medicolegal Issues in Prenatal Testing

Antima Rathore, Sujjanna AL Manuel

INTRODUCTION

Prenatal testing is the aspect of prenatal care that focusses on detecting genetic/ structural abnormalities in the conceptus (zygote/embryo or fetus). Certain women have increased risk of having abnormalities in their babies—women with advanced age, family history/past history of fetal anomaly, history of drug ingestion (anticonvulsants/ warfarin/substance abuse), advanced partner's age. However, 95% of abnormalities occur in fetuses born to mothers who have no risk factors.[1] Hence, routine screening should be offered to all pregnant women.

Prenatal testing may be a screening procedure or a confirmatory test. These tests may be conducted in embryos before implantation (*Preimplantation Testing*) or during pregnancy (*Prenatal*); may be noninvasive (*Ultrasound, NIPT*) or invasive (*Chorion Villous Sampling, Amniocentesis, Fetal Blood Sampling*).

Aim of Prenatal Testing

1. Identify the fetal malformation thereby facilitating counseling and making informed choice regarding further management.
2. Avail in-utero treatment when feasible that can improve fetal condition prior to birth and improve survival.
3. To plan safe management of delivery. To decide and facilitate appropriate timing, place (*Tertiary hospital with neonatal unit*), and care providers (*multidisciplinary teams—neonatologists, pediatric surgeons*) for safe delivery.
4. Decrease maternal morbidity and perinatal mortality rates by enabling fetal terminations prior to viability.

NONINVASIVE PRENATAL TESTS

Ultrasonography (USG)

Certain aneuploidies, especially Trisomy 13 and 18, are associated with higher incidence of major structural anomalies. Although ultrasound cannot diagnose aneuploidies, yet it detects structural anomalies which urges further evaluation to rule out aneuploidies.

First Trimester Scan

The first trimester ultrasound is invaluable in determining the site, viability, number, fetal anomalies, and best assessment of gestational age of a pregnancy. However, there is a considerable grey zone with a single ultrasound evaluation, irrespective of operator expertise, which is attributed to the developmental window and evolving nature of fetal anatomy and anomalies that are inherent of early pregnancy.

Gestational Age

First trimester ultrasound is the most accurate way for estimating the gestational age of the fetus by assessing the CRL and has an accuracy of +/– 5 days.

Site and Viability

A definitive diagnosis of a viable intrauterine pregnancy can be made when an intrauterine gestational sac containing an embryo with cardiac activity is visualized. Follow-up ultrasounds (10 days–2 weeks) and serial beta-hCG estimations are appropriate in early pregnancies to determine viability and to rule out ectopic and pregnancy of unknown location when unable to visualize a viable intrauterine pregnancy. The presence of "Intra Decidual sign" (IUGS eccentrically located in the decidua anterior or posterior to the white line that represents the collapsed intrauterine cavity) and "Double Sac Sign" (two concentric echogenic rings surrounding an IUGS) can be reassuring features of an early intrauterine pregnancy.

Sonographic Features Diagnostic of Missed Miscarriage[2]

1. Embryo with no cardiac activity when Crown-Rump Length (CRL) is >7 mm.
2. Gestational sac containing no embryo with heartbeat when mean sac diameter (MSD) is >2.5 cm.
3. When the CRL and MSD do not reach the cut-off of 7 and 25 mm, respectively.
   a. No embryo with heartbeat on a follow-up USS 2 weeks after the initial scan that showed a gestational sac without a yolk sac.
   b. No embryo with heartbeat on follow-up scan after 11 days following an initial scan that showed a gestational sac with a yolk sac.

The most definitive way of ruling out an ectopic when an adnexal mass is seen but an extrauterine fetal pole with cardiac activity or fluid in the Pouch of Douglas are absent, is by noting the "Sliding Sign" (observing the movement of the adnexal mass relative to the ovary when pressure is applied by the transvaginal transducer). If the mass and ovary move together it is likely to be a corpus luteum and if the mass slides along the ovary it is extraovarian and ectopic needs to be ruled out. Other features of an ectopic pregnancy are—an extraovarian mass with an anechoic center surrounded by an echogenic ring with prominent flow with Doppler—"Ring- of-Fire" appearance.

Number

Pregnancy number assessed prior to 6 weeks gestation may subsequently decrease due to the 'Vanishing Twin', or increase due to the "Appearing Twin" phenomenon, viz. monochorionic twins can be missed prior to the visualization of 2 Yolk sacs and monoamniotic twins missed as they have only a single yolk sac.[3] Other factor that leads to erroneous assessment of multifetal pregnancies in the early first trimester is suboptimal visualization secondary to high maternal BMI, uterine myomas and uterine orientation.

Aneuploidy Scan/NT Scan[4]

Testing timeframe: 11–13 weeks + 6 weeks

It includes assessment of viability, accurate dating, screening for Trisomy 21 (increased Nuchal translucency >2.5 mm) and diagnosing major structural defects (anencephaly, holoprosencephaly, encephalocele, Dandy-Walker syndrome, cardiac anomalies, gastroschisis, exomphalos, megacystis, diaphragmatic hernia, multidysplastic kidney, skeletal dysplasias, etc.)[3] with high resolution probes and a combination of transabdominal and transvaginal assessment. It is usually combined with serum markers for prenatal screening. The overall detection rate of first trimester fetal structural abnormalities varies from 17 to 90%.[5]

The accuracy of fetal anatomical survey is limited by the operator's expertise, physiological variation and development of pregnancy. There are certain anomalies which are detected in early gestation, but they resolve as pregnancy advances, e.g., resolution of physiologic herniation of midgut seen at 9–10 weeks by the middle of 10th through 11 weeks, resolution of tricuspid regurgitation in certain fetuses. On the other hand, certain anomalies evolve as pregnancy advances like congenital diaphragmatic hernias, skeletal dysplasia, congenital heart defects such as cardiomyopathy, etc.

Detection Rate of Fetal Anomalies in First Trimester[6]

- *Neck:* 92%
- *Abdomen:* 88%
- *Brain and Spine:* 51%
- *Heart:* 48%
- *Limbs:* 34%
- *Genitourinary:* 34%
- *Face:* 34%

Medicolegal Implication

The erroneous reporting, although rare but in few cases the reports are found to have errors, and it might lead to distrust in the service provision and may involve repercussions varying from complaint to malpractice litigation and unjustified termination of normal pregnancies if the patient opted for the same after the report. It can be prevented by following standard procedures, having proper and updated training, adequate counseling of the patient regarding the limitations of an ultrasound scan. For example, when diagnosing the miscarriage, take second opinion or repeat scan to confirm the diagnosis when CRL and MSD are not meeting the criteria.

Second Trimester—Detailed Fetal Anomaly Scan[7]

Testing timeframe: 18–22 weeks

It involves assessment of fetal viability, number, fetal age, and size; placenta (site, any masses, accessory lobe), and amniotic fluid volume. Parameters measured for assessing gestational age and fetal biometry are biparietal diameter (BPD), head circumference (HC); abdominal circumference (AC) or diameter; femur diaphysis length (FDL). All anomalies diagnosed in the first trimester (skeletal, cranial, cardiac, GIT, urinary tract) can be diagnosed in the second trimester, and additional anomalies can also be picked up.

Medicolegal Implication

Missing fetal abnormalities, especially the lethal defects and conditions that result in long-term physical and mental comorbidities that result in need for extensive health or supportive care and cost are the most common reasons for medical litigation. Hence, it is sentinel to be open about the suboptimal examination (document in the report notify the patient and referring clinician of the same) and offer other fail-safe measures—serial evaluation, referral for a second opinion or referral to a center with appropriate equipment and expertise.

Other Investigations

Doppler ultrasound is used for studying most of the major fetal circulatory systems particularly helpful in evaluating the fetal cardiovascular system, fetoplacental and uteroplacental blood flow, assessment of fetal well-being in growth restricted fetuses, evaluation of fetal anemia by assessment of peak systolic flow in the middle cerebral artery, evaluation of maternal-placental interface in the diagnostic evaluation of the placenta accrete spectrum and evaluation of suspected vasa previa. Several modalities are available-continuous wave, pulsed wave (spectral Doppler) color flow mapping. The first trimester use of fetal Doppler has concern of adversely affecting organogenesis and hence avoided upto 10+6 weeks. It can be used at 11 weeks, when organogenesis is complete but the T1 should be <1 and exposure time be kept to 5–10 minutes.[8]

3D sonography: It can reduce scanning time while providing adequate fetal imaging and enables better visualization of facial, skeletal, and CNS anomalies.

4D sonography: Also called dynamic 3D sonography refers to 3D that can be viewed in real time and can be used to study the fetal heart/movement and behavioral states.

Role of disclaimer/information in ultrasound report related to limitation of ultrasound (False positives and negatives): Though ultrasound is an invaluable in assessing fetal morphology, and wellbeing, this does have the caveat of false positives—detection of soft markers, that may imply fetal abnormality which after prenatal diagnostic work-up would rule out an anomaly. However, such reports cause considerable maternal anxiety, negatively impact maternal fetal attachment and lead to further prenatal work-up and their cost implications. On the other hand, one may fail to detect fetal anomalies due multiple factors like maternal habitus, gestational age, fetal movements, position, amount of liquor, evolving nature of anomalies, type of equipment and operator's expertise.[9] Missing out the fetal anomaly negates the primary aim of planning optimal management of the fetus with abnormality as well as parental preparation through counseling and may be grounds for medical litigation. Hence, it is paramount to counsel patients and document in the written report of the limitations of ultrasound the need for further testing if needed as well as the chance of unexpected fetal abnormality at birth.

Noninvasive Prenatal Testing (NIPT) (Cell-free DNA)[10,11]

Timeframe: 9–10 weeks onwards

It is the most sensitive and specific screening test (sensitivity and specificity—99%) for the aneuploidy screening in fetus. It involves the analysis of fetal fraction (derived from placental trophoblast) of cell-free DNA fragments in the mother's blood, which consists of about 3–13% of the total cell-free DNA in maternal blood. The quantity of the fetal fraction is affected by gestational age (increase with gestation), maternal BMI, medication, race, aneuploidy in mother, fetal or maternal mosaicism, and multiple gestation. It can be offered if patient refuses diagnostic test after positive serum screening. However, there is a 2% residual risk of chromosomal abnormalities even if results are negative. A baseline ultrasound must be performed before offering NIPT as the findings may affect the timing of the test. Patients with fetal anomalies should be offered genetic counselling and diagnostic testing instead of genetic screening. A false-positive results may be seen in cases of fetal/maternal mosaicism, a duplicated chromosomal region, a vanishing twin, or an underlying maternal condition such as malignancy. A diagnostic test is required in such cases.

Cell free-DNA can also be used to identify fetal sex. In organ transplant recipients, results are affected by the sex of the organ donor. It may also incidentally pick up medical conditions affecting the patient herself such as chromosomal aneuploidy, mosaicism, or malignancy.

Use of NIPT as routine screening tool varies from country to country depending upon the recommendation of governing body, and financial implications on service provider as well as the service receiver. Some prefer to offer NIPT as routine screening test to all pregnancies irrespective of age or risk factors (ACOG, 2020)[10], while some prefer to keep it reserved for the patients who have intermediate risk[12] on combined screening as a tool to avoid invasive diagnostic tests. In both cases, invasive tests are advised to confirm the diagnosis if NIPT is positive.

INVASIVE PRENATAL TESTS[13-15]

Indications

- Positive screening for chromosomal anomaly (NIPT/biochemical)
- Ultrasound detected fetal abnormality
- Parental balanced translocation
- Previous baby with chromosomal abnormality
- Risk of X-linked disease in male fetus
- Facilitate diagnosis of certain congenital infections (CMV/Toxoplasmosis) with amniocentesis/fetal blood sampling

All invasive procedures can lead to Rh-sensitization therefore, all Rh-negative mothers with Rh-positive fetus must be given Anti-D immunoglobulin. They also involve associated with infection and pain.

Chorionic Villous Sampling (CVS)

Testing time frame: 10–13 weeks

Method: Samples placental tissue which is derived from the same fertilized egg as the fetus and can be done transabdominally or transcervically. Choice of route is dependent on operator expertise, placental location, and uterine axis. It is called placental biopsy when it is done after the first trimester.

Transabdominal: An 18–20-gauge needle is introduced under ultrasound guidance through the maternal abdomen to the placenta and aspirating placental tissue via a syringe attached to the needle.

Transcervical: Done in posterior low-lying placenta where transabdominal CVS is not possible, using aseptic technique the cervix is visualized with a speculum. Transabdominal ultrasound is used to visualize the cervical canal and a needle/catheter, or a biopsy forceps which is introduced through the cervix to the placenta and sample is taken.

Advantage: Early diagnosis and possible 1st trimester termination.

Risks:

- Fetal limb defects when done before 10 weeks
- Miscarriage—1%
- Cytogenetically ambiguous resulting from maternal cell contamination or mosaicism

Amniocentesis

Testing time frame: 15–18 weeks

Method: Aspiration of 15–20 mL of amniotic fluid that contains fetal cells (shed from fetal bladder, skin, GI tract and amnion) through a 22-gauge needle transabdominally under real-time ultrasound using aseptic technique. Puncturing placenta can lead to fetal blood contamination, giving erroneous results.

Risks: (1) Miscarriage—1%

(2) Failure of cell culture—0.5% (necessitating further invasive testing)

Fetal Blood Sampling (FBS)[16]

Indications:

- Rapid karyotyping
- Management of fetal hemolytic disease
- Work-up of severe early onset fetal growth deficiency
- To confirm suspected congenital infection

Testing time frame: 20 weeks and onwards

Method: Introduction of a 20-gauge needle under ultrasound guidance with aseptic technique and fetal blood aspirated from umbilical vein either at the placental insertion/fetal insertion (umbilical) or free loop of cord. Fetal cardiac puncture or intrahepatic venepuncture are alternative sites. If fetal movements are a concern injection of 0.3 mg/kg pancuronium (maximum 0.6 mg) may be given intravenously or intramuscularly in the fetal buttock with a 25-gauge needle, which will provide neuromuscular blockade for 1–2 hours.

Advantages:
- Rapid fetal karyotyping in 48–72 hours
- Facilitate fetal blood transfusion

Risks: Fetal bradycardia, umbilical cord bleeding/hematoma, fetomaternal hemorrhage and sensitization, prolabor rupture of membranes, preterm labor, placental abruption, fetal death 1–2%, amnionitis/maternal sepsis, emergency C-section, failure to obtain sample.

Prenatal Diagnosis: Medicolegal Aspects

Obstetrics and gynecology is the branch of medicine with one of the highest litigation rate, and prenatal diagnosis is one of the most regulated practice in this field. It is vital to understand the medicolegal aspects related to prenatal diagnostics to avoid inconvenience of being dragged into legal battles. One must acquaint themselves with the historic PC-PNDT Act, which is the most important law regulating the field of prenatal tests. Understanding the governing laws is of utmost importance, and so is the proper documentation and paperwork.

Most Common Issues Leading to Medicolegal Litigation

- *Substandard care (leading to harm):* A procedure must be performed by a competent person following standard procedure. If a person performing the procedure is not competent as per the standard or if standard protocols are not followed while performing the procedure, the person is liable to pay compensation if anything goes wrong.
- *Missed diagnosis:* Missing a crucial diagnosis often brings litigation charges. However, the inherent margin of error in case of any procedure is acceptable provided that the care provided was up to the standards.
- *Failure to communication:* Communication is crucial before, during, and after conducting any procedure. It not only helps to build a rapport with the patient but also decreases the changes of patient turning towards the court for the explanation/grievance.
- *Improper consent:* Taking proper informed consent is one of the important things which reflects proper care and vigilance.
- *Inadequate documentation:* Proper documentation of everything is extremely important because that is the only proof of the care provided. "If it is not documented, it means that it has not been done." Keeping this in mind one must ensure that they have documented every discussion/advice.

How to Avoid Malpractice Litigation?

- Detailed and complete history—always obtain complete clinical history including the history of presenting illness, past-history, and occupational and drug history.

- Establishing a good rapport with the patient—it is important to build confidence and comfort in doctor-patient relationship. It reduces the chances of complaint by the patient.
- Obtain a valid consent—always take an informed written consent after explaining the risks and benefits of the procedure. A valid consent is one which is obtained without coercion and in language, which patient understands. Explain the limitations of that procedure and available alternatives, if any. Signature/ thumb impression of the patient must be taken. One must countersign the consent. In case, a patient is deemed incapable of giving valid consent, consent must be obtained from immediate family member/guardian of the patient.
- Date and time of the examination should always be documented.
- Always follow the recommended standard protocols
- While performing an imaging procedure:
    - Obtain a proper and adequate number of images.
    - Compare with previous images if needed.
    - Document the noted abnormality in the report and reach a conclusion.
    - Always proofread the report. Correcting typographical errors is also important. The quality of written reports determine the standard of care.
- Offer a chaperone—make sure that a chaperone is present especially while examining or conducting procedure on a female patient. It is good medical practice even if the doctor is also a female.
- Updated yourself with the new technologies and current practice guidelines.
- Preserve the documents in the departmental records.

PRE-CONCEPTION AND PRE-NATAL DIAGNOSTIC TECHNIQUES ACT (PCPNDT ACT) [17,18]

The Pre-natal Diagnostic Techniques (Regulation and Prevention of Misuse) Act (PNDT Act), 1994 was enacted to provide for the regulation of: *'the use of pre-natal diagnostic techniques for the purpose of detecting genetic or metabolic disorders or chromosomal abnormalities or certain congenital malformations or sex-linked disorders; for the prevention of the misuse of such techniques for the purpose of pre-natal sex determination leading to female feticide; and for matters connected there with or incidental thereto.'* It came into force on January 1st, 1996. It was amended in 2003 to bring the new technologies under the Act and was renamed the *Pre-conception and Pre-natal Diagnostic Techniques (Prohibition of Sex Selection) Act* or PCPNDT Act. I became effective from February 14, 2003. The Act was again amended in 2012 with steps towards stronger, rigorous, and effective implementation of the Act.

The PNDT Act prohibits sex selection before or after conception and misuse of *pre-natal diagnostic techniques* for determination of the sex of the fetus, leading to female feticide as also advertisements in relation to such techniques for detection or determination of sex. The Act also specifies the punishment for violation of its provisions. The offence under the Act shall be tried only in a court of the Metropolitan Magistrate or a Judicial Magistrate of the First Class.

The Act further permits the use of such techniques only under certain conditions by the registered bodies.

A. For the detection of:
   a. Chromosomal abnormalities
   b. Genetic metabolic diseases
   c. Hemoglobinopathies
   d. Sex-linked genetic diseases
   e. Congenital anomalies or other abnormalities or diseases as specified by the Central Supervisory Board
B. If any of the following conditions exist:
   a. Age of the pregnant woman is above thirty-five years
   b. Pregnant woman has undergone two or more spontaneous abortions or fetal loss
   c. Pregnant woman has been exposed to potentially teratogenic agents such as drugs, radiation, infection, or chemicals
   d. The pregnant woman or her spouse has a family history of mental retardation or physical deformities such as, spasticity or any other genetic disease
   e. Any other condition specified by the Central Supervisory Board.

Registration of all bodies mentioned under the PNDT Act, whether the body is government, private, voluntary, honorary, part-time, contractual, or consultative, is mandatory. They can register either separately or jointly when a body is for instance both a center and a clinic. Registration can be subjected to cancellation in case of any serious charges/misconduct.

The offences under the Act are:

Cognizable: This means that for such an offence the police officer may arrest without warrant.

Non-bailable: This means that the police cannot grant bail in such a case.

Non-compoundable: This means that the parties to the case cannot settle the case and decide not to prosecute.

Who can make a complaint?

a. Any officer authorized on this behalf by the Central Government or State Government or the Appropriate Authority.
b. Any public-spirited person/social organization/lawyer—alone or together.

Once the complaint is made in the Court the public prosecutor will take on from there and the complainant need not be present on every date of hearing.

Good Faith

The Central or State Government or the Appropriate Authority or any officer authorized by them cannot be prosecuted or have any legal proceedings against them for anything which is in *good faith* done or intended to be done under the Act. Thus, the Appropriate Authority can perform its duties under the Act without any fear of any type of legal proceeding being initiated against him/her.

DEFINITIONS RELATED TO PRENATAL TESTING[17,18]

Techniques

Pre-natal diagnostic techniques include all pre-natal diagnostic procedures and pre-natal diagnostic tests.

A. Pre-natal diagnostic procedures mean all gynecological or obstetrical or medical procedures such as:
   a Ultrasonography
   b. Fetoscopy
   c. Taking or removing samples of: Amniotic fluid, chorionic villi, blood, any tissue or fluid of a man or a woman before or after conception for being sent to a Genetic Laboratory or

Genetic Clinic for conducting any type of analysis or pre-natal diagnostic tests for selection of sex before or after conception.

B. Pre-natal diagnostic test means:
   a. Ultrasonography
   b. *Test or analysis of amniotic fluid, chorionic villi, blood, any tissue or fluid of any pregnant woman or conceptus conducted to detect:* Genetic disorders, metabolic disorders, chromosomal abnormalities, congenital anomalies, hemoglobinopathies, sex-linked diseases.

C. *Sex selection:* Procedure, technique, test, administration, prescription or provision of anything for the purpose of ensuring or increasing the probability that an embryo will be of a particular sex.

Places

A. *Genetic counseling centre:* An institute, hospital, nursing home, or any place by whatever name called which provides *genetic counseling to patients.*

B. *Genetic Clinic means:* A clinic, institute, hospital, nursing home or any place by whatever name called which is used for *conducting* pre-natal diagnostic procedures.

   By an amendment to the Act of 1994, a genetic clinic includes a vehicle, where ultrasound machine or imaging machine or scanner or other equipment capable of determining sex of the fetus or a portable equipment which has the potential for detection of sex during pregnancy or selection of sex before conception, is used.

C. *Genetic laboratory:* A laboratory; and includes a place where facilities are provided for *conducting analysis or tests of samples* received from genetic clinic for pre-natal diagnostic test.

The amendments of 2002—"Genetic laboratory includes a place where ultrasound machine or imaging machine or scanner or other equipment capable of determining sex of the fetus or a portable equipment which has the potential for detection of sex during pregnancy or selection of sex before conception, is used."

Qualified Persons

A. Gynecologist means a person who possesses a postgraduate qualification in gynecology and obstetrics.

   For a genetic counseling center, the gynecologist must have *6 months' experience* in genetic counseling; or *4 weeks training* in genetic counseling.

   For a genetic clinic, the gynecologist should have adequate experience in pre-natal diagnostic procedures, i.e., should have performed *at least 20* procedures in chorionic villi aspirations per vagina or per abdomen, chorionic villi biopsy, amniocentesis, cordocentesis fetoscopy, fetal skin or organ biopsy or fetal blood sampling, etc. under supervision of an experienced gynecologist in these fields.

B. Medical geneticist includes a person who possesses: Degree, or Diploma in Genetic Science in the fields of sex selection and pre-natal diagnostic techniques or has experience of not less than two years in any of these fields after obtaining. Any one of the medical qualifications recognized under the Indian Medical Council Act, 1956; or A postgraduate degree in biological sciences. Under the amended definition, possessing a certificate does not make one a qualified medical geneticist.

C. Pediatrician means a person who possesses a postgraduate qualification in pediatrics. For a genetic counseling center, the pediatrician must have *6 months' experience* in genetic counseling; or *4 weeks' training* in genetic counseling.

D. Registered Medical Practitioner means a medical practitioner who possesses any recognized medical qualification as defined in clause (h) of Section 2 of the Indian Medical Council Act, 1956; and whose name has been entered in a State Medical Register. The Rules framed under the Act further *qualify* the qualifications by providing additional requirements for a registered medical practitioner when employed by a genetic clinic. For the purposes of a genetic clinic the registered medical practitioner should have a postgraduate degree or diploma or six months training or one year experience in sonography or image scanning.

Besides, the Act and the Rules also refer to other types of personnel.

For a genetic laboratory, there should be:

a. *Laboratory technician* having BSc Degree in Biological Sciences; or Degree or; Diploma, in Medical Laboratory course; and At least *one year's experience* in conducting appropriate pre-natal diagnostic techniques, tests or procedures.
b. Radiologist
c. Sonologist or Imaging Specialist means a person who possesses: Any one of the medical qualifications recognized under the Indian Medical Council Act, 1956; or a postgradute qualification in Ultrasonography or Imaging Techniques or Radiology.

PROHIBITIONS AND PENALTIES

On Places

No genetic counseling center or genetic clinic or genetic laboratory shall:

a. Conduct; or associate with; or help in conducting pre-natal diagnostic techniques unless registered. Moreover, the Registration certificate must be displayed prominently on board in such places.
b. Employ or cause to be employed or take services of any person, whether on an honorary basis or on payment who does not possess prescribed qualifications **(Table 1)**.

Every genetic counseling center or genetic clinic or genetic laboratory is required to display prominently a notice in english and in the local language or languages that conduct of sex-determination tests/disclosure of sex of the fetus is prohibited.

On Persons

1. A person shall not open any genetic counseling center, genetic clinic or genetic laboratory (including clinic, laboratory or center) having ultrasound or imaging machine or scanner or any other technology capable of undertaking of sex of fetus and sex selection unless such center, clinic or laboratory is duly registered separately or jointly.
2. A qualified person providing/helping services covered by the act shall work only at the place registered under the act.
3. No person (including a relative or husband of the pregnant woman) can ask/encourage the use of any pre-natal diagnostic techniques on her except for the purposes specified in clause of Section 4 of the Act.
4. No person (including a relative or husband of a woman) can ask/encourage to conduct of any sex-selection technique on her or him or both.
5. No person shall conduct or cause to be conducted any pre-natal diagnostic technique including ultrasonography for purpose of sex determination.

TABLE 1: Screening tests.[10]

Test	*Timeframe (weeks)*	*Component*	*Detection rate for Down syndrome (%)*	*False pos-itive (%)*	*Comments*
First Trimester screening	10–13 weeks + 6 weeks	Nuchal translucency (NT) + PAPP-A, free β-hCG, +/– AFP (Alpha-fetoprotien)	85%	5%	• Provides risk for Trisomies 21, 13, and 18 • Superior to 2nd Trimester Serum screening in detecting Trisomy 21 • Does not screen for open NTD
Quad Screening	15–22 weeks	AFP + β-hCG + Unconjugated Estriol (uE3) + Dimeric Inhibin A (DIA)	76%	5%	• Provides risk for Trisomy 21, 18 and Open NTD • *Serum markers level:* – Decrease—Insulin dependent diabetes, high maternal BMI – Increase—multiple gestations – high AFP – Afro - Caribbean ethnicity, Smokers
Integrated or combined (1st trimester and 2nd trimester) screening	10–13 weeks + 6 weeks, then 15 to 22 weeks	(NT + PAPP-A) + quad test	5%	5%	• First and second trimester tests are combined, and results are revealed after second trimester only • Delays management
Serum integrated	10–13 weeks + 6 weeks, then 15 + 2 weeks	PAPP-A + Quad screen	88%	5%	• Ultrasound not required • Two samples needed • First trimester results not revealed

Contd...

Contd...

Test	***Timeframe (weeks)***	***Component***	***Detection rate for Down syndrome (%)***	***False positive (%)***	***Comments***
Sequential: Stepwise	10–13 weeks + 6 weeks, then 15–22 weeks	NT+ free β- hCG + PAPP-A +/– AFP, + Quad screen	95%	5%	• High risk—offer diagnostic test • Low risk—offer 2nd trimester screening test • Only few women need 2nd trimester tests
Contingent screening	10-13 weeks + 6 weeks, then 15 to 22 weeks	NT + β-hCG + PAPP-A +/- AFP, then quad screen	88–94%	5%	• If first-trimester test result: – *Positive*: Offer diagnostic test or cell-free DNA – *Negative:* No further testing – *Intermediate:* Offer second trimester screening • Final risk assessment incorporates first- and second-trimester results
Nuchal translucency alone	10–13 weeks + 6 weeks	Ultrasound	70%	5%	• Useful in multifetal gestations • Also rules out fetal anomalies • Poor sensitivity and specificity when used alone
Triple screening	15–20 weeks	AFP + β-hCG + uE3	69%	5%	Same as Quad test

6. No person, including a specialist or a team of specialists in the field of infertility, shall conduct or cause to be conducted or aid in conducting by himself or by any other person, sex selection on a woman or a man or on both or on any tissue, embryo, conceptus, fluid, or gametes derived from either or both of them.
7. No person shall, by whatever means, cause or allow to be caused selection of sex before or after conception.
8. No person including the person conducting a pre-natal diagnostic procedure shall *communicate* to the pregnant woman concerned or her relatives or any other person the sex of the foetus by words, signs or in any other manner whatsoever.

Miscellaneous

No person, organization, Genetic Counseling Center, Genetic Laboratory or Genetic Clinic, including clinic, laboratory or center having ultrasound machine or imaging machine or scanner or any other technology capable of undertaking determination of sex of fetus or sex selection shall *issue, publish, distribute, communicate*, or cause to be issued, published, distributed or communicated *any advertisement, in any form, including Internet, regarding* facilities of pre-natal determination of sex or sex selection before conception available at such center, laboratory, clinic or at any other place; by any means whatsoever, scientific or otherwise.

No person shall sell, distribute, supply, rent, allow, or authorize the use of any ultrasound machine or imaging machine or scanner or any other equipment capable of detecting sex of fetus whether on payment or otherwise to any Genetic Counselling Centre, Genetic Laboratory, Genetic Clinic or any other person or body not registered under the Act.

"Person" includes manufacturer, importer, dealer, or supplier of ultrasound machines/imaging machines or any other equipment capable of detecting sex of fetus as also any organization including a commercial organization.

PRESCRIPTIONS AND REGULATIONS

a. The person conducting the tests shall keep a complete record (Form F—ultrasonography, Form G—Prenatal/pre-conceptional genetic tests).
b. Informed consent should be taken, in the prescribed format in a language which she understands. Copy of the consent form to be given, if asked. A distinction has been made between invasive and noninvasive techniques for the purpose of obtaining consent and the consent is required in the case of invasive techniques.
c. In case of ultrasonography, any person conducting ultrasonography/image scanning on a pregnant woman shall give a declaration on each report on ultrasonography/image scanning that he/she has neither detected nor disclosed the sex of fetus of the pregnant woman to anybody. The pregnant woman before undergoing ultrasonography/image scanning declare that she does not want to know the sex of her fetus.
d. A *Genetic Laboratory* cannot accept for analysis or test any sample, unless referred to it by a *Genetic Clinic.*
e. Every *pre-natal diagnostic procedure* has to be immediately preceded by locating the fetus and placenta through ultrasonography.
f. The *pre-natal diagnostic procedure* shall be done under direct ultrasonographic monitoring to prevent any damage to the fetus and placenta.

PENALTIES

Offence by Persons

I. For *advertisement* (as mentioned earlier)—Sections 22(1) and 22(2)
First instance: *Imprisonment* which may *extend to 3 years;* and *Fine* which may *extend to ₹10,000.*
Any subsequent conviction: *Imprisonment* which may *extend to 5 years;* and *Fine* which may extend to ₹50,000.

II. *A person seeking* sex selection or for conducting pre-natal diagnostic techniques on any pregnant woman for the purposes other than those specified in Section 4(2).
First instance: Imprisonment which may extend to *three years;* and *Fine* which may extend to *₹50,000.*
Any subsequent conviction: *Imprisonment* which may extend to *5 years;* and *Fine* which may extend to *₹1 lakh.*
Husband and relatives of the pregnant woman are presumed to have compelled the woman to undergo the pre-natal diagnostic technique *unless the contrary is proved;* and are held liable and are punished for the offence under Section 23(3). If the contrary is proved, the woman can also be likewise punished. The woman who was compelled to undergo such diagnostic techniques or such selection is not liable/punished.

III. A *registered medical practitioner* involved in activity illegal as per the act—reported by the Appropriate Authority to the State Medical Council who will:
- Suspend the registration if charges are framed by the court and till the case is disposed of
- Remove his name from the register of the council on conviction
  - Five years for the first offence
  - Permanently for the subsequent offence

VI. If any person contravenes any provision of the Act or the Rules made there under for which no penalty has been specified, he will be liable to be punished with: *Imprisonment* which may *extend to three months*; or *Fine* which may *extend to ₹1000*, or with both. Any subsequent contravention entails an *additional fine* which may extend to ₹500 for every day during which such contravention continues after conviction for the first such contravention.

V. *Minor offences:*
a. Non-availability of copy of PNDT
b. Act in the registered center
c. Non-display of registration certificate
d. Non-display of the board in English and local language

For first offence: Imprisonment for *3 months* or fine up to ₹*1000*
For subsequent offence. Additional fine up to ₹500 per day for the period of contravention
Or Show cause notice for temporary suspension of registration

VI. *Unregistered centers*—the equipment to be seized and sealed by Appropriate authority; Registration at 5 times fees as penalty after undertaking as per PCPNDT Act.

VII. *Irregularities at registered center*—suspension or cancellation of registration with/without Show Cause Notice.

VIII. *Irregularities in record keeping (as per revised Form F)*—It is a major offence.

Offence by a Company

A company means any corporate body; includes a firm or other association of individuals. In case of offence by a company: every person In-charge of; and every person responsible for the conduct of the business of the company (Director, manager secretory) at the time the offence was committed, shall

all be deemed to be guilty and accordingly proceeded against and punished. Unless if any such person proves that the offence was committed without his knowledge or that he had exercise due diligence to prevent the commission of such offence, he may not be so liable.

GUIDELINES FOR THE USE OF ULTRASOUND IN GENETIC CLINIC UNDER THE ACT

1. Centers where ultrasound is intended to be carried out should get registered, at least 30 days in advance.
2. All ultrasound machines available at that center along with the qualified doctors performing USG should be registered on the certificate.
3. No doctor other than the one registered in that center is allowed to use the machine.
4. In the case of a locum doctor, the doctor's name and personal details, state council registration number, and his/her degree certificate need to be sent to the appropriate authority (AA)/ward office, requesting permission for the use of the machine by the locum on the specified dates.
5. The USG machine should not be shifted from one center to another.
6. Any changes in the center (e.g., change in machine or place of use) should be intimated to the AA 30 days in advance of the expected date of such change.
7. Portable ultrasound machines should be used as a part of the registered mobile medical unit, offering other health and medical services. It cannot be used in a vehicle not registered under the Act.
8. Registration and practice of sonography by a radiologist/sonologist is restricted to two clinics/facilities within a district. The consulting hours by such medical practitioner should be specified by each clinic/center.
9. Renew the certificate of registration every five years, with application of renewal being applied 30 days before the date of expiry to the AA.
10. A copy of PC-PNDT registration certificate should be displayed in reception area and the USG room.
11. A copy of PC-PNDT Act booklet should be made available in both the waiting room and USG room.
12. Sign in English and in the local language must be displayed, indicating that fetal sex is not disclosed in the clinic.
13. Form F must be filled completely. The signed consent of the patient as well as the radiologist signature who performed the procedure should be obtained. A hard copy with patient signature must be preserved at the clinic when form 'F' is submitted online.
14. A monthly report should be submitted to the AA regularly, before the 5th of every month.
15. All the records need to be maintained for a minimum of 2 years. If there is any legal proceeding pending in the court of law, then these records should not be destroyed till the proceedings have been disposed of.

RELEVANT JUDGMENTS

Case 1: G Vijayashankar & Anr. Ms Chitra Vijayashankar vs. Madras Medical Mission & Ors:[19]

The couple conceived by IUI after 15 years of marriage and multiple failed IVF cycles. Baby was born with Down syndrome, and couple filed the case against the institute for providing substandard care (re-advanced maternal age) resulting into birth of child with Down syndrome causing mental agony to the couples. However, the medical records showed that mother had vanishing twin in early pregnancy and had received all the care as per standard (2002) which included NT scan, discussion about Triple screening, and invasive prenatal diagnostic tests, anomaly scan by experienced radiologist. The couple had, however, decided not to opt for invasive tests due to risk of miscarriage as the pregnancy was precious. The appeal was dismissed as they failed to prove any deficiency in care and medical negligence.

This case shows the importance of providing care as per standard and proper documentation which proved to be the main factor in deciding the result. On contrary, there has been instances where court has ordered lakhs in compensation where doctor did not discuss or offer aneuploidy screening. In some of these cases, although the doctors were working in the government hospital but patient consulted them in their private practice, and there was no mention of screening tests or counseling of screening on medical records.

Case 2: Dr Ashishkumar Govindrao Wagh vs. The Competent Authority and Anr[20] on 27 September 2016

The doctor was accused of doing TVS in patient who had miscarriage without completing Form 'F', and surnames of some of the patients were incorrect. Based on these allegations, a process was issued by the Magistrate which was then challenged by the doctor. As per the doctor, there was no TVS probe available at the institute (as mentioned in registration), and he has written PS not TVS. Moreover, regarding the error with surnames of other patients, they did not come under the PCPNDT Act. The case was considered to be based on speculations and the court ruled in favor of the doctor. This case highlights the importance of proper documentation and presenting facts in the court.

Case 3: Dr Vijaymala vs. The State of Maharashtra[21] on 9 May 2014

The doctor was charged under the PCPNDT Act as the authority found certain lacunae in maintaining records, and the sonography machine was sealed and registration suspended. The Form 'F' filled by the doctor were not as per the Act, and there was no referral slip attached for some of the forms. However, the writ was discarded as any deficiency in record maintenance is unacceptable under the law.

Case 4: Ravindra Dnyaneshwar Patil & Anr vs Dr Vinay Tule[22] on 17 July 2017

The couple were sickle cell carriers and undergone CVS during the pregnancy. The report did not show sickle SS pattern, and they continued the pregnancy. On birth, child was pale, and test revealed that the child was suffering from *SS Pattern Sickle Cell Trait*. They accused doctors and the laboratory of negligence and wrong report as the report suggested that fetus is carrier of sickle cell and doctor took it as conclusive. However, the court ruled in the favor of the doctor in view following points—doctor had appropriate experience to conduct invasive prenatal test and to manage the pregnancy; all documents were correct including the Form 'G', except the typographical error in the date of the results; tests were conducted using standard procedures; maternal cell contamination is a known cause of error in such tests.

REFERENCES

1. Whittle M. Ultrasound Screening for Fetal Abnormalities. Report of the RCOG Working Party. London: RCOG Press 1997.

2. Doubilet PM, Benson CB, Bourne T, et al. Early First trimester diagnostic criteria for nonviable pregnancy. N Eng J Med. 2013;369:1443-51.
3. Doubilet PM, Benson CB. The appearing twin: undercounting of multiple gestations on early first trimester sonograms. J Ultrasound Med. 1998;17:199-203.
4. Whitlow BJ, Chatzipapas IK, Lazanakis ML, et al. The value of sonography in early pregnancy for detection of fetal abnormalities in unselected population. Br J Obstet Gynecol. 1999;106:929-36.
5. Farraposo S, Montenegro N, Matias A. Evaluation of role of 1st trimester obstetric ultrasound in the detection of major anomalies: a systematic review. J Perinat Med. 2014;42(2):141-9.
6. Rossi AC, Prefumo F: Accuracy of ultrasonography at 11–14 weeks of gestation for detection of fetal structural anomalies: a systematic review. Obstet Gynecol. 2013;122(6):1160-7.
7. Salomon LJ, Alfirevic Z, Berghella V, Bilardo C, Hernandez-Andrade E, Johnsen SL, et al. ISUOG Clinical Standards Committee. Practice Guidelines for Performance of the Routine Mid-trimester Fetal Ultrasound Scan. Ultrasound Obstet Gynecol. 2011;37(1): 116-26.
8. Salvesen K, Abramowicz J, Ter Haar G, et al. ISUOG statement on safe use of Doppler for fetal ultrasound examination in the first 13+6 weeks of pregnancy. Ultrasound Obstet Gynecol. 2021;57:1020.
9. Edvardsson K, Small R, Persson M, et al. Ultrasound an invaluable third eye, but it cannot see everything: a qualitative study with Obstetricians in Australia. BMC Pregnancy Childbirth. 2014;14,363.
10. American College of Obstetricians and Gynaecologist's Committee on Practice Bulletins—Obstetrics; Committee on Genetics; Society for Maternal-Fetal Medicine. Screening for Fetal Chromosomal Abnormalities: ACOG Practice Bulletin, Number 226. Obstet Gynecol. 2020;136(4): e48-69.
11. Non-Invasive Prenatal Testing for Chromosomal Abnormality using Maternal Plasma DNA Scientific Impact Paper No. 15 March 2014, Royal College of Obstetricians and Gynaecologists. Available from: https://www.rcog.org.uk/media/gecpbqau/sip_15_04032014.pdf.
12. Ashoor AMG, Nicolaides KH. Evolution in screening for Down syndrome. The Obstetrician and Gynaecologist. 2019;21: 51-7.
13. Ghi T, Sotiriadis A, Calda P, Da Silva Costa F, Raine-Fenning N, Alfirevic Z, McGillivray G. International Society of Ultrasound in Obstetrics and Gynecology (ISUOG). ISUOG Practice Guidelines: invasive procedures for prenatal diagnosis. Ultrasound Obstet Gynecol. 2016;48(2):256-68.
14. Navaratnam K, Alfirevic Z. Royal College of Obstetricians and Gynaecologists. Amniocentesis and chorionic villus sampling: Green-top Guideline No. 8. BJOG, 2021.
15. Alfirevic Z, Mujezinovic F, Sundburg K. Amniocentesis and CVS for prenatal diagnosis. Cochrane database Syst Rev, 2009.
16. Henderson J, Weiner. Needle-guided technique shows needle in umbilical vein confirmed with Doppler. Glob Libr Women's Med; 2008 (ISSN: 1756-2228).
17. Handbook on Pre-Conception & Pre-Natal Diagnostic Techniques Act and Rules with Amendments. Ministry of Health and Family Welfare Government of India, 2006.
18. Prashant Onkar and Kajal Mitra. Important points in the PC-PNDT Act. Indian J Radiol Imaging. 2012;22(2):141-3.
19. G Vijayashankar & Anr. Ms Chitra Vijayashankar vs Madras Medical Mission & Ors. Available from: https://indiankanoon.org/doc/121275882/.
20. Dr Ashishkumar Govindrao Wagh vs. The Competent Authority and Anr. Available from: https://indiankanoon.org/doc/51582652/.
21. Dr. Vijaymala vs The State of Maharashtra. Available from: https://indiankanoon.org/doc/103509774/.
22. Ravindra Dnyaneshwar Patil & Anr. vs Dr. Vinay Tule. Available from: https://indiankanoon.org/doc/76855873/.

CHAPTER 17

Anemia in Pregnancy

Sangeeta Pahwa

INTRODUCTION

Anemia, the most common hematologic abnormality, is a reduction in the concentration of erythrocytes or hemoglobin in blood.[1] It is a major public health problem in our country. India has the highest prevalence in the world. The most common cause is nutritional anemia due to iron deficiency. There has been marginal decrease in prevalence of anemia in pregnant women in India from 58% in NFHS-3 (National Family Health Survey, 2005–2006) to 50% in NFHS-4 survey (2015–2016).[2]

DEFINITION

WHO defines anemia in pregnant women as hemoglobin below 11 gm/dL and a hematocrit of less than 33% whereas Centre for Disease Control (CDC) defines: Anemia as Hb conc. <11 g% in 1st and 3rd trimesters and <10.5 g% in 2nd trimester. According to FOGSI, Hb level <10 g/dL.[3]

EPIDEMIOLOGY

WHO has classified the world into different zones according to prevalence of anemia:

- *High prevalence:* >40%
- *Medium:* 15–39%
- *Low:* 5–14.9%
- *Not a problem:* <5%

In developing countries and India, the prevalence is around 40–90%, compared to 10–20% in developed countries. Sub-Saharan Africa and Southeast Asia come in high prevalence zone. Globally, the incidence of anemia is about 30%.[3]

PHYSIOLOGICAL ANEMIA OF PREGNANCY

During normal pregnancy, there is a greater expansion of plasma volume relative to the increase in the red cell mass, which results in dilutional anemia, termed as the physiologic anemia of pregnancy. Although this type of anemia is mild (hemoglobin of 10–11 g/dL), there is no specific hemoglobin or hematocrit value that can distinguish physiologic anemia from other causes of anemia in pregnancy.[4]

Causes of Anemia

- Increased demand ~1,000 mg (growing fetus + placenta + blood loss during labor)
- Low bioavailability of iron in food
- Inadequate intake of iron rich foods
- Inadequate intake of folate and vitamin B_{12}
- Excess consumption of coffee/tea
- Chronic infections like malaria, TB, UTI
- Worm infestation
- Chronic diarrhea and excessive vomiting
- Intake of antiepileptic drugs (resulting in folic acid deficiency)
- Hemolytic anemia.

Signs of Anemia

- Pallor of mucous membrane or nailbed

- Undernourished, lack of luster of hair
- Conjunctiva, nailbeds, larynx, palate, tongue (glossitis and absence of papilla), stomatitis may be present.
- *Palms:* Spoon-shaped nails, pedal edema, jaundice
- *CVS:* Tachycardia, ejection systolic murmurs, crepts in pulmonary CHF
- Hepatomegaly, splenomegaly, increased JVP, postural hypotension.

WORK-UP OF PREGNANCY WITH ANEMIA

Detailed history should be taken—age, race, parity, dietary habits, history of passing worms in stools, history of bleeding PR, hematuria, hyperemesis, malabsorption, chronic diseases like TB, malaria, bleeding disorders, etc. History of drug intake, repeated blood transfusions, history of anemia in previous pregnancy, abruption, low birth weight baby, PPH, blood transfusions, spacing (if pregnancy occurs within 2 years of last child birth more iron requirement), history of any gastrojejunostomy, family history of thalassemia, sickle cell anemia.

Patient may present with following symptoms: Weakness, fatigue, palpitations, dyspnea, lack of concentration, light headedness, PICA, CHF if severe anemia, irritability.

Examination Findings

- Undernourished, lack of luster of hair.
- Pallor of mucus membrane and nailbed.
- Glossitis and absence of papilla, cheilitis, stomatitis may be present.
- *Palms:* Spoon-shaped nails
- Pedal edema, jaundice
- Increased JVP, postural hypotension
- *CVS:* Tachycardia, ejection systolic murmurs, crepts in pulmonary CHF
- Hepatomegaly
- Splenomegaly—hemolytic anemia
- Jaundice—hemolytic anemia
- Purpura—bleeding disorder
- Leg ulcers—sickle cell anemia
- Neurological deficit—megaloblastic anemia
- Anasarca and signs of cardiac failure in severe case

Lab Investigations

- To determine the severity of anemia, blood test (Hb & hematocrit) should be done. To determine the type of anemia: PBF, red cell indices should be tested.
- *Bone marrow activity:* reticulocyte count (N-0.2-2%).
- Platelet count, BT, CT

Normal Red Cell Values

- *Hemoglobin:* 11.5–15.5 g/dL.
- *RBC count:* 3.9–5.6 million/mL
- *MCH:* 27–34 pg
- *MCV:* 80–95 Fl
- *MCHC:* 30–35 g/dL
- *Reticulocyte count:* 0.5–1.5%

Iron Indices

- *Serum ferritin:* Abnormal if <20 ng/mL (normal range = 40–160 ng/dL). Assess the iron stores, if <15 μg/dL, virtual absence of iron stores
- *Serum iron:* Normal range = 65–165 μg/dL (it is not considered a good indicator)
- *Serum iron binding capacity:* It reflects the availability of iron binding sites. Normal range = 300–360 μg/dL, increases with severity of anemia
- *Percentage saturation of transferrin:* Ratio of S. Fe/TIBC 35–50%, decreases to less than 20% in Fe deficiency anemia. Most sensitive test.

- *RBC protoporphyrin*: 30 μg/dL, it doubles or triples in Fe deficiency anemia (substrate to bind with Fe, cannot be converted into Hb in Fe deficiency)
- *Electrophoresis:* To exclude thalassemia and sickle cell anemia
- Red cell folate assay is better indicator than serum folate levels.
- *Soluble transferrin receptor:* It is the only measurement to accurately reflect the iron deficit between the point of storage iron depletion and development of anemia.

Table 1 provides iron indices for diagnosis of type of anemia.

Peripheral Blood Film (PBF) Findings

- *Normal smear:* Normocytic (normal size RBC), normochromic (normal color RBC)
- *Iron deficiency:* Microcytic (small RBC), hypochromic (pale RBC), anisocytosis (variation in size), poikilocytosis (variation in shape), with or without target cells
- Malarial parasites can be seen.
- Aplastic anemia shows low/no counts.
- Sickle cells can be demonstrated.
- Triad of oval macrocytes, Howell-Jolly bodies and hypersegmented neutrophils seen in megaloblastic anemia
- Abnormal blast cells
- Target cells in thalassemia

Other Investigations

- BUN/Serum creatinine (renal disease)
- LFT (Hepatic disease)
- Urine examination (RBC, casts)
- Stool examination (Occult blood, ova)
- Bone marrow examination (refractory anemia)
- X-ray chest (Pulmonary TB)
- USG whole abdomen

Routine screening with serum ferritin in patients with pregnancy associated anemia is not yet proven to be a cost-effective strategy to diagnose IDA.

While bone marrow stainable iron store is the gold standard for diagnosing IDA, the test is invasive and impractical to use during pregnancy.[8] Serum ferritin is a more sensitive and specific marker for ID than serum iron, transferrin saturation (TSAT), and erythrocyte protoporphyrin values. Currently, low serum ferritin values are regarded as the best test for confirmation of iron deficiency in pregnancy. When compared to bone marrow iron stores a threshold of <12 μg/dL is only 25% sensitive to diagnose ID, a cut-off of <30 μg/dL is 92% specific and 98% specific in diagnosing ID.[9]

TABLE 1: Iron indices for diagnosis of type of anemia.[5-7]

Test	*Iron deficiency*	*Chronic disease*	*Thalassemia*	*Sideroblastic*
Hb	Decreased	Normal/decreased	Decreased	–
Ferritin	Decreased	Normal/increased	Normal/increased	Normal/increased
Serum iron	Decreased	Normal /decreased	Normal /increased	Normal /increased
TIBC	Increased	Slight decrease	Normal	Normal
TS	Decreased	Normal/decreased	Normal/increased	Normal/increased
MCV	Decreased	Normal /decreased	Decreased	Normal
Reticulocytes	Decreased	Normal /decreased	Increased	–

(MCV: mean corpuscular volume; TIBC: total iron-binding capacity; TS: transferrin saturation)

Effect of Anemia on Mother and Fetus

During pregnancy, iron deficiency anemia adversely affects the maternal and fetal well-being, as it is associated with increased morbidity and fetal death. Pregnant ladies with anemia may experience breathing difficulties, fainting, tiredness, palpitations, and sleep difficulties. They are prone to the adverse effects of anemia as follows:

Antepartum Complications

- Intercurrent infection
- Preeclampsia
- Abortions
- APH
- Preterm labor
- Cardiac failure

Intrapartum Complications

- Uterine inertia
- Dysfunctional labor patterns
- Increased risk of instrumental deliveries
- Fetal distress
- Shock

Postpartum Complications

- Puerperal sepsis
- Subinvolution of uterus
- Failing lactation
- Puerperal venous thrombosis
- Pulmonary embolism
- Delayed wound healing

Harmful Effect on Fetus

- IUGR
- Prematurity
- Congenital malformation
- Stillbirth
- Intrauterine deaths (severe maternal anoxemia)
- Increased neonatal death/perinatal mortality
- Increased risk of iron deficiency anemia in early infancy

IRON DEFICIENCY ANEMIA

Pregnancy costs an approximate 630 mg of extra iron to the mother. In the hierarchy of iron usage, the fetus takes priority, followed by maternal hematocrit while the maternal iron stores are the poor last and are often depleted during the course of pregnancy. Majority of iron transfer to the fetus occurs during the second and third trimesters. The average daily requirement of iron has been calculated as 0.8 mg/day in the first trimester and increases to 7.5 mg/day in the third trimester. And form Indian diet availability varies from 0.8 mg/day to 4.5 mg/day depending on the type of staple used.[10]

The recommended dietary allowance (RDA) of iron in third trimester is 30 mg/day. The average iron density in an average Indian diet is 8.5 mg/1,000 kcal and the average iron absorption from a rice-based and wheat-based Indian diet in pregnancy is 13.3 and 5.3% respectively:

Role of deworming: WHO recommends routine deworming using single dose albendazole (400 mg) or mebendazole (500 mg) in all pregnant patients after first trimester.

TREATMENT OF IRON DEFICIENCY ANEMIA

Oral Iron

All pregnant women should be instructed to take oral iron, empty stomach or 1 hour after meals for better absorption preferably with vitamin C rich product such as orange juice or guava. In general, ferric salts (III) have a superior GI tolerability than ferrous (II) salts at the cost of reduced iron absorption. Gastrointestinal side effects (nausea, constipation, diarrhea, indigestion, and metallic taste) are reported in 70% of pregnant patients owing to the progesterone-induced decreased GI motility and effect of gravid uterus. Measures such as reducing the frequency, content of oral iron and changing it to an alternative preparation or taking the iron with meals may be employed to reduce GI side effects.

Iron Rich Diet

Meat and eggs: Ham, chicken, beef, pork, liver, eggs, seafood—oysters, tuna, sardines, shrimps

Bread and cereals: Whole wheat bread, wheat products, corn meal, oats, rye bread, brown rice, *Lobhia*, soybeans

Fruits: Strawberries, figs, watermelon, dried apricots, dried peaches, raisins, dates

Beans and other foods: Beans, tomato products, molasses, dark chocolate, vegetables, potatoes, spinach, sweet potatoes, peas, broccoli.

Prophylactic Dose

Daily iron supplementation (60–100 mg) of iron and folic acid (500 µg) for all non-anemic pregnant women at first antenatal visit is recommended for primary prevention of anemia with repeat hemoglobin at least once in each trimester.

- In pregnant women with established mild-to-moderate anemia, with a period of gestation less than 30–32 weeks, and those who respond to a trial of oral iron, the treatment should continue with 100 mg elemental iron twice daily and 500 µg of folic acid with an assessment for the rise in hemoglobin. Repeat hemoglobin is recommended after 4 weeks of oral iron.[9]
- After achieving the normalization of hemoglobin, a prophylactic daily iron supplementation (60–100 mg and 500 µg of folic acid) is recommended for at least 6 month during pregnancy and should be continued in postpartum for another 6 months.
- Pregnant women on oral iron supplements should be counseled about steps to reduce gastrointestinal side effects. These include consuming the tablet at least about one hour before a meal, along with absorption enhancers (like vitamin C).
- Parenteral iron is recommended for pregnant women with anemia who do not respond or are intolerant to oral iron. Among the newer intravenous formulation, iron sucrose is approved for use during pregnancy though it is better avoided during the first trimester.
- Parenteral iron is also recommended for pregnant women with severe anemia who require rapid restoration of iron stores in the second and early 3rd trimester of pregnancy.
- Packed red cell transfusion should be reserved for those with severe anemia at any period of gestation.

Parenteral Therapy Indications

- Contraindications of oral therapy
- Patient not co-operative to take oral iron
- Cases seen for the first time during the last 8–10 weeks with severe anemia
- Malabsorption
- Small bowel resection

Side effects of parenteral therapy

- Fever, arthralgia, skin rashes, lymphadenopathy local pain and black staining, anaphylactic reaction.
- It has been found that, the rise in Hb levels after parenteral therapy is 0.7–1 g per week which is same as seen with oral therapy.

The main advantage of parenteral therapy is certainty of its administration.

Calculation of iron requirement

- 250 mg × Hb% deficit + another 50% for replenishment of stores or
- 2.4 × pre-pregnancy weight (kg) × Hb deficit + 1,000 mg (for storage)
- (1,000 mg is taken for complete restoration of the stores in patients with continuing blood loss otherwise 500 mg is adequate)
- Hb deficit = Desired Hb - Actual Hb

Elemental Iron IM Preparations

- Iron Dextran (Imferon) 50 mg/mL
- Iron sorbitol citric acid complex (Jectofer) 50 mg/mL

Drawbacks: Painful injection, skin discoloration, local abscess, allergic reaction, Fe overload, category C drug, gluteal sarcoma. Acute anaphylactic reactions may occur.

Epinephrine should be given immediately in a dose of 0.5 mL of a 1:1,000 solution by SC or IM injection. A test dose of 0.5 mL should be given at the injection site. The full dose should be given at least after 1 hour, if there is no adverse reaction to the test dose. The drug should be injected deeply with a 2″ or 3″ 20–22 gauze needle with Z-track technique.

Intravenous Preparations

Iron dextran: The advantage of iron dextran is the possibility of giving larger doses of iron, up to 1,000 mg in one sitting. A test-dose should be given before every infusion. 25 mg of iron dextran is added to a 50 mL bag of NS and run over 10–15 minutes. Patients should be monitored for another 15–20 minutes. If there are no signs of adverse reactions the rest of the dose diluted in a 500 mL bag of S should be administered over 2–6 hours; the rate of infusion should not exceed 500 mg per hour.

Adverse reactions: Arthralgia, backache, chills, dizziness, moderate-to-high fever, headache, malaise, myalgia.

Iron sucrose: It is commonly used. Preferred in cases of chronic kidney diseases. *How to give:* Dilute 200 mg to be diluted with 200 mL NS, infuse at least 20 minutes. It is to be given three times, weekly. 200 mg max dose per sitting. Rate of administration should not be more than 20 mg/min.

Adverse reactions: Experienced in >5% of patients: Hypotension, cramps/leg cramps, nausea, headache, vomiting, diarrhea.

Newest Fast Acting IV Molecules

Ferric carboxymaltose: It is a novel iron complex that consists of ferric hydroxide core stabilized by a carbohydrate shell, allow for controlled delivery of iron to target tissues. Rapidly taken up by the RE cells, liver, spleen on intravenous route. $T_{1/2}$: 16 hrs. *Dose:* Single dose of 1,000 mg over 15 minutes (maximum 15 mg/kg by injection or 20 mg/kg by infusion). There is a rapid increase in Hb and stores, less antigenic.

Management Protocol of Anemia during Pregnancy

Management of iron deficiency anemia includes dietary modification, oral iron supplementation, intravenous iron and blood transfusion. **Flowchart 1** provides the management protocol of anemia during pregnancy.[11]

Management during Labor in Case of Severe Anemia

First stage: The patient should be in bed or propped up. Oxygen inhalation, intermittent chest auscultation. Strict asepsis Labor monitoring by partograph, CTG monitoring, sedation and analgesic, fluid restriction.

Flowchart 1: Management protocol of anemia during pregnancy.[9]

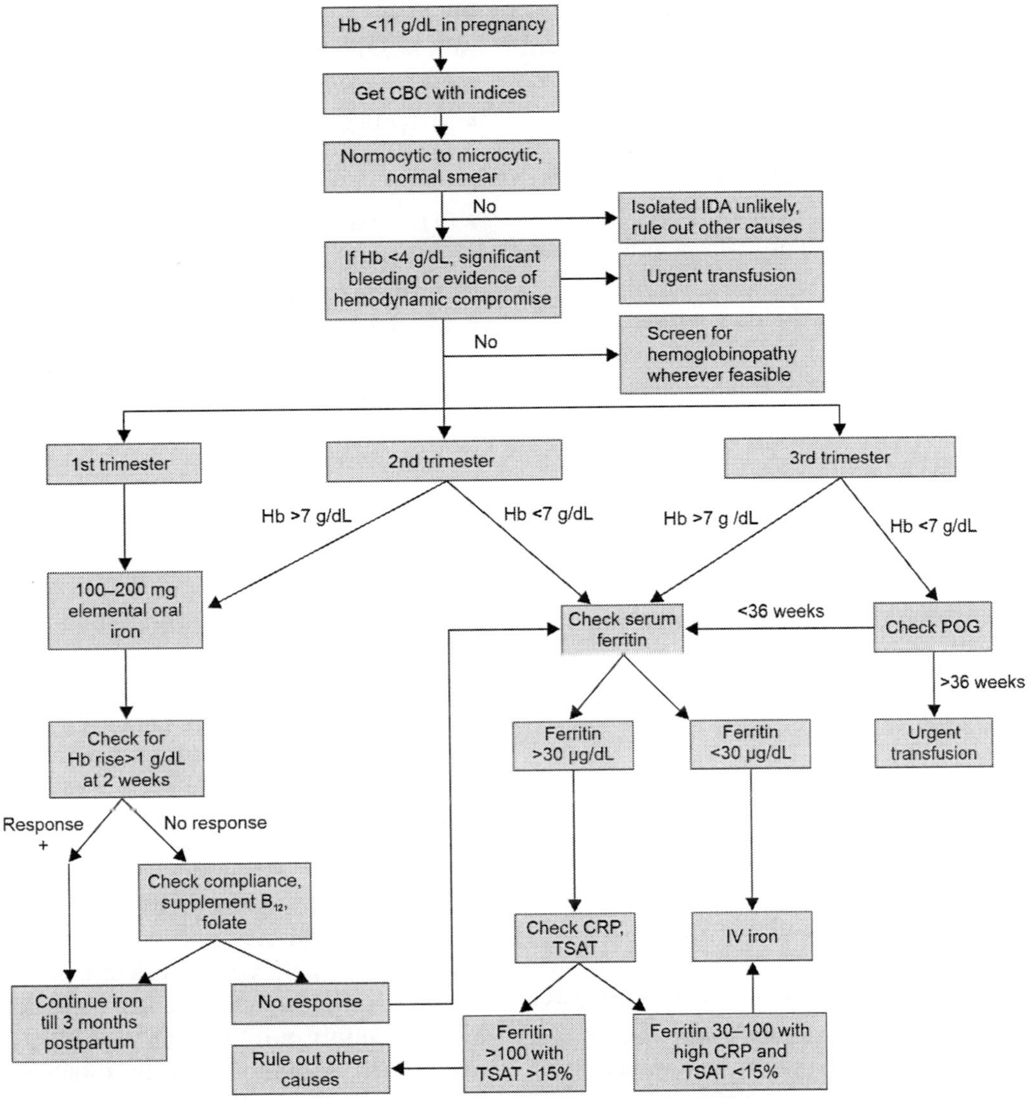

(CBC: complete blood count; CRP: C-reactive protein; IV: intravenous; SAT: transferrin saturation)

Second stage: Asepsis oxytocin-concentrated form, restrict fluid prophylactic low forceps or vacuum delivery to cut short second stage of labor.

Third stage: Active management of 3rd stage. Blood loss with fresh packed cell transfusion, diuretics prior to transfusion, close monitoring of vitals look for any genital trauma.

Management – Puerperium

- Prophylactic antibiotics
- Iron therapy for at least 3 months
- Contraception advice

POSTPARTUM ANEMIA

It is a common problem throughout the world and the prevalence is high in developing countries around 15–20%.

Risk factors:

- Iron deficiency anemia in 3rd trimester
- Acute bleeding at delivery
- Infections such as malaria and intestinal worms
- Diseases conditions such as hemoglobinopathies, poor socioeconomical conditions and nutritional deficiency.

Diagnosis: Hb <10 g/dL, S. ferritin <15 μg/dL in 24–48 hours post-delivery.

Severe postpartum anemia has a negative impact on both mother and child health, it is associated with increased risk of PPH, depression, reduced cognitive functions and urinary tract infections, fatigue and exhaustion, insufficient milk syndrome and reduced breast milk quality.

MEGALOBLASTIC ANEMIA

Derangement in red cell maturation due to impaired DNA synthesis.

Etiology: Folate deficiency, vitamin B_{12} deficiency

Folic acid is necessary for the synthesis of purines and pyrimidines, which ultimately take part with vitamin B_{12} in the synthesis of nucleic acid and nucleoproteins.

Incidence: 0.2–5%

In pregnancy cause is almost always folate deficiency.

Folate stores last for 2–4 months, vitamin B_{12} for 2–3 years, vitamin B_{12} deficiency occurs only in pure vegetarians. Pernicious anemia associated with infertility.

Sign and symptoms: Anorexia and occasional diarrhea, Pallor of varying degree, ulceration in mouth and tongue, hemorrhagic patches under the skin and conjunctiva, enlarged liver and spleen.

Lab investigations:

- HB <10 gm%
- Hypersegmented neutrophil
- MCV >100
- Oval macrocytes and pancytopenia
- MCH >33 pg
- S Folate <3 ng/mL
- Serum iron is normal or high
- Bone marrow shows megaloblasts
- Serum vitamin B_{12} <100 pg/mL
- Red cell folate assay is better indicator than serum folate levels.

Treatment:

Prophylactic: All woman of reproductive age should be given 400 μg of folic acid daily.

Curative: Daily administration of folic acid 5 mg orally continued for at least 3 months postpartum. *Vitamin B_{12}:* 1 mg IM on alternate days for 2 weeks followed by 1 mg IM once a month for 6 months.

THALASSEMIA

Two classes of abnormality of Hb A synthesis can result in a decreased portion of Hb A:

1. Quantitative defect (thalassemia)
2. Qualitative defect (sickle cell disease)

The synthesis of globin chain is partially or completely suppressed resulting in reduced Hb. content in red cells, which have shortened life span. The result is ineffective erythropoiesis, hemolysis and varying degree of anemia.

Incidence: 1 in 300–500 pregnancies

Types of thalassemia:

- Alpha-thalassemia (impaired production of alpha chain)
- Beta-thalassemia (impaired production of beta chains)
- Thalassemia intermedia and minor

Low MCV, MCHC, near normal or normal MCHC.

Diagnosis is confirmed by a raised concentration of HbA2.

If patient is found to have thalassemia partner should be tested if both have thalassemia trait the couple is offered prenatal diagnostic testing. Pregnancy termination can be offered if fetus is found to be thalassemia major. In thalassemia minor, oral iron and folate prescribed but never parenteral preparations.

α-Thalassemia

- Four types—alpha major, intermediate form or HbH disease and two minor traits
- Alpha major is usually incompatible with life and pregnancy ends in a hydropic fetus.
- Alpha-thalassemia trait—no/mild anemia in pregnancy, no abnormal Hb found.
- HbH disease—chronic hemolytic anemia, moderate anemia, 5–30% HbH on electrophoresis, transmitted as alpha-thalassemia trait
- Management of carrier state is as in case of beta-thalassemia minor.
- They should receive routine iron and folate supplements.

β-Thalassemia Major

- It is rarely encountered.
- Both beta chains are missing.
- Severe anemia occurs.
- It is diagnosed in pediatric age.
- Hypogonadotropic hypogonadism, diabetes and thyroid diseases, so reduced fertility. Screening of the husband is necessary followed by genetic counseling.
- Thalassemia patients have poor cardiac reserve and are at risk for acute fatty liver of pregnancy and HELLP syndrome.
- They are prone to cholelithiasis due to hemolytic anemia and subsequent cholecystitis.
- *Follow-up during pregnancy:* It is recommended that there should be monthly follow-up till 28 weeks then every 2 weeks. Aim is target Hb >10 gm%.
- *Treatment* is blood transfusion, iron therapy is contraindicated.
- Desferrioxamine discontinued during pregnancy due to possible harmful effect on fetus and risk of iron deficiency in neonate. During pregnancy chelation can be used in second and third trimesters for cases where potential benefit outweighs the potential fetal risk.
- *Intrapartum management*: Time and mode of delivery is individualized. However, most cases undergo C-section because of cephalopelvic disproportion, mainly due to short maternal stature and skeletal deformity.
- If vaginal delivery is decided, then active management of third stage of labor.
- *Postpartum management*: There is high risk of thromboembolism so low molecular weight heparin prophylaxis should be administered.

HEMOLYTIC ANEMIA

Hemolytic anemia is a disorder in which red blood cells are destroyed faster than they can be made. It may occur because of erythrocyte defects such as abnormalities of hemoglobin structure, membrane abnormalities or metabolic disturbances. Hemolytic anemia can be inherited or acquired:

Inherited hemolytic anemia occurs when parents pass the gene for the condition on to their children. Almost all erythrocyte defects causing hemolysis are hereditary in nature.

Acquired hemolytic anemia is not something you are born with. You develop the condition later. Some types of acquired hemolytic anemia are short-term (temporary) and go away over several months. Other types can become lifelong (chronic). Acquired anemia may happen because of:

- Certain infections, which may be viral or bacterial.
- Medicines, such as penicillin, sulfa-medicines, antimalarial medicines, or acetaminophen
- Blood cancers
- Autoimmune disorders, such as lupus, rheumatoid arthritis, or ulcerative colitis
- An overactive spleen (hypersplenism)
- Mechanical heart valves that may damage red blood cells as they leave the heart
- A severe reaction to a blood transfusion

Classification of Hemolytic Anemia

Hemolytic anemia can be classified in various ways as follows:

- *Primary hemolytic anemia:* Various types are
  - Sickle cell disease
  - Hereditary spherocytosis
- *Secondary hemolytic anemia:*
  - Lupus erythematosus
  - Preeclampsia syndrome

Hemolytic anemia can also be classified as:

- *Intrinsic defects:*
  - Hemoglobinopathy
  - Red cell membrane defect
  - Red cell enzymes effect
- *Extrinsic defects:*
  - Autoimmune hemolytic anemia
  - Paroxysmal nocturnal hemoglobinuria (PNH)
  - Disseminated intravascular coagulation (DIC)
  - HELLP syndrome
  - Thrombotic thrombocytopenic purpura (TTP)
  - Acute fatty liver of pregnancy

SICKLE CELL DISEASE

There are different variants of sickle cell disease, more common during pregnancy are homozygous sickle cell (SS) disease and sickle cell hemoglobin C (SC) disease.

Etiology

Sickle cell trait is caused by abnormal hemoglobin called sickle hemoglobin or HbS. Sickle hemoglobin is as a result of a point mutation in the beta-globin chain. This point mutation replaces A with T at codon 6 of beta-hemoglobin chain. This causes the switch from glutamic acid to valine amino acid. The valine-type hemoglobin causes red cells to sickle when exposed to a low oxygen threshold. Patient with sickle cell trait inherits HbS from one parent and HbA from the other parent making them heterozygous.[11]

Sickle cell trait is more prevalent in people who are of African-descent and also whose ancestors come from tropical and sub-tropical regions where malaria is endemic. The prevalence rates of sickle cell trait in the United States is 9% among African American which is about 3 million people, and 0.2% among Caucasians. Worldwide, it is estimated that there are 300 million people with sickle cell trait and one-third of this number are in sub-Saharan Africa. The prevalence of sickle cell trait is higher in areas where malaria is endemic.[12]

Pathophysiology

Conditions that favor sickling:

- Severe hypoxia
- Dehydration
- Increase in sympathetic outflow

- Hypothermia/hyperthermia, high 2,3-DPG levels, and release of inflammatory cells.

The HbS will result in the clogging of tiny capillary vessels, especially in the bones by sickled red blood cells. Apart from the sickling of the cells, other cells interact to cause more adhesion of the red blood cells including inflammatory cells, and platelets. This could occur in multiple organs in the body including the chest, heart, lungs, abdomen, kidneys, and extremities. Due to the repeated attacks, organ damage may happen due to constant ischemia. This reduces the average lifespan of RBCs to only 17 days in contrasts to 120 days of normal erythrocytes. This results in chronic compensated anemia with Hb ranging from 6 to 9 g/dL. Due to excessive red cell destruction, there is associated splenomegaly and gallstone formation.[12]

Clinical Features of Sickle Cell Disease

- Painful crisis
- Chronic hemolytic anemia
- Higher infection rate
- Chest syndrome
- Hyposplenism
- Avascular bone necrosis

Effect of Sickle Cell Disease on Pregnancy

- Miscarriage
- Infection
- Pre-eclampsia
- Prematurity
- Fetal growth restriction
- Maternal morbidity
- Stillbirth
- Perinatal mortality

Diagnosis of Sickle Cell Disease

1. Peripheral blood film shows anisocytosis, poikilocytosis, Howell–Jolly bodies, target cells and sickle cells.
2. Sickling test
3. High performance liquid chromatography (HPLC)
4. Hemoglobin (Hb) solubility test
5. Increased reticulocytes counts if severe sickling occurs.

SICKLE CELL CRISIS

Vaso-occlusive Crisis

Sickle cells have altered motion due to distorted erythrocyte membranes resulting in vascular stasis and hypoxia. This leads to metabolic acidosis which further aggravates tissue hypoxia and sickling. Also, there is interaction of sickled erythrocytes with capillary endothelial membrane and microvascular injury. It causes a prothrombotic state and ischemic necrosis and infarction of various organs. All this leads to painful, vaso-occlusive sickle cell crisis resulting in end organ damage.

Hematologic Crisis

Rarely aplastic crisis can happen in these patients during pregnancy with malnutrition and multiple pregnancies.

Acute chest syndrome: It is a serious complication resulting from sickling in lungs compounded by infection, infarction, pulmonary sequestration and fat embolization from bone marrow with development of restrictive chronic lung disease.

Sickle cell trait patients may have hematuria and rhabdomyolysis.

Antenatal Evaluation

Unlike other developing and some developed world countries, parents in the United States are offered genetic testing when the female is pregnant. Also, there is a requirement for newborn screening in all 50 states for the sickle cell trait before a baby is discharged from the hospital.

To evaluate this disease, the sickling test can be used as a primary screening procedure. A drop of blood is placed on a slide and then prepared to be inspected under the microscope. If sickling is observed, hemoglobin electrophoresis is used to confirm the diagnosis. The hemoglobin electrophoresis gives a percentage of each hemoglobin type that is present in a sample. In sickle cell trait, patients have a mixture of both the normal hemoglobin A and hemoglobin S.

Treatment/Management

Sickle cell trait patients usually do not require any treatment. Treatment is only indicated if a patient presents with medical conditions including the ones that have been associated with the trait. It is important for clinicians to recognize the complications associated with sickle cell trait so that prompt management can be started once patients present with symptoms.

Pregnancies with sickle cell disease are high-risk pregnancies. Iron supplementation is avoided and given only for proven iron deficiency.

First trimester:

1. Low-dose aspirin 75 mg once daily
2. Low molecular weight aspirin during hospital admission
3. Prophylactic graduated compression stockings
4. Prenatal testing can be done using chorion villus sampling or amniocentesis for DNA of abnormal Hb.

Second and third trimester

USG for fetal growth to rule out fetal growth restriction.

The patient should be given folate supplementation and penicillin prophylaxis to prevent infections like pneumonia. kidney and liver function tests should be regularly done.

Management of Adverse Events in Pregnancy with Sickle Cell Disease

Six major adverse events need planning with effective management for better maternal and neonatal outcomes, as described here:

1. *Painful crisis:* Pregnant women presenting with vaso-occlusive crises should be hospitalized, adequate bed rest and fluid intake should be ensured. For pain relief, paracetamol and other NSAIDs should be given.
2. *Acute chest syndrome (ACS):* Pregnant women with SCD presenting with complaints of severe cough and chest pain should be evaluated for ACS. Pulmonary infiltrates on chest X-ray, leukocytosis, blood, and sputum cultures is done to ascertain infectious complications. Treatment includes appropriate antibiotics, oxygen support, hydration, analgesics and if required blood transfusion.
3. *Pulmonary embolism:* Women presenting with chest pain and respiratory distress with normal chest X-ray should be suspected to have pulmonary embolism. Treatment should be started with LMWH awaiting the confirmation of the diagnosis.
4. *Strokes:* Infarctive and hemorrhagic strokes should be suspected in any female presenting with acute neurological impairment.
5. *Hematological complication:* Anemia is the most common complication of pregnancy. Blood loss, bone marrow suppression by parvovirus infection and nutritional deficiencies are the causes.[2] However, RCOG guidelines (Royal College of Obstetrician and Gynaecologists) do not recommend the same. HELLP syndrome can develop in

up to 10% of women with pre-eclampsia. It can be managed conservatively or by urgent delivery depending on gestational age.[13]

6. *Infections:* The major sites of infection are the urinary tract and the respiratory system. Less often, puerperal endometritis, hepatitis, transient bacteremia, osteomyelitis, and HIV have been encountered. Antibiotics and symptomatic management, followed by elective cholecystectomy, is advised in the postpartum period.

Prenatal Diagnosis

Prenatal diagnosis remains an important option for couples at-risk of having a child with SCD. With increasing awareness in the community, more couples are opting for prenatal diagnosis. First-trimester prenatal diagnosis by chorionic villus sampling at 10–12 weeks of gestation and DNA analysis is the method of choice. Often couples at risk are identified late in the second trimester, and they can still be offered amniocentesis at 14–15 weeks gestation and DNA analysis or fetal blood sampling by cordocentesis at 18–19 weeks gestation and HPLC analysis of the fetal blood to look for the percentage of adult and sickle hemoglobin present.

Celocentesis for aspiration of celomic fluid at 7–9 weeks gestation allows earlier prenatal diagnosis for monogenic disorders like beta-thalassemia and sickle cell anemia. However, there is a problem of maternal cell contamination. It has been recently shown that this can be overcome through embryofetal erythroid precursors selection using anti-CD71 Microbeads or by direct micromanipulator pick up of the cells selected based on their morphology.[14]

Pregnancy Management in Sickle Cell Disease

Preconceptual Care

- All women with SCD in reproductive age should be provided with relevant information on how SCD affects pregnancy and what measures should be taken for better maternal and fetal outcomes. It is during this period that she should be made aware of the importance of partner screening and the options for prenatal screening.
- A complete medical and social history of the mother should be obtained, including her vaccination status, current medications, any other co-morbid condition, and any drug abuse. Vaccination against all encapsulated organism, including *Neisseria meningitides*, *Streptococcus pneumonia*, and *Haemophilus influenza* should be updated. In addition, hepatitis B and influenza vaccine should be given.
- Folic acid (5 mg) should be given once daily both preconception and throughout pregnancy. Iron is recommended if there is evidence of iron deficiency, but most of the women have iron overload.
- Most of the women are on hydroxyurea. It is recommended that drugs like hydroxyurea, ACE (angiotensin-converting enzyme) inhibitors, and iron chelators should be discontinued at least 3 months before conception due to the risk of teratogenic side effects.
- Screening for complications like pulmonary hypertension by 2D echocardiography, retinal screening for proliferative retinopathy, iron overload, renal and liver function studies to rule out sickle nephropathy and hepatic involvement should be done yearly.

Antenatal Care

- The first prenatal visit should be a comprehensive assessment. Routine blood investigations like complete blood count, HIV, HBs Ag, HCV should be done along with urine examination. Mother should be explained the importance of a regular antenatal visit; it is recommended to visit obstetrician every other week during the first two trimesters. Blood pressure and urinalysis should be performed at each consultation, and midstream urine for culture performed monthly as these women are prone to pre-eclampsia and increased risk of urinary tract infections.
- Mothers should be explained to avoid precipitating factors of sickle cell crises such as exposure to extreme temperatures, dehydration, and overexertion. Also, repeated vomiting can cause dehydration and precipitate crisis. Hence, she should seek medical advice at the earliest.
- Women who are at increased risk of pre-eclampsia are advised to take low-dose aspirin 75 mg from 12 weeks of gestation unless they have aspirin sensitivity.
- Transfusion is indicated in case of severe anemia, and exchange transfusion is recommended in case of stroke and acute chest syndrome.

Intrapartum Care

- Delivery of SCD mother should be conducted in a center equipped with all healthcare facilities to manage high-risk pregnancies. Pregnant women with SCD who have a normally growing fetus should be offered elective birth through induction of labor at 38–40 weeks of gestation, as SCD by itself is not a contraindication to attempt vaginal delivery or vaginal birth after cesarean section.
- If there is any indication or impending complications, cesarean delivery should be considered.
- Women should be kept warm and given adequate fluid during labor. Pain can be managed with adequate use of analgesics. Epidural anesthesia is particularly useful in this regard, and efforts should be made to shorten the duration of labor as well.
- Continuous intrapartum electronic fetal heart rate monitoring is recommended owing to the increased risk of fetal distress.
- Blood should be cross-matched and kept ready at the time of delivery.

Postpartum Care

- In the postpartum period, it is crucial to assess the degree of anemia aggravated by blood loss during labor and delivery, and replacement instituted when indicated.
- Hydration and oxygenation should be maintained, and early mobilization encouraged. Crises should be managed as for non-pregnant women.
- NSAIDs are routinely administered in the postpartum period and can be used during breastfeeding.
- Breastfeeding should be encouraged, as in women without SCD.
- Thromboprophylaxis in the form of low-molecular-weight heparin is recommended for seven days following vaginal delivery or a period of 6 weeks following cesarean section.
- Antithrombotic stockings are also recommended.
- Screening of newborns for sickle hemoglobin is recommended.
- Mother should be advised regarding contraception, progestogen-containing contraceptives such as the progesterone-only pill, injectable contraceptives, and the levonorgestrel intrauterine system

are safe and effective in SCD. Estrogen-containing contraceptives should be used as second-line agents. Barrier methods are as safe and effective in women with SCD as in the general population.

APLASTIC ANEMIA

Aplastic anemia causes a deficiency of all blood cell types: Red blood cells, white blood cells, and platelets.

Aplastic anemia can be definitively diagnosed by bone marrow biopsy. Normal bone marrow has 30–70% blood stem cells, but in aplastic anemia, these cells are mostly gone and are replaced by fat.

It is characterized by pancytopenia and bone marrow hypocellularity.

1. Hereditary—Fanconi's anemia
2. Acquired—Radiation

Viruses: Parvovirus, hepatitis, Epstein-Barr virus, systemic lupus erythematosus (SLE).

Many other conditions can cause aplastic anemia, including:

- Autoimmune diseases, such as rheumatoid arthritis or lupus
- Cancer
- Chronic infections, such as HIV/AIDS and tuberculosis
- Chronic kidney disease
- Inflammatory bowel disease (IBD), such as Crohn's disease or ulcerative colitis
- Other chronic diseases that involve inflammation, such as diabetes and heart failure.

Treatment

- Terminate pregnancy in first trimester after counseling
- *Second and third trimester:* 1st line—erythropoietin and granulocyte transfusion
- Thymocyte gamma-globulin, high-dose steroids, cyclosporine
- The disease has a serious prognosis, and the maternal mortality is about 30%.

Massive Blood Transfusion

Various definitions of massive blood transfusion (MBT) have been published in medical literature such as:[15-17]

a. Replacement of one entire blood volume within 24 hours
b. Transfusion of >10 units of packed red blood cells (PRBCs) in 24 hours
c. Transfusion of >20 units of PRBCs in 24 hours
d. Transfusion of >4 units of PRBCs in 1 hour when on-going need is foreseeable.
e. Replacement of 50% of total blood volume (TBV) within 3 hours

1. The cornerstone of massive blood transfusion is balanced transfusion with PRBCs, platelets, and fresh-frozen plasma (FFP). Blood products in a 1:1:1 ratio of PRBC: FFP: Platelets.[18] Avoid crystalloid resuscitation. For hemorrhagic shock with ongoing bleeding, crystalloid administration may dilute out coagulation factors and erythrocyte concentration. Ultimately blood products will be needed (to achieve target hemoglobin concentrations and coagulation factor levels), so front-loading your resuscitation with crystalloid may eventually serve to promote *volume overload.*[19]
2. Fibrinogen may become depleted in massive transfusion, due to dilution. There is some fibrinogen in fresh-frozen plasma, but not necessarily enough. Fibrinogen can be supplemented via the administration of fibrinogen concentrates or cryoprecipitate.
3. Tranexamic acid has a proven benefit in obstetric hemorrhage and early traumatic bleeding. Typical dosing is one gram IV given immediately, which may be followed by infusions of 1 g over 8 hours repeatedly for 24 hours.

4. *Reversal of other coagulopathies:* The MTP protocol is designed to avoid *causing* dilution coagulopathy, but it would not *correct* a pre-existing coagulopathy. So, consideration is warranted regarding any underlying coagulopathies that the patient may have. Warfarin or oral anticoagulation require immediate reversal, e.g., with PCC (prothrombin complex concentrate).[19]

   Platelet dysfunction: This is commonly caused by antiplatelet agents or uremia. The most common emergency treatment is *desmopressin* (DDAVP; 0.3 µg/kg IV to a maximum dose of 21 µg).
5. Hypocalcemia is problematic because it causes coagulopathy. When administering one round of MTP (containing 6 units PRBCs), it is probably reasonable to add either 1–2 g of IV calcium chloride or 3–6 g of IV calcium gluconate.
6. *Avoid acidosis*: Acidosis impairs the interaction between calcium and negatively charged phospholipids, blocking the initial steps in the coagulation cascade.
7. *Avoid hypothermia:* Patients undergoing massive transfusion tend to develop *hypothermia*, which will impair blood clotting. This is promoted by rapid administration of cooled or room-temperature blood products and fluids. Hypothermia may be avoided or treated by:
   - Providing warmed blood products (e.g., via a Level 1 or Belmont infusers with in-line warming)
   - Preemptive use of warming blankets, in response to any evidence of hypothermia or shivering
   - With intubated patients, warming the inhaled gas as much as possible (some ventilators may allow control of the degree of warming)
   - Monitoring the patient's temperature[19]

Key Points

- Anemia in pregnancy is a major public health problem in India since it is direct cause for 20% of maternal death and indirect cause for 20% of maternal death.
- According to WHO, Hb <11 g/dL, is considered as anemia in pregnancy; according to FOGSI: Hb <10 g/dL is considered as anemia in pregnancy and according to CDC: Hb <11 g/dL in the first trimester and third trimester and <10.5 g/dL in the second trimester.
- Most common anemia during pregnancy is iron deficiency and it can be dual, both iron and folic acid deficiency.
- There is an increased iron requirement during pregnancy for fetus, placenta, for RBC expansion, blood loss during pregnancy. Net requirement during pregnancy is 1,000 mg.
- Due to physiological changes in pregnancy, there is increase in plasma volume to 50% and RBC cell mass increases only to 20%, there is a fall in hemoglobin concentration and hematocrit resulting hemodilution termed as physiological anemia of pregnancy.
- Symptoms may be easy fatigue, breathlessness, palpitations, pedal edema and signs are pallor, glossitis, tachycardia, hemic murmur ad may result in CCF.
- Effects of anemia during pregnancy on mothers are pre-eclampsia, abruptio, pre-term labor and on fetus are IUGR, IUD, prematurity, LBW.
- Often, the root cause of anemia holds back in infancy and childhood. Treating the anemia in childhood can prevent anemia in pregnancy by correcting the nutrition in childhood and adolescent age group.[1,4,6] Instead of increasing bank balance, we should create iron balance in adolescents and reproductive age group females. Blood can be replaced only with blood. We cannot create blood bank in every corner of India but we can treat anemia.

REFERENCES

1. Anaemia in Pregnancy. ACOG Practice Bulletin No. 233. American College of Obstetricians and Gynaecologists. Obstet Gynecol 2021;138:e55-64.
2. Ministry of Health and Family Welfare (2015–2016) Govt. of India, National Family Health Survey (NFHS-4), State Fact Sheet. Mumbai: International Institute for Population Sciences.
3. World Health Organization. Anaemia. [Internet]. Geneva: World Health Organization; [updated 2023; cited 2023]. Available from: https://www.who.int/data/nutrition/nlis/info/anaemia.
4. American College of Obstetricians and Gynaecologists. ACOG Practice Bulletin No. 95: Anaemia in pregnancy. Obstet Gynecol. 2008;112(1):201-7.
5. Thomas C, Thomas L. Biochemical markers and hematologic indices in the diagnosis of functional iron deficiency. Clin Chem. 2002;48:1066-76.
6. Wallach JW. Hematologic diseases. Interpretation of Diagnostic Tests, 8th edition. Lippincott Williams & Wilkins; 2006. pp. 385-419.
7. Carley A. Anemia: When is it iron deficiency? Pediatr Nurs. 2003;29(2):127-33.
8. Pavord S, Myers B, Robinson S, et al. UK Guidelines on the management of iron deficiency in pregnancy. Br J Haematol. 2012;156(5):588-600.
9. FOGSI General Clinical Practice Recommendations. Management of Iron Deficiency Anemia in Pregancy, May 2016.
10. Stevens GA, Finucane MM, De-Regil LM, et al. Global, regional, and national trends in haemoglobin concentration and prevalence of total and severe anaemia in children and pregnant and non-pregnant women for 1995–2011: a systematic analysis of population-representative data. Lancet Glob Health. 2013;1(1):e16-25.
11. Tandon R, Jain A, Malhotra P. Management of iron deficiency anemia in pregnancy in India. Indian J Hematol Blood Transfus. 2018;34(2):204-15.
12. Mitchell BL. Sickle Cell Trait and Sudden Death. Sports Med Open. 2018;4(1):19.
13. Rogers ZR. A Pediatrician's Quick Guide to Sickle Cell Trait. Pediatr Rev. 2023;44(4):240-2.
14. Boga C, Ozdogu H. Pregnancy and sickle cell disease: a review of the current literature. Critical Reviews in Oncology/Hematology. 2016;98:364-74.
15. Giambona A. Embryo-fetal erythroid cell selection from celomic fluid allows earlier prenatal diagnosis of haemoglobinopathies. Prenat Diagn. 2016;36(4):375-81.
16. Raymer JM, Flynn LM, Martin RF. Massive transfusion of blood in the surgical patient. Surg Clin North Am. 2012;92:221-34.
17. Chidester SJ, Williams N, Wang W, Groner JI. A pediatric massive transfusion protocol. J Trauma Acute Care Surg. 2012;73:1273-7.
18. Massive transfusion protocol (MTP) for hemorrhagic shock ASA committee on blood management. Available from: https://www.asahq.org/For-Members/About-ASA/ASA-Committees/Committee-on-Blood-Management.aspx.
19. Pacheco LD, Saade GR, Costantine MM, et al. An update on the use of massive transfusion protocols in obstetrics. Am J Obstet Gynecol. 2016;214(3):340-4.

CHAPTER 18

Intrauterine Fetal Death and its Medicolegal Implications

Sarika Gautam, Pooja Sinha

INTRODUCTION

When a woman gets pregnant, she hopes to have a healthy baby when she gives birth, but some women regrettably do not have this happy ending and instead experience intrauterine fetal death, which adds to their mental strain. The loss of an intrauterine fetus is distressing for the couple and the attending obstetrician. A thorough approach that should be used by the obstetrician to treat the condition, including counselling before and after birth, the choice of delivery mode, emotional support during delivery, and advice for the necessary investigation to identify the etiology of intrauterine fetal death (IUFD).

DEFINITION AND TYPES

Early IUFD: Early IUFD is defined as IUFD occurs between 20-to-28-week gestation age. As per International Classification of Disease Revision 10 (ICD-10), an early fetal death is defined as a death with fetal weight at least of 500 g or crown-rump length of 25 cm or more.

Late IUFD: as per ICD 10, An IUFD beyond 28 weeks or crown-heel length more than 35 cm.[1]

Type According to Time of Death

Fresh still birth: Defined as stillbirths occurring after the onset of labor in less than 12 hours before delivery with no skin changes weighing more than 1,000 g and more than 28 weeks of gestation but excludes severe lethal congenital abnormalities.

Macerated stillbirth: Antepartum stillbirth is a baby born with all the changes which occur in a fetus retained in utero after death and the death occurred before the initiation of labor. A "macerated" fetus shows skin and soft-tissue changes (skin discoloration or darkening, redness, peeling, and breakdown).[2]

Definition

The intrauterine fetal death defined as per World Health Organization (WHO), "Fetal demise (fetal death) refers to situations in which the fetus is no longer alive, but the uterus has not yet started to expel its contents and the cervical os remains closed.[1] WHO further suggested definition of late fetal death for international comparison as "fetal death of ≥1000 g birth weight, ≥28 completed weeks of gestation and ≥35 cm body length, with birth weight given priority over gestational age".[3]

It has been recommended by WHO that birth weight can vary as per region and gender so use of gestational age is more appropriate than birth weight. Information regarding gestational age can be retrieved easily than the birth weight. In recent decades, viability also increased because of better intensive care in high income countries and they need to record the outcomes.[3]

The Perinatal Mortality Surveillance Report (CEMACH) defined stillbirth as "a baby delivered with no signs of life known to have died after 24 completed weeks of pregnancy'. Intrauterine fetal death refers to babies with no signs of life in utero.[4]

DIAGNOSIS

Symptoms

Female patients frequently complain that they are not feeling fetal movement, but a doctor should not base their diagnosis simply on this symptom because loss of fetal movement can also be caused by other conditions, such as anomalies in the amniotic fluid. The absence of fetal movement cannot be assumed to be an indication of IUFD, but it must be taken seriously as a warning indicator, and the cause must be thoroughly investigated.

Signs

Regression of pregnancy related changes like breast changes (but non-specific in cases of multiparous lady, decreased fundal height, all these signs are only useful in booked cases), Decrease tone of uterus, non-audible fetal heart on auscultation. Real-time ultrasonography is the investigation of choice to confirm IUFD. Fetal heart should be checked at least for 2–3 minutes before giving the diagnosis of IUFD associated findings with IUFD should also mention in the ultrasound report like amount of liquor, placental position, no of fetus (if multiple gestation), findings suggestive of hydrops fetalis. Any associated important findings like overlapping of skull bones (Spalding sign), Deuel's halo sign, gross distortion of fetal anatomy (maceration), soft-tissue edema: skin >5 mm, few uncommon findings may be thrombus in fetal heart, gas shadow in fetal heart, Deuel's halo sign.[5]

Obsolete Signs/Very Less Used (Academic Use)[6]

- X-ray of maternal abdomen
- Crowding of fetal ribs
- Hyperflexion of fetal spine
- skull bones (Overriding of fetal Spalding sign)
- Deuel's Halo sign
- Gas in umbilical arteries (Helix sign)
- Gas shadow in heart (Robert's sign)

Ultrasonographic Signs of IUFD[5]

- Absent fetal heart
- Absent fetal parts movement
- Skin edema >5 mm

Signs of Older IUFD

- Halo sign
- Robert's sign
- Thrombus in fetal heart
- Gas shadow in fetal heart
- Gross distortion of fetal anatomy (Advanced)

MRI Signs of IUFD

Although USG is a definitive economic choice to confirm the diagnosis but MRI also plays an important role to search the cause of IUFD.

Two main MRI sequences are being used in IUFD one is T2-like two-dimensional balanced steady state-free precession, a white blood sequence, or T2-weighted single shot fast spin echo (SSFSE), a black blood sequence. Specific signs of IUFD are:

- Constricted fetal heart with poorly delineated heart chamber
- Global brain ischemia, abnormal globes, effusions, body wall edema, and umbilical cord thrombosis.[7]

Etiology

Stillbirth could be due to various risk factors which can be broadly divided into:

- Maternal
- Placental
- Fetal
- Unexplained

Despite rigorous investigation to find out the root cause of the IUFD in majority of cases etiology remain unexplained in approximately 25–72% cases.[8]

Risk factors of IUFD broadly divided into maternal, fetal, and placental causes.

Risk Factors[9]

The risk factors of intrauterine fetal death can be multiple as depicted in **Table 1**.

Medicolegal Causes Related to Fetal Death

- Abdominal trauma
- Homicidal violence
- Suicide
- Sexual assault
- Poisoning or substance abuse

MANAGEMENT OF IUFD

- Pre-delivery counseling and investigation
- Type of management (expectant vs. induction of labor)
- Delivery
- Fetal and placental evaluation
- Post-delivery counseling
- Breast care and management
- Follow-up visit

TABLE 1: Risk factors of intrauterine fetal death.[9]

Maternal risk factor			
Medical conditions	***Obstetric conditions***	***Placental risk factor***	***Fetal risk factor***
• Obesity • Maternal age • Infections (sepsis, malaria, syphilis, influenza, COVID-19) • Hyperpyrexia • Smoking • Substance abuse • Maternal preexisting diabetes • Hypertension • Red cell isoimmunization • Thyroid disorder • Systemic lupus erythematosus • APLA • Cholestasis of pregnancy • Liver disorders, AFLP, acute liver injury • Thrombophilias • Maternal trauma	• Abruption placenta • Obstetric hemorrhage • PPROM • Multifetal gestation • Shoulder dystocia • Unattended prolonged labor • Obstructed labor • Uterine rupture	• Cord accidents • Placenta previa and Placental abruption • Chorioamnionitis • Twin-to-twin transfusion • Discordant twins • Iatrogenic (external cephalic version, drug overdoses)	• Multiple pregnancy • PROM/PPROM • Congenital anomalies • Genetic disorders • Immune/Nonimmune hydrops • Congenital infections

Pre-delivery Counseling

Meticulous couple counseling plays a major role in management while dealing with the case of IUFD, tender empathetic counseling leads to build-up confidence in couples to deal with all the stages of labor and post-delivery void of their life.

It should be done in private room, if hospital premises permits, they should be well informed about the options available for investigations and management, post-delivery baby handover, whether mother want to see the baby, awareness of burial as per their religion and belief to be discussed.

Investigations

The aim of investigations is to rule out known etiology and find out any other specific individual reason of IUFD, it includes thorough maternal and fetal evaluation.

Maternal Evaluation

Complete maternal evaluation needed to find out the etiology of IUFD, a detailed history which includes medical, obstetric history, drug, substance, radiation exposure, working culture, family history in detail with three generation pedigree analysis.

Detailed obstetric history for previous child if any and their developmental profile should be asked to rule out any genetic causes. Consanguineous Marriage history should also be sought to rule out autosomal recessive disorders which are running in family.

Menstrual history should be enquired and gestational age to be confirmed by LMP.

In medical history, always rule out chronic medical, infectious, and genetic disorders such as diabetes mellitus, chronic hypertension, heart diseases, venous thromboembolism, malaria, syphilis, COVID-19, dengue, *Listeria*, TORCH infections, GBS, *E. coli*, hereditary thrombophilia, autoimmune disorders.[10]

Investigations to be Sent before Delivery

- Complete hemogram with absolute platelet count
- Liver function test
- Renal function test
- ABO-Rh if not done till now
- Rh-isoimmunization
- Bleeding time, clotting time, prothrombin time and INR
- Rule out various bacterial infections by urine culture
- Blood culture
- High vaginal swab
- Cervical swab
- VDRL
- Viral hepatitis's screen
- Human immunodeficiency virus screen
- Serum thyroid-stimulating hormone (STSH)
- Oral glucose tolerance test
- HbA1C
- Thrombophilia screening

Investigations to be Sent Post-Delivery

These tests should be sent only after parents pre-delivery counseling along with written and informed consent:

- Fetal blood
- Fetal swab
- Placental swab
- Fetal and placental tissue for karyotyping
- Post-mortem X-ray, MRI
- Fetal height, weight, visible gross congenital malformation

Management of Labor and Delivery

- Grieved parents need to be offered that management can be done by expectant vs. induction of labor.
- All the advantages and disadvantages need to be discussed. Vaginal birth is the most preferred method until unless LSCS is indicated due to some obstetric or medical conditions.[10]

Expectant Management

if there is no risk of preeclampsia, vaginal bleeding, infection, or rupture of membrane than the risk for next 48 hours is low and if women opt for expectant management for more than 48 hours, she should be advised to get DIC profile twice a week.[10]

Induction of Labor

Induction of labor to be done by combination of mifepristone and misoprostol safely.[11]

Mifepristone needs to be given orally either in single-dose regimen or multi-dose regimen.

Single-dose regimen: Mifepristone to be given orally 200 mg stat followed by prostaglandins.

Multi-dose regimen: If prostaglandins need to be avoided than mifepristone can be given as 200 mg three times a day for 48 hours.

Prostaglandins: Tablet Misoprostol and Prostaglandin E2 gel both can be tried but tablet is preferred over gel to decrease the cost and better results by tablet than gel.

Misoprostol: As per International Federation of Gynecology and Obstetrics (FIGO) guidelines, misoprostol regimen for fetal death, doses are different for defined gestational as shown in **Table 2.**[12]

FIGO and WHO both recommend that wherever mifepristone is available, it should be given 24–48 hours prior to misoprostol with minimum recommended interval between the two should be 24 hours.

TABLE 2: Misoprostol regimen for fetal death.

13–26 week	*27–28 week*	*>28 week*
200 µg Misoprostol sublingual/ buccal/per vaginal	100 µg SL/ PV/buccal every four hours	25 µg PV every 6 hours or 25 µg po every 2 hours

Prostaglandin E2 Gel

Prostaglandin E2 gel can be used both for 2nd trimester and 3rd trimester IUFD cases. It is more preferred in third trimester IUFD because of its safety.[13]

Induction of Labor in Previous Cesarean Cases

Induction in scarred cases to be tried by mechanical methods preferably by intra-cervical Foley insertion especially in those cases who are near term but as per RCOG recommendation, there is risk of ascending infection in cases of IUFD and need to be avoided[10] while South Australian Perinatal Practice Guidelines[14] advised transcervical balloon ripening of cervix in cases of >1 LSCS and in cases where ripening with misoprostol is contraindicated. Use of prostaglandin is seen more in cases less than 28-week gestational age.[13] Induction of labor in scarred cases to be done cautiously with good clinical monitoring.

Mifepristone can be used alone in cases of scarred uterus in doses as described above. [10]

Labor and Management

Labor to be monitored as usual, antibiotic prophylaxis is not recommended until there is rupture of membrane.

In cases of IUFD, artificial rupture of membrane (AROM) is not suggested until unless it is a case of fresh IUFD due to abruption placenta because in these cases AROM suggested to decrease the intrauterine pressure because of intrauterine hemorrhage.

Labor analgesia to be offered as usual but the risk of disseminated intravascular coagulation needs to be rule out.

Signs of scar rupture to be monitored carefully in case of scarred uterus like maternal tachycardia vaginal bleeding, hematuria, and sudden deterioration of vitals.

Oxytocin augmentation needs to be supervised in cases of scarred uterus to avoid rupture of uterus.[10]

Post-delivery Care and Counseling: Shift to Ward

After observation of fourth stage of labor, woman can be shifted to postnatal ward under care of nursing staff. Few females may still require critical care because of under lying medical condition. Parents who are willing to take photographs of the baby, hospital premises should allow them and the baby need to be handed over by nurse on duty with utmost care. Patient needs to be discharged after proper counseling regarding post-delivery care, nutrition, appropriate contraception, and breast care.[1]

Breast Care and Management after IUFD

After the unfortunate incident of IUFD obstetrician or attending doctor need to give careful advice regarding breast care and lactation suppression. Although in the absence of physical stimulation, breast milk naturally stops but in cases of IUFD while caring for the emotion of mother a good clinical advice is to suppress the milk expression.

Suppression of Lactation

Nonpharmacological methods:

- Breast binding
- Avoidance of unnecessary breast stimulation
- Application of cooling agent if soreness occurs.

Pharmacological methods: Cabergoline is a dopamine agonist and directly stimulate D_2 dopamine receptors on pituitary lactotrophs and inhibits the secretion of prolactin which in-turn suppress the lactation.

Doses: Cabergoline should be advised on Day 1 postpartum in the dosage of 1 mg. In the market, preparation of 0.25 and 0.5 mg are available according to those four or two tablets to be advised. It must be kept in mind not to advise with D_2 antagonist drugs like metoclopramide or phenothiazines as it may affect prolactin suppression effect.

Caution to be taken in cases of preeclampsia and eclampsia. Women can experience hypotension, headache, and dizziness.[15]

Management of Next Pregnancy

Counseling for the next pregnancy can be decided as per the current status of bereaved mother and at least 6-month interval (preferably one year) should be recommended and appropriate contraception to be offered to cope up with mother from recent loss.[16]

If case received at different physician next time, the detailed prenatal counseling is recommended with following points keeping in mind:

- Detailed medical and obstetric history
- To check and do evaluation of previous stillbirth
- Rule out recurrent causes
- Obesity control and weight loss
- Diabetes and hypertension screening
- Thyroid status
- APLA screening
- Genetic counseling
- Due respectful care and assurance

Antenatal work-up: Detailed anatomic, genetic sonogram and biochemical markers, genetic screening.

Medical management as per the requirement, case-to-case individualization is a better approach.

Growth scan to be offered at 28 weeks to rule out fetal growth restriction, fetal surveillance to be started at 32 weeks or 1–2 week prior to previous loss.

Plan of delivery is to be individualized as per the medical and obstetric indication.

Labor and delivery: Delivery to be planned at 39 weeks to 39+6 weeks gestational age, or earlier as per the obstetric and medical history.

Medicolegal Implication of IUFD

It is very crucial to identify whether found fetus for autopsy was born live or an IUFD. The postmortem examination can be very helpful in planning appropriate management and caution for the future.

Key Points of Fetal Autopsy

External Examination

Fetal height should include crown-rump length and crown-heel length. *Head circumference:* Thorax circumference at the level of nipples, abdominal circumference at the level of umbilicus. Foot length which is found more reliable even in case of macerated stillbirth. Assessment regarding the baby is large for gestational age or growth restricted.[17]

Radiological Examination

- A full body X-ray (skeleton X-ray)
- MRI

Histopathological Examination

Lungs, brain, and Kidneys need to be examined by expert forensic pathologists to comment upon approximate gestational age of fetus.

Estimation of time of death:[18] An estimation of time of death can be measured by as shown in **Box 1**.

BOX 1: Postmortem findings to determine time since death.[18]

12 hours: Slippage of skin noted
24 hours: Skin bleb formation
48 hours: Sloughing of skin, rupture of blebs, and hemolysis in viscera
5 days: Liquefaction of brain and Spalding sign
7 days: Bone joint got lax

Photographic records: It is a wise decision to collect photographic evidence of postmortem for gross examination. These are valuable if a second opinion is required further.

Examination of Placenta

If placenta is made available for examination, it needs to be examined thoroughly by gross and histopathologic examination.

Gross Examination

During gross examination, the weight of placenta, measurement of diameter, site of insertion of the cord, length of available cord, number of vessels in umbilical cord, coiling of cord, knots in cord any false or true. Placenta complete or incomplete, placental swab, status of attached membrane all to be noted.

Microscopic Examination

Either the whole placenta or at least 1 × 1 inch block of placenta need to be sent for microscopic examination. Samples need to be taken from fetal surface near the cord insertion (Especially in those cases where parents consented to know the cause of IUFD).

CONCLUSION

Intrauterine fetal death is still underreported in developing nations and we all should work under notion that every birth counts.

REFERENCES

1. Institute of Obstetricians and Gynaecologists, Royal College of Physicians of Ireland and Directorate of Strategy and Clinical Programs, Health Service Executive. Investigation And Management Of Late Fetal Intrauterine Death And Stillbirth [Internet]. 2011. Available from: https://rcpi-live-cdn.s3.amazonaws.com/wp-content/uploads/2016/05/4.-Investigation-and-Management-of-Late-Fetal-Intrauterine-Death-and-Stillbirth.pdf.
2. Operational Guidelines for Establishing Sentinel Stillbirth Surveillance System [Internet]. www.nhm.gov.in. 2016. Available from: https://www.nhm.gov.in/images/pdf/programmes/RBSK/Operational_Guidelines/Operational_Guidelines_for_establishing_Sentinel_Stillbirth_Surveillance_System.pdf.
3. Making every baby count [Internet]. www.who.int. Geneva 27, Switzerland: WHO Press; 2016. Available from: https://www.who.int/publications/i/item/9789241511223.
4. Weindling AM. The confidential enquiry into maternal and child health (CEMACH). Archives of Disease in Childhood. 2003;88(12):1034-7.
5. Refaey M, Yap J, Weerakkody Y, et al. Fetal death in utero. Reference article, Radiopaedia.org https://doi.org/10.53347/rID-4877.
6. Gajbhiye R. Intrauterine fetal death [Internet]. 2015 Mar 9. Available from: https://www.slideshare.net/RajeshGajbhiye/iud-final.
7. Tan E, Zhou JC, Mahmood O, Ong CL, Ng CH. MRI signs of intrauterine fetal demise. Abdominal Radiology. 2021;46(7):3365-77.
8. Maslovich MM, Burke LM. Intrauterine fetal demise. InStatPearls [Internet]. 2021 Nov 5. StatPearls Publishing.
9. Dutta DC, Konar H. Preterm labor, preterm rupture of the membranes, postmaturity, intrauterine death of the fetus, 7th edn. Textbook of Obstetrics DC Dutta's including Perinatology and Contraception. 2013; pp. 322-323, ISBN 978-93-5152-067-2.
10. D Siassakos, R Fox, T Draycott, C Winter. Late intrauterine fetal death and stillbirth [Internet]. www.rcog.org.uk. 2010 [cited 2022 Nov 21]. Available from: https://www.rcog.org.uk/media/0fefdrk4/gtg_55.pdf.
11. Inducing labour [Internet]. https://www.nice.org.uk/guidance/ng207. 2021. Available from: https://www.nice.org.uk/guidance/ng207/resources/inducing-labour-pdf-66143719773637.
12. Morris JL, Winikoff B, Dabash R, Weeks A, Faundes A, Gemzell-Danielsson K, Kapp N, Castleman L, Kim C, Ho PC, Visser GH. FIGO's Updated Recommendations for Misoprostol used alone in Gynecology and Obstetrics. Int J Gynaecol Obstet. 2017;138(3):363-6. doi: 10.1002/ijgo.12181. Epub 2017 Jun 23.
13. Amin KV, Chauhan AR, Goel A. Current Practices of Cervical Ripening, and Induction of Labour in Intrauterine Foetal Demise: An Observational Study. The Journal of Obstetrics and Gynecology of India. 2019;69(1):37-42.
14. South Australian Perinatal Practice Guidelines Medical Management of Late Intrauterine Fetal Death [Internet]. www.sahealth.sa.gov.au.
15. Literature Summary for Lactation Suppression Treatment for Post-Partum Women [Internet]. http://www.bcwomens.ca/. 2015 Available from: http://www.bcwomens.ca/Professional-Resources-site/Documents/Oak%20Tree/Immediate%20Suppression%20of%20Lactation%20Appendix%201%20-%20Lit%20summary.pdf
16. Management of Stillbirth [Internet]. www.acog.org. [cited 2022 Nov 21] Available from: https://www.acog.org/clinical/clinical-guidance/obstetric-care-consensus/articles/2020/03/management-of-stillbirth.
17. Cohen MC, Scheimberg I. Forensic aspects of perinatal deaths. Academic sathology. 2018;8(3):452-91.
18. Sharma L. Autopsy in foetal infant deaths. In: Criminology and Post-Mortem Studies: Analyzing Criminal Behaviour and Making Medical Decisions. 2020, Jun 9. DOI: 10.5772/intechopen.92673.

CHAPTER 19

Preterm Labor and Birth

Kavita Mandrelle, Sahir Bhatti, PV Varughese

INTRODUCTION

Preterm birth is the leading cause of neonatal mortality and the most common reason for antenatal hospitalization. Preterm births account for approximately 70% of neonatal deaths. Infant death is seen in 36% of preterm deliveries and 25–50% of preterm babies may have long-term neurologic impairment.[1]

DEFINITION AND CLASSIFICATION

- Preterm birth is defined as babies born before 37 weeks of pregnancy.
- Preterm labor (PTL) is defined as presence of regular uterine contractions that result in cervical dilation and effacement between 24+0 to 36+6 weeks of gestation.

There are subcategories of preterm birth, based on gestational age shown in **Table 1**.[2]

ETIOLOGY

Preterm labor can be because of the following cause:

- Spontaneous labor with intact membranes
- Preterm premature rupture of the membranes (PPROM)
- Iatrogenic—Labor induction or cesarean delivery for maternal or fetal indications
- Idiopathic

TABLE 1: Category of preterm birth.

Category of preterm birth	*Gestational age*
Extremely preterm	<28 weeks
Very preterm	<32 weeks
Moderate-to-late preterm	32 to <37 weeks

PATHOLOGY/PATHOGENESIS

Preterm labor may involve the following pathogenic processes:

- Activation of the maternal or fetal hypothalamic-pituitary-adrenal axis associated with maternal anxiety and depression or fetal stress
- Infection
- Decidual hemorrhage
- Pathological uterine distention such as in polyhydramnios and multiple order pregnancy
- Cervical insufficiency

PREDICTIVE/RISK FACTORS

Risk Factors

- Low socioeconomic status
- Anxiety, stress related to life events such as death of near ones, separation and divorce
- Depression, use of selective serotonin reuptake inhibitors
- Abdominal surgery during pregnancy
- Occupational hazards (physical exhaustion, mental or environmental stress related to work conditions)
- Multiple order pregnancy
- Polyhydramnios
- Uterine anomaly, including diethylstilbestrol-induced changes in uterus

- Space occupying uterine lesions such as leiomyomas
- Preterm premature rupture of membranes
- Previous second-trimester abortion
- Previous cervical surgery such as trachelorrhaphy
- Premature cervical dilatation or effacement (short cervical length)
- *Vaginal infections:* Sexually transmitted infections
- Systemic infections
- Pyelonephritis, appendicitis, pneumonia
- Bacteriuria
- Periodontal disease
- Placenta causes such as placenta previa and placental abruption
- Vaginal bleeding, especially if it occurs in more than one trimester
- Previous preterm delivery
- Substance abuse
- Smoking
- Maternal age (<18 or >40 years)
- African American race
- Poor nutrition and low body mass index
- Inadequate prenatal care
- Anemia (hemoglobin <10 g/dL)
- Fetal anomaly
- Fetal growth restriction
- Environmental factors
- Iatrogenic causes such as fetal anomaly, fetal growth restriction, intrauterine fetal demise before 37 weeks

The two most significant risk factors include a prior history of preterm birth and multiple gestation.

PRIMARY PREVENTION

- Short cervical length or ultrasound examination between 16–24 weeks of gestation in the current pregnancy is a risk factor for preterm labor. Progesterone supplementation may prolong gestation.
- Prevention of multifetal gestations using single embryo transfers and controlled stimulation cycles in infertile couples can prevent preterm deliveries.

SECONDARY PREVENTION

Progesterone supplementation with or without cervical cerclage placement in certain circumstances may be helpful to prevent preterm labor in the current pregnancy.

DIAGNOSIS OF PRETERM LABOR

Clinical Criteria

History

- *Prodromal signs and symptoms of preterm labor:*
  - Menstrual-like cramping
  - Mild, irregular contractions
  - Low backache
  - Pressure sensation in the vagina or pelvis
  - Vaginal discharge of mucus, which may be clear, pink, or slightly increased vaginal discharge.
- Present and past obstetrical history of preterm birth, gynecologic, surgical, and medical history. History of intercourse, travel, exercise, and trauma.
- Regular painful uterine contractions accompanied by cervical change (dilation and/or effacement).

Physical Examination

- Assessment of uterine contraction frequency, duration, and intensity
- Digital and speculum examination of the cervix to look for effacement and dilatation
- Ultrasound evaluation of the fetus for gestational age

Speculum Examination

- Estimate cervical dilation. Cervical dilation ≥3 cm is diagnostic of preterm labor
- Presence of show
- Confirm presence or absence of fetal membranes
- Sample for fetal fibronectin (fFN) test can be obtained.

Digital Cervical Examination

- Cervical dilation and effacement are assessed by digital examination after speculum examination
- Evaluate the cervix for its consistency, location and effacement
- Placenta previa and rupture of membranes should be excluded prior to examination.

Confirmatory Findings in Preterm Labor[1]

- Uterine contractions (≥4 every 20 minutes or ≥8 in 60 minutes) AND
- Cervical dilation ≥3 cm

OR

- Documented cervical change or cervical effacement ≥80% or cervical dilation >2 cm
- If transvaginal cervical length evaluation is available, then consider:
    - Cervical length <20 mm on transvaginal ultrasound or
    - Cervical length 20–30 mm on transvaginal ultrasound and positive fetal fibronectin

Diagnostic Tests

- Uterine contraction monitoring (i.e., tocodynamometer) and fetal heart rate assessment
- Speculum examination with fFN testing in women <34 weeks of gestation
- Fetal fibronectin (fFN) should be performed if available when the diagnosis of PTL is doubtful.
- A fFN concentration ≥50 ng/mL in cervicovaginal fluid between 22+0 and 34+6 weeks of gestation in women with intact membranes correlates with an increased risk of preterm delivery within seven days
- Evaluation for preterm rupture of membranes with tests like nitrazine, litmus test and ferning
- Rectovaginal group B streptococcal culture if not done within the previous 5 weeks; antibiotic prophylaxis depends on the result.
- Urine culture because asymptomatic bacteriuria is associated with and increased risk of preterm labor and birth.
- Drug testing in patients with risk factors for substance abuse, given the link between cocaine use and placental abruption
- Testing for sexually transmitted infections (e.g., *Chlamydia, Gonorrhea*) depends on the patient's risk factors for these infections.

Imaging Technique

- Transvaginal ultrasound (TVU) measurement of cervical length—a short cervix ≤2.5 cm prior to 34 weeks of gestation is predictive of preterm labor.
- A long cervix has a high negative predictive value for preterm birth.

PREVENTION OF PRETERM LABOR AND BIRTH

- Asymptomatic women with singleton gestation are at high risk of preterm birth. Women at high risk of preterm birth (a prior spontaneous preterm birth and/or ultrasound diagnosed short cervix) with a singleton gestation should be offered daily vaginal progesterone or weekly 17-OH progesterone treatment to prevent preterm birth. Effectiveness of progesterone in women with previous spontaneous preterm birth with normal cervical length (>25 mm at mid-trimester ultrasound) is uncertain.

- *Asymptomatic women with a singleton gestation without a prior history of preterm birth or short cervical length:* Progesterone therapy is not recommended for the prevention of preterm birth in women with singleton gestation without a prior history of preterm birth or short cervical length.
- *Asymptomatic women with multiple pregnancy:* For women with multiple pregnancies, progesterone therapy is not recommended for the prevention of preterm birth. For women with multiple pregnancies and a history of previous preterm birth, it is not known whether progesterone therapy is effective.
- *Type of progestogen*: Daily vaginal progesterone or weekly 17-OH progesterone can be used for the prevention of preterm birth. The type of progesterone preparation used should be at the discretion of the woman and her clinician.[3]
- *Cervical cerclage for prevention of preterm birth:*[4] Cervical cerclage is a commonly performed intervention for women at risk of preterm birth and second-trimester fetal loss. Cervical cerclage can be categorized by the indication for insertion:
  1. *History of the patient*: In asymptomatic women with risk factors that increase the risk of preterm birth. A history indicated cerclage can be offered to women who have had three or more preterm deliveries and/or mid-trimester losses.
  2. *Ultrasound findings:* In asymptomatic women with ultrasound finding of cervical shortening. An ultrasound-indicated cerclage should be offered to women with a cervical length <25 mm if they have had one or more spontaneous preterm birth and/or mid-trimester loss. In women who have no previous mid-trimester loss or preterm birth but with short cervix on ultrasound, there is no clear benefit of cervical cerclage. For twin pregnancy, cervical cerclage may benefit in shorter cervical lengths (<15 mm).
- *Rescue cerclage:* Where the cervix is dilated, and membranes prolapsed into vagina. In women who present with exposed membranes prolapsing through the cervical os, a rescue cerclage can be considered on an individual case basis, taking into account the high risk of infective morbidity to mother and baby.
- An abdominal cerclage can be offered in women who have had a failed cerclage. Removal of cervical stitch is considered at 36–37 weeks of gestation.

Treatment

- An accurate identification of women in true preterm labor allows appropriate management that can improve neonatal outcome. These include:
  - Antenatal corticosteroid therapy[5]
  - Group B streptococcal infection prophylaxis
  - Magnesium sulfate for neuroprotection
  - Transfer to a facility with an appropriate level nursery (if necessary)

Triage of women in false preterm labor can avoid unnecessary interventions and associated costs for ≥50% of patients with suspected preterm labor who will go on to deliver at term without treatment. Hospitalization is required for patients with diagnosis of preterm labor.

TREATMENT OF PRETERM LABOR

Antenatal Corticosteroids

A single course of corticosteroids is recommended for pregnant women between 24 weeks and 34 weeks of gestation who are at risk of delivery within 7 days.

One repeat "rescue" course may be administered as long as they have not had a course of antenatal corticosteroids at least 14 days previously and are at ≤34 weeks of gestation.[5]

The American College of Obstetricians and Gynecologists recommends administration of antenatal steroids for women with a singleton pregnancy at 34+0 to 36+6 weeks of gestation at imminent risk of preterm birth within 7 days who have not received a prior course of antenatal corticosteroids (Committee on Obstetric Practice 2017; Lockwood 2018).

Contraindication: Chorioamnionitis

Remarks

Betamethasone suspension 12 mg intramuscularly every 24 hours for two doses or four doses of 6 mg.

Dexamethasone intramuscularly 12 hours apart

1. Transient maternal hyperglycemia, the steroid effect begins approximately 12 hours after the first dose and may last for 5 days.
2. Transient fetal heart rate (FHR) and behavioral changes that typically return to baseline by 4–7 days after treatment: most consistent FHR finding is a decrease in variability on days 2 and 3 after administration, reduced fetal breathing and body movements have also been reported.

Tocolytic Drugs

Evidence supports the use of first-line tocolytic treatment for short-term prolongation of pregnancy (up to 48 hours) to allow for the administration of antenatal steroids.

Maintenance therapy with tocolytics is ineffective for preventing preterm birth and improving neonatal outcomes and is not recommended for this purpose.

Contraindications

- Intrauterine fetal demise
- Lethal fetal anomaly
- Non-reassuring fetal assessment
- Severe intrauterine growth restriction
- Chorioamnionitis
- Maternal hemorrhage with hemodynamic instability
- Severe preeclampsia or eclampsia

Remarks

- *Indomethicin:* 50–100 mg loading dose (orally or per rectum), followed by 25 mg orally every 4–6 hours.

Maternal effects: Nausea, esophageal reflux, gastritis, and emesis

Fetal effects: Oligohydramnios, fetal ductus arteriosus closure

- *Nifedipine (calcium channel blocker):* Initial loading dose of 20–30 mg orally, followed by an additional 10–20 mg orally every 3–8 hours for up to 48 hours, with a maximum dose of 180 mg/day.

Maternal effects: Nausea, flushing, headache, dizziness, and palpitations

- *Terbutaline (Beta-2 agonist):* 0.25 mg can be administered subcutaneously every 20–30 minutes for up to 4 doses or until tocolysis is achieved. Once labor is inhibited, 0.25 mg can be administered subcutaneously every 3–4 until the uterus is quiescent for 24 hours.

Maternal effects: Tachycardia, palpitations and lower blood pressure, hypokalemia, hyperglycemia, and lipolysis.

Fetal effects: Hyperinsulinemia, hypoglycemia

- *Atosiban:*

Dose: Administered intravenously beginning with a bolus of 6.75 mg over 1 minute followed by a 300 µg/min (18 mg/hour) infusion for three hours, and then 100 µg/min (6 mg/hour) for up to 45 hours (to a maximum of 330 mg).

Side effects: Minimal side effects in the form of hypersensitivity and injection site reactions. No adverse maternal cardiovascular effects have been reported.

Contraindications: No absolute contraindications

- *Nitric oxide (NO) donors (Nitroglycerin, NTG patch):*

Dose: 10 mg nitroglycerine patch is applied to the skin of the abdomen. After one hour, if there is no reduction in contraction frequency or intensity, an additional patch is applied; a maximum of two patches are administered simultaneously. The patches are left in situ for 24 hours, after which they are removed, and the patient reassessed.

Side effects: Dizziness, flushing, palpitations, and maternal hypotension

Contraindications: No donors should not be used in women with hypotension or with preload-dependent cardiac lesions, such as aortic insufficiency.

Antibiotic for Group B *Streptococcus* chemoprophylaxis

Intrapartum antibiotic prophylaxis is most effective if administered at least 4 hours before delivery.

Remarks

Penicillin G: 5 million units intravenously initial dose, then 2.5–3 million units intravenously every 4 hours until delivery.

Ampicillin: 2 g intravenously initial dose, then 1 g every 4 hours until delivery. Patients with penicillin allergy

Low risk: Cefazolin 2 g intravenously initial dose, then 1 g every 8 hours until delivery

High risk: Clindamycin 900 mg intravenously every 8 hours until delivery.

OR vancomycin 2 g intravenously initial and then 1 g every 12 hours thereafter until delivery.

Magnesium Sulfate

For pregnancies at 24–32 weeks of gestation who are likely to deliver within 24 hours.

Remarks

4 gm loading of *magnesium sulfate* over 20 minutes and a maintenance dose of 1 g/hour.

In-utero exposure to magnesium sulfate provides neuroprotection against cerebral palsy and other types of severe motor dysfunction in offspring born preterm. Magnesium sulfate infusion given to a maximum of 24 hours, even if delivery has not occurred.

Retreatment of the full dose of magnesium sulfate if delivery is again considered imminent may be given if the pregnancy is still <32 weeks gestation and the initial magnesium infusion had been discontinued for more than 6 hours.

Fetal effects: Decrease in baseline fetal heart rate (generally remains within the normal range) and a decrease in fetal heart rate variability, which may be absent or minimal.

Maternal effects: Diaphoresis, flushing, warmth, low blood pressure, nausea, vomiting, headache, muscle weakness, visual disturbances and palpitations.

Dyspnea or chest pain may be symptoms of pulmonary edema, which is a rare side effect.

It is contraindicated in women with myasthenia gravis, should be avoided in women with known myocardial compromise and used cautiously in women with impaired renal function.

PREVENTION OF COMPLICATIONS WITH MEDICATION

- Indomethacin can cause premature constriction of the ductus arteriosus and oligohydramnios especially if the duration of indomethacin exposure exceeded 48 hours and is given after 31–32 weeks. Therefore, Indomethacin is not recommended after 32 weeks of gestation. If the duration of indomethacin administration exceeds 48 hours between 24-32 weeks of gestation a fetal echocardiographic evaluation is useful for monitoring ductal effect.
- Calcium channel blockers are contraindicated in women with hypotension, preload-dependent cardiac lesions, and known hypersensitivity to the drugs. It should be used with caution in women with left ventricular dysfunction or congestive heart failure.
- The concomitant use of a calcium channel blockers and magnesium sulfate is not recommended as a synergistic effect may lead to suppression of muscular contractility and result in respiratory depression and cardiac complications.
- Pulmonary edema is an uncommon side effect of beta-agonist therapy. It probably results from increased heart rate, fluid overload from excessive intravenous crystalloid infusion and increased plasma volume of pregnancy. Myocardial ischemia is a rare complication. Terbutaline should not be used in pregnant women for prolonged (beyond 48–72 hours) treatment of preterm labor or prevention of recurrent preterm labor because of the potential for serious maternal heart problems and death. The FDA has opined that oral terbutaline should not be used for prevention or treatment of preterm labor because it has not been shown to be effective and has similar safety concerns (US-FDA 2011).
- Tocolytics should be discontinued 48–72 hours after administration of the first corticosteroid dose if contractions subside. There is no evidence to support their use for longer duration. Tocolytics should also be stopped if labor progresses despite treatment.

OTHER THERAPIES

- Antibiotic therapy has no role in the treatment of acute preterm labor in the absence of infection or GBS prophylaxis.
- Progesterone supplementation has no role in the treatment of acute preterm labor.[4]
- There is no evidence-based role of bed rest, hydration, or sedation in preterm labor.

Approach to Triage: Singleton Pregnancies

- *≥34 weeks of gestation:* Women in preterm labor at ≥34 weeks are admitted for delivery. After an observation period of four to six hours, women without progressive cervical dilation and effacement are discharged. Confirm fetal well-being and rule out obstetric complications such as abruptio placentae, chorioamnionitis, and preterm rupture of membranes before discharge.

- *<34 weeks of gestation:* In women <34 weeks with uterine contractions and cervical dilation ≥3 cm initiate treatment of preterm labor in these women to reduce neonatal morbidity and mortality.
- *Cervical length 20 to <30 mm:* Symptomatic women with cervical dilation <3 cm and cervical length 20 to <30 mm are at increased risk of preterm birth. A significant proportion of patients in this group are at low (<5 percent) risk of preterm delivery within seven days therefore a cervicovaginal sample for fFN testing will help in diagnosis.
- *Cervical length <20 mm:* Symptomatic women with cervical length <20 mm are at high risk (>25%) of delivery within seven days. Fetal fibronectin testing does not significantly improve the predictive value of cervical length measurement alone in these women.
- *Cervical length ≥30 mm:* Approximately 50% of women with symptoms of preterm labor have a transvaginal ultrasound cervical length ≥30 mm. The addition of fFN testing does not significantly improve the predictive value of cervical length measurement in this group of women.

Approach to Triage: Twin Pregnancy

- The prediction of preterm birth based on cervical length measurement is different for twin pregnancies.
- *≥34 weeks of gestation*: Triage is same as for singletons.
- *<34 weeks of gestation*: For women with twin pregnancies <34 weeks with uterine contractions, cervical dilation ≥3 cm supports the diagnosis of preterm labor; further diagnostic evaluation is not warranted. Instead, treatment of preterm labor should be initiated.
- In women with contractions and cervical dilation <3 cm a transvaginal ultrasound measurement of cervical length is done.
- Women with cervical length >35 mm and no cervical change on digital examination can be discharged home after a four- to six-hour period of observation. Confirm fetal wellbeing before discharge.
- Women with cervical length <25 mm are at high risk of preterm delivery. Start treatment to prevent neonatal morbidity and mortality due to prematurity.
- Women with cervical length 25–35 mm on transvaginal ultrasound examination should undergo fFN testing. If the test is positive, begin interventions to reduce morbidity associated with preterm birth.
- If the labor progresses, and preterm delivery is imminent:
  - Avoid early amniotomy unless indicated.
  - Mode of delivery is decided by the obstetric indications.
  - Selective use of episiotomy
  - Instrumental delivery only if indicated. Use of vacuum is to be limited to deliveries ≥34 weeks of gestation because of the risk of intraventricular hemorrhage.
  - Neonatologist to be informed prior to delivery.
  - Active management of third stage of labor and delayed cord clamping are recommended.

Preterm Newborn Intensive Care

The recent advancements in perinatal and neonatal care have led to improvement in outcomes in extreme preterm babies and also increasing the long-term morbidities, hence raising issues related to ethics and ethical dilemmas. It has now become very important for a neonatologist to become familiar with these ethical dilemmas. There are no legal guidelines in India that are adopted when we know. Resuscitation is unlikely to be beneficial. The infant may remain on prolonged ventilation, in a persistent vegetative state, may be a burden to the parents but in spite of these, no guidelines are there on withdrawal of care or end-of-life decisions. The progression from birth to death may occur in such a short time that it gives a very little time period to doctors and family members to make such critical decisions.

Challenging Situations

- Extremely preterm peri-viable neonates (23–25 weeks)
- Neonates with multiple anomalies, chromosomal defects
- Infants with long-term lethal prognosis or predicted poor quality-of-life (e.g., HIE/ progressive neuromuscular paralysis, bilateral periventricular leukomalacia/ Grade 4 intraventricular hemorrhage).

ETHICS IN NEWBORN INTENSIVE CARE [6-10]

The recent advancements in perinatal and neonatal care have led to improvement in outcomes in extreme preterm babies and also increasing the long-term morbidities, hence raising issues related to ethics and ethical dilemmas. It has now become very important for a neonatologist to become familiar with these ethical dilemmas.

There are no legal guidelines in India that are adopted when we know. Resuscitation is unlikely to be beneficial. The infant may remain on prolonged ventilation, in a persistent vegetative state, may be a burden to the parents but in spite of these, no guidelines are there on withdrawal of care or end-of-life decisions. The progression from birth to death may occur in such a short time that it gives a very little time period to doctors and family members to make such critical decisions.

Basic Principles

- *Non-maleficence (Avoid Harm):* Do no harm in basic principle of medical care; harm not to be inflicted intentionally and should be closely linked to care.
- *Beneficence (acting for patients benefit):* A moral obligation to act for the benefit of patients, helping them to further their legitimate interests and at times preventing and removing possible harm.
- *Autonomy (Rights to make choices):* Individuals are entitled to make their own choices and decisions; hence neonates rely on their parents to make decisions for them.
- *Distributive justice (Truthful and fair):* Prescribe actions that are fair to those involved. Suggest that similar clinical situations should be treated alike and that variations in management must be justified by relevant clinical/evaluative conditions.

Approach to Preterm Babies at Peri-viable Age [11-13]

- *Uncertain gestation:* Initiate life-sustaining interventions until clinical course is clearer and initiate decision-making protocols.
- *24–24 weeks +6:* Life-sustaining interventions are not recommended but if baby is stable at delivery room do appropriate counseling and if family agrees then provide care.
- *25–27 weeks +6:* Life-sustaining interventions are recommended, if family does not agree for treatment, then provide palliative care.
- *RCPCH Criteria (Royal College of Paediatrics and Child Health):* The

situations in which it is appropriate to limit treatment:
- When treatment is unlikely to prolong life (brainstem death, imminent death, inevitable death).
- When treatment may be able to prolong life significantly, but burdens outweigh any potential or actual benefits (burdens on treatment, burdens child underlying condition, lack of ability to benefit)

- *Informed competent refusal of treatment—antenatal counseling:* It should be done with parents. The team should consist of pediatrician and obstetrician. They should be told about the outcomes of similar babies of the Institute in the past. Other things which should be informed as mentioned hereunder:
  - *Complications:*
    1. *Immediate:* Asphyxia, shock, surfactant requirement for respiratory distress, hypoglycemia, and apnea
    2. *Short term:* Sepsis/prolonged ventilation/jaundice
    3. *Long term*: Cerebral palsy/Hearing, visual, learning problems/chronic lung disease, germinal matrix hemorrhage
  - Cost of treatment (For ventilation/ CPAP/Surfactant/IV nutrition/ NICU care)
  - Parents should be explained that the effect of resuscitation will not be same in all babies.
  - Parents should be assured that every effort will be put to save the baby, but decisions may be modified in the delivery room after seeing baby's condition at birth and gestational age assessment.
- All the babies that are peri-viable/extreme preterm/moderate preterm/ term babies should be resuscitated equally.
- *Do Not Resuscitate (DNR):* No clear-cut guidelines for DNR in India. According to IAP-NNF, it is recommended to encourage only comfort care for babies at 24 weeks.
- Prognosis explained should be recorded, written down and signed by one of the parents.

After Birth Counseling

- The parents should be counseled regularly after birth.
- Counseling by more than one consultant helps family members in making better decisions.
- Complications already faced by the neonate and their effects.
- Cost of treatment to be explained to the relatives.
- Once or twice a week up-to-date billing to be done and to be given to the relatives.
- We cannot predict the outcome too early because complications occur at time in the hospital before discharge which can hamper the prognosis.
- *Decision making:* After the counseling let the parents decide the best for their child and document that in file.
- Baby will be screened for TSH/hearing screen/retinopathy of prematurity (ROP) screening. The parents can be told about other screening tests like G6PD, congenital adrenal hyperplasia (CAH), galactosemia.
- Cranial ultrasound to be done for preterm babies within first week.
- Rickets panel to be done for preterm babies at 1 month of age
- Discharge to be planned only when baby is stable, fully on breastfeed. For very low

birth babies discharged to be planned when baby is on breastfeeds and spoon feeds, gaining weight (around 1500 g).

- According to RBSK guidelines,[14] ROP screening to be done for:
  - Birth weight less than 200 g
  - Gestational age less than 34 weeks
  - Gestational age between 34–36 weeks but with risk factors such as cardiorespiratory support, prolonged oxygen therapy, respiratory distress syndrome, chronic lung disease, fetal hemorrhage, blood transfusion, neonatal sepsis, exchange transfusion, intraventricular hemorrhage, apnea, poor postnatal weight gain.
  - Infants with an unstable course who are at high risk
- For babies who are discharged early, ROP screening has to be done from OPD around 3 weeks.
- Many litigations have occurred due to non-screening for ROP so in case the preterm babies who are discharged early and advised for ROP screening from OPD do not turn up for follow-up, the documentation should be done in the file.

RECENT UPDATES

The combination of quantitative fetal fibronectin testing and cervical length measurement will help in the prediction of preterm labor. A model consisting of quantitative fFN, cervical length, demographic information, and obstetric history (previous spontaneous preterm birth/preterm prelabor rupture of membranes or suspected preterm labor) has been incorporated into an App (QUiPP) for prediction of spontaneous preterm birth.

Other laboratory tests like placental alpha-microglobulin-1 (PAMG-1) or phosphorylated insulin-like growth factor binding protein-1 (pIGFBP-1) in vaginal or cervical secretions are potential markers of an increased risk of preterm birth. The utility of these newer tests require validation.

Medicolegal Aspects

When the fetal prognosis is uncertain, decisions regarding obstetric management must be made by the parents and their physicians and documented in the obstetric records. The active participation of parents in discussions regarding delivery, maternal transport, and other management decisions is important. The obstetric-neonatal physician team must approach the patient in a nonjudgmental fashion and provide objective data about the maternal risks involved in various treatment plans and likely neonatal outcomes at certain gestational ages. The parents and obstetrician-neonatal team should be involved in a shared decision making for the treatment option.

CONCLUSION

There are many risk factors for preterm labor and delivery. Prior PTB is the strongest risk factor for future PTB, and recurrences often occur at the same gestational age. For women with a history of spontaneous preterm birth, progesterone supplementation reduces the risk of recurrence in present pregnancy. Short cervical length on transvaginal ultrasound examination between 16 and 24 weeks of gestation in the current pregnancy is a risk factor for PTB and is the basis for screening for a short cervix in the mid trimester and placement of a cerclage may prolong gestation. The major goals of treatment of acute preterm labor are to delay delivery by at least 48 hours so that antenatal corticosteroids administered to the mother have time to achieve their maximum neonatal effects. Provide time for safe transport of the mother, if indicated, to a facility that has an appropriate level of neonatal care if she delivers preterm. For women at risk for imminent preterm delivery confer with the neonatology team and jointly counsel families about possible management strategies.

REFERENCES

1. Lockwood CJ. Preterm labor: Clinical findings, diagnostic evaluation, and initial treatment. [Internet]. UpToDate; [2022] [cited 2024 Jul 2]. Available from: https://pro.uptodatefree.ir/Show/6798.
2. American College of Obstetricians and Gynecologists. Practice bulletin no. 171: management of preterm labor. Obstetrics and gynecology. 2016;128(4):e155-64.
3. Shennan A, Story L, Jacobsson B, Grobman WA, FIGO Working Group for Preterm Birth, Simpson JL, Norman J, Bianchi A, Munjanja S, González CM, Mol BW. FIGO Good Practice Recommendations on Cervical Cerclage for Prevention of Preterm Birth. International Journal of Gynecology & Obstetrics. 2021;155(1):19-22.
4. Shennan A, Suff N, Leigh Simpson J, Jacobsson B, Mol BW, Grobman WA, FIGO Working Group for Preterm Birth, Norman J, Grobman W, Bianchi A, Munjanja S. FIGO Good Practice Recommendations on Progestogens for Prevention of Preterm Delivery. International Journal of Gynecology & Obstetrics. 2021;155(1):16-8.
5. Society for Maternal-Fetal Medicine (SMFM). Electronic address: pubs@smfm.org; Reddy UM, Deshmukh U, Dude A, Harper L, Osmundson SS. Society for Maternal-Fetal Medicine Consult Series #58: Use of antenatal corticosteroids for individuals at risk for late preterm delivery: Replaces SMFM Statement #4, Implementation of the use of antenatal corticosteroids in the late preterm birth period in women at risk for preterm delivery, August 2016. Am J Obstet Gynecol. 2021;225(5):B36-42.
6. Tiwari S, Kuthe A. Care at edge of viability: legal and ethical issues. New Indian J Pediatr. 2016;5(2):76-80.
7. Nimbalkar SM, Bansal SC. Periviable Birth: The Ethical Conundrum. Indian Pediatr. 2019;56(1):13-7. PMID: 30806353.
8. Institute of Medicine (US) Committee on Understanding Premature Birth and Assuring Healthy Outcomes; Behrman RE, Butler AS, editors. Preterm Birth: Causes, Consequences, and Prevention. Washington (DC): National Academies Press (US); 2007. C, A Review of Ethical Issues Involved in Premature Birth. Available from: https://www.ncbi.nlm.nih.gov/books/NBK11389/.
9. Lancet T. The ethics of premature delivery. The Lancet. 2006;368(9550):1844.
10. Seubert DE, Huang WM, Wasserman-Hoff R. Medical legal issues in the prevention of prematurity. Clin Perinatol. 2007;34(2):309-18, vii. doi: 10.1016/j.clp.2007.03.008. PMID: 17572237.
11. Janvier A, Barrington KJ, Aziz K, Lantos J. Ethics ain't easy: do we need simple rules for complicated ethical decisions? Acta Paediatr. 2008;97(4):402-6.
12. Fanaroff AA. Extremely low birthweight infants: the interplay between outcomes and ethics. Acta Paediatr. 2008;97:144-5.
13. Beauchamp TL, Childress JF. Principles of biomedical ethics, 7th edn. New York: Oxford University Press; 2013.
14. Reproductive and Child Health (RCH) Division, Ministry of Health and Family Welfare, Government of India. Revised Operational Guidelines for Rashtriya Bal Swasthya Karyakram (RBSK). [Internet]. New Delhi: National Health Mission; 2017 [cited 2024 Jul 18]. Available from: https://nhm.gov.in/images/pdf/programmes/RBSK/Resource_Documents/Revised_ROP_Guidelines-Web_Optimized.pdf.

CHAPTER 20

Medicolegal Aspects of Postpartum Collapse

Panchampreet Kaur, Manpreet Kaur, Divyanee Gulati

INTRODUCTION

Maternal collapse is a potentially fatal occurrence with a wide variety of etiologies affecting the cardio-respiratory and central neurological systems that results in a decreased or absent state of consciousness during pregnancy or up to 6 weeks postpartum. The result, which is critical for both mother and fetus, is contingent upon timely and successful resuscitation.[1] The maternal mortality rate (MMR) in India in 1990 was 556 per 1,00,000 live births, and the target of MDG (millennial development goal) was to reduce it to 139 per 1,00,000 live births by the year 2015. Maternal Mortality Ratio (MMR) of India for the period 2016-18, as per the latest report of the National Sample Registration System (SRS) data is 113 per 1,00,000 live births, declining by 17 points, from 130/ 1,00,000 live births in 2014-16. Despite a reduction, India remains one of the significant contributors to maternal deaths in the world.[2]

Early Detection in the Key!

It is crucial to recognize a case of postpartum collapse as it plays a significant role in maternal morbidity and mortality. An obstetric early warning score chart (EWS) should be used consistently for all women to enable early detection of a woman who is getting dangerously sick.[3] Maternal collapse can occur without notice in certain situations, however pre-existing risk factors may make it more likely. Antenatal assessment and management of women, who are at risk of collapse, should involve collaboration with a multidisciplinary team and the establishment of a pregnancy and delivery management plan.

ETIOLOGY

There are several etiological factors of the postpartum collapse, which may be pregnancy-related or develop from non-pregnancy related problems that may have existed prior to pregnancy. A systematic examination of reasons of the collapse in a hospital environment enables the trained rescuers to determine the cause and if reversible, improve the survival.[4]

Causes of Postpartum Collapse

4 H's

- *Hypovolemic:* Bleeding may be revealed/ concealed (Obstetric/other reasons); or relative hypovolemic of dense spinal block; septic or neurogenic shock
- *Hypoxia:* Pregnant patients can become hypoxic more quickly
- *Hypo/hyperkalemia and other electrolyte disturbances*
- *Hypothermia*

4 T's

- *Thromboembolism*: Amniotic fluid embolus, pulmonary embolus, air embolus, and myocardial infarction

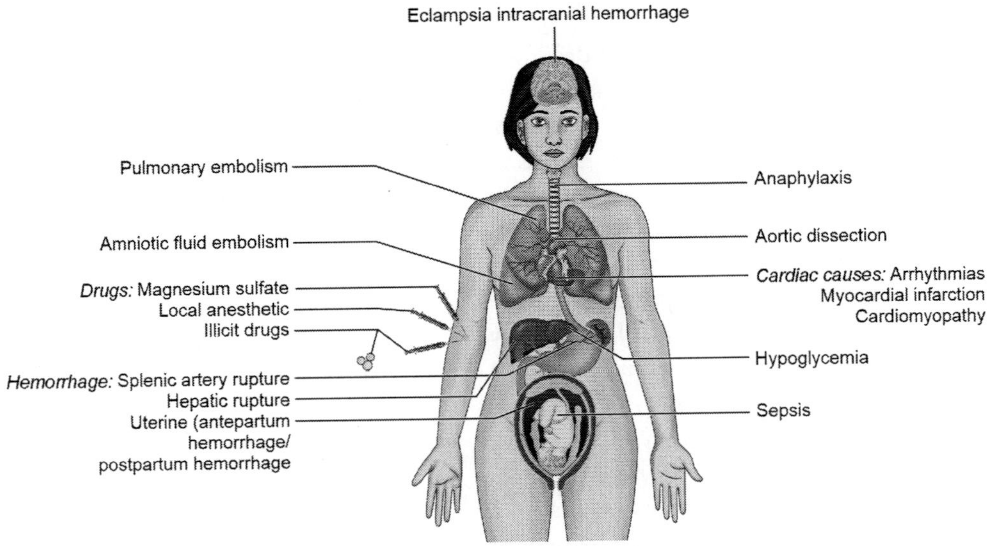

Fig. 1: The etiological factors of postpartum collapse.[1]

- Toxicity
- Tension pneumothorax
- Tamponade (cardiac)

Cardiac Events:

- Peripartum cardiomyopathy
- Myocardial infarction
- Aortic dissection
- Large-vessel aneurysms

Others: Eclampsia, pre-eclampsia, and anaphylaxis

- *Hemorrhage:* This is the most common cause of maternal collapse. The causes of major obstetric hemorrhage include postpartum hemorrhage, antepartum hemorrhage from placenta previa, placenta accreta spectrum, placental abruption, uterine rupture and ectopic pregnancy.
- *Hypoxia:* Hypoxia is common in pregnant females and may occur due to cardiac as well as respiratory factors. Common causes include peripartum cardiomyopathy, myocardial infarction, aortic dissection, and large-vessel aneurysms.
- *Electrolyte imbalance:* Hypokalemia and hyperkalemia can be seen due to several factors such as hyperemesis gravidarum, renal disorders, diabetic ketoacidosis, burns, and trauma resulting in postpartum collapse.
- *Hypothermia:* Commonly due to excessive cold exposure
- *Thromboembolism:* Pregnancy is associated with several physiological changes including hypercoagulability, increased venous stasis, and decreased venous outflow, which increases the risk of thromboembolism. Venous thromboembolism includes deep venous thrombosis (DVT) and pulmonary embolism. Half of these events occur during pregnancy while the other half is seen in the postpartum period[5] and it is an important cause of postpartum collapse.
- *Amniotic fluid embolism:* Amniotic fluid embolism manifests as collapse during labor or delivery or within 30 minutes of delivery, characterized by severe hypotension, respiratory distress, and

hypoxia. Seizures and cardiac arrest are possible complications.

- *Cardiac disease:* Myocardial infarction, aortic dissection and cardiomyopathy are the three leading cardiac causes of mortality.[6] Primary cardiac arrest in pregnancy is extremely rare, occurring in around 1/30,000 maternities. The majority of cardiac events are preceded by signs and symptoms. These patients should be addressed by a multidisciplinary team that is adequately qualified and experienced. Additional cardiac reasons include coronary artery dissection, abrupt left ventricular failure, infectious endocarditis, and pulmonary edema.
- *Sepsis:* Sepsis is a leading cause of maternal morbidity and mortality. Inadequate treatment can be fatal.[6] Bacteremia, which can occur in the absence of pyrexia, or an elevated white cell count can rapidly progress to severe sepsis and septic shock, which can result in death. The most frequently implicated organisms in obstetrics are streptococcal groups A, B, and D, *Pneumococcus*, and *Escherichia coli*.
- *Drug toxicity/overdose:* Magnesium sulphate toxicity is prevalent in the context of renal impairment. Accidental administration of anesthetic drugs can also lead to disastrous consequences. Substance abuse or illegal drug consumption can also result in maternal morbidity and death.
- *Eclampsia:* Eclampsia, as a consequence of pre-eclampsia, is also a significant cause of maternal collapse.
- *Intracranial hemorrhage:* Intracranial hemorrhage is a common consequence of uncontrolled hypertension, particularly systolic hypertension. It can also occur as a result of burst aneurysms or arteriovenous malformations. Although maternal collapse is frequently the primary manifestation, severe headache frequently precedes this.
- *Anaphylaxis:* Anaphylaxis is a severe, potentially fatal systemic hypersensitivity reaction that manifests as respiratory, cutaneous, and circulatory abnormalities, as well as gastrointestinal disruption and collapse. There is substantial shift of intravascular volume, which might result in reduced cardiac output. Acute ventricular failure and myocardial ischemia are also possible complications. Occlusion of the upper airways due to angioedema, bronchospasm and mucus clogging of smaller airways all lead to severe hypoxia.

Anaphylaxis is likely when all of the following three criteria are met:

1. Sudden onset and rapid progression of symptoms.
2. Life-threatening airway and/or breathing and/or circulation problems.
3. Skin and/or mucosal changes (flushing, urticaria, angioedema).

RISK FACTORS

Postpartum collapse is a catastrophic condition which can occur without any significant risk factor, but some of the predisposing factors are:[7]

Predisposing factors: Maternal malnutrition, anemia, hypertensive disorders, coagulation disorders, sepsis, prolonged labor, previous cesarean section, antepartum hemorrhage, and morbidly adherent placenta

Pre-existing conditions: Poor socioeconomic condition, chronic hypertension, diabetes mellitus, cardiac diseases, epilepsy, chronic liver disease, and chronic renal disease

MANAGEMENT

The woman who is critically ill and in shock requires special expert management due to various physiological changes that occur in pregnancy.

Managing a Patient with Postpartum Collapse: Important Points

- Changes in lung function, diaphragmatic splinting and increased oxygen consumption make the pregnant woman become hypoxic more readily and make ventilation more difficult.
- Weight gain in pregnancy, large breasts inhibiting the working space and laryngeal edema can all contribute to make intubation more difficult.
- The pregnant woman is at a significantly higher risk of regurgitation and aspiration secondary to the progesterone effect relaxing the lower esophageal sphincter and delayed gastric emptying, along with the raised intra-abdominal pressure secondary to the gravid uterus.
- Gestational aortocaval compression significantly reduces venous return hence reducing the efficacy of CPR.
- A left lateral tilt of 15 on a firm surface relieves the aortocaval compression in the majority of pregnant women and allows effective chest compressions to be performed.

MANAGEMENT OF SPECIFIC CONDITIONS

Hemorrhage

The most common cause of maternal death in India is hemorrhage. Four main causes are *Tone, Tissue, Trauma, and Thrombin*. Early diagnosis and prompt management are the mainstay of the treatment. Hemorrhage is the most common cause of maternal collapse and a consequence of other causes of collapse. Awareness of the limitations of clinical signs must be kept in mind and caution must be exercised in the presence of severe pre-eclampsia and eclampsia, where fluid overload can contribute to poor outcome.

HAEMOSTASIAS

Table 1 provides "HAEMOSTASIS" algorithm for management of massive postpartum hemorrhage.[8]

Placenta Accreta Spectrum

Placenta accreta spectrum (PAS) or morbidly adherent placenta is a term that refers to a variety of diseases in which the placenta or a portion of it is adhered to the uterine wall. It is a leading cause of postpartum hemorrhage (PPH) and obstetric hysterectomy, which is linked with considerable morbidity and death.

TABLE 1: HAEMOSTASIS algorithm for management of massive postpartum hemorrhage.

H	Ask for help
A	Asses vital parameters and blood loss
E	• Establish etiology (4Ts: Trauma, Tissue, Tone, and Thrombin) • Ensure availability of blood
M	Massage uterus
O	Oxytocin infusion
S	• Specific surgical management • Shift to OT (bimanual compression)
T	Tamponade (balloon and uterine packing)
A	Apply compression sutures
S	Systematic pelvic devascularization (uterine, ovarian, and internal iliac)
I	Intervention radiology—UAE
S	Subtotal and total abdominal hysterectomy

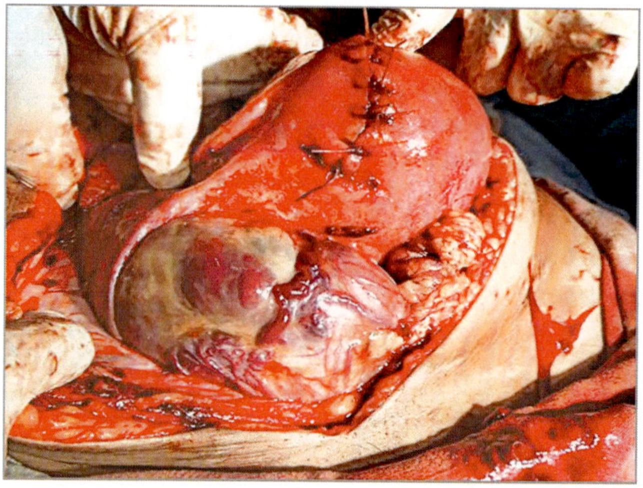

Fig. 2: Image showing placenta percreta. Placenta was occupying the hole in the lower uterine segment and was extending into leaves of broad ligament. Classical cesarean section was done, and placenta was left in situ (Image obtained by Authors during their clinical practice).

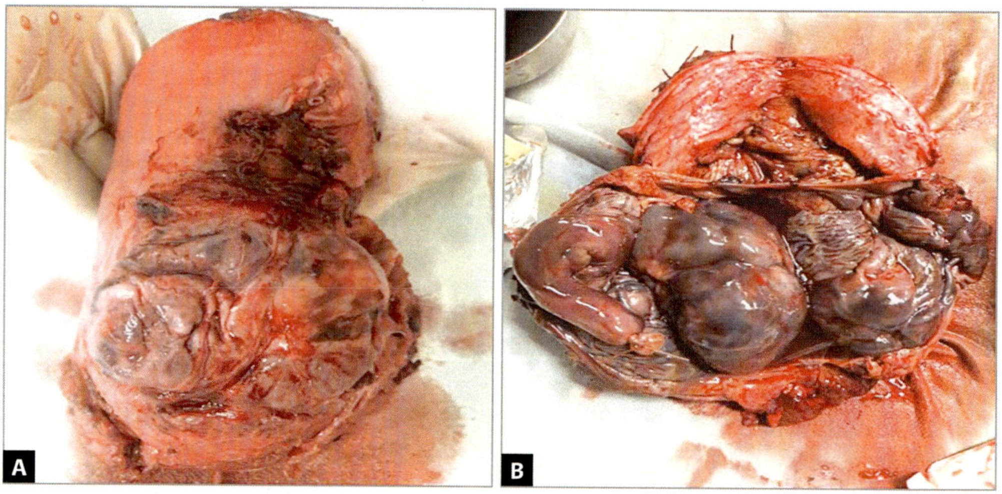

Figs. 3A and B: Image showing hysterectomy specimen which was done on later date with placenta in situ (Image obtained by authors during their clinical practice).

Morbidly adherent placenta is mostly asymptomatic antenatally, and the diagnosis is only established by ultrasound during antenatal period or after unsuccessful attempts to remove the placenta at delivery. Postpartum hemorrhage is the most common complication, which further results in postpartum collapse.

Management[9]

- Management of a woman with a morbidly adherent placenta/PAS should be multidisciplinary, with surgery conducted ideally electively under controlled settings.
- *Surgical management includes* Triple P procedure—upper border of placenta is

delineated preoperatively and delivery of fetus by transverse incision above the placental border, pelvic devascularization; and placental non-separation with myometrium excision and reconstruction of uterine wall.

- *Definitive treatment:* Peripartum hysterectomy

Acute Uterine Inversion

Acute uterine inversion is a rare, but life-threatening complication of third stage of labor with an estimated incidence of 1:2,000–1:50,000 deliveries.

Types

- *Incomplete:* Fundus of uterus inverted, but not descended through the cervix.
- *Complete:* Fundus of uterus inverted and lying in the vagina or outside introitus.

Risk Factors

- Fundal placental implantation
- Uterine atony
- Cord traction applied before placental separation
- Abnormally adhered placentation such as the accreta spectrum
- Connective tissue disorder
- Abnormally Short Cord

Clinical Features

1. Large boggy mass appearing at introitus
2. Shock is out of proportion to blood loss, mostly neurogenic
3. Hypogastric pain

Management

- Immediate recognition of uterine inversion improves the chances of a quick resolution and good outcome.
- Once any degree of uterine inversion is recognized, several steps must be taken urgently and simultaneous resuscitation of patient must be done.
- Immediately call for help including obstetrical and anesthesia team.
- Blood (MTP) is arranged
- Large-bore intravenous infusion systems are secured to begin rapid crystalloid infusion to treat hypovolemia while awaiting arrival of blood products.
- If the recently inverted uterus has not contracted and retracted completely and if the placenta has already separated, then the uterus may often be replaced simply by pushing up on the inverted fundus with the palm of the hand and fingers in the direction of the long axis of the vagina.
- If the placenta is still attached, then attempts are made to reposition the uterus with the placenta in situ with steady pressure with the fist, palm, or fingers applied to the inverted fundus in an attempt to push it up into and through the dilated cervix.
- Once the uterus is restored to its normal configuration, oxytocin is infused.
- *O'Sullivan's technique:* Hydrostatic replacement by infusing 3–5 L of fluid into the upper vagina (only after ensuring there are no vaginal or cervical lacerations), seal the introitus by hand or vacuum cup to achieve desired result.

Surgical Intervention

a. *Huntington's operation:* Stretch the cervical ring, gradually pull the myometrium just inside the uterine dimple and revert the inversion.
b. Hysterectomy is the last resort in management of recurrent inversion.
c. Uterotonics are to be continued for at least 8 hours.
d. Broad-spectrum antibiotics should be given.

Sepsis

Puerperal sepsis refers to the infection of the genital tract occurring at any time between the rupture of membranes or labor and the 42nd day postpartum, of which two or more of the following are present.[10]

- Pelvic pain
- Fever 38.5°C or more
- Abnormal vaginal discharge
- Delay in reduction of size of uterus (<2 cm a day during the first 8 days).

Definitions Related to Sepsis

Systemic inflammatory response syndrome (SIRS): SIRS with a suspected source of infection is termed sepsis. Sepsis with one or more end organ failure is called severe sepsis, and with hemodynamic instability despite intravascular volume replacement is called septic shock. SIRS is defined by presence of any two of these five criteria:

1. Temperature >38° C (100.4°F) or <36°C (96.8°F)
2. Heart rate >90 beats/min
3. Respiratory rate >20 breaths/min or
4. $PaCO_2$ <32 mm Hg
5. WBC count >12,000/cumm or <4,000/cumm.

Sequential organ failure assessment (SOFA): SOFA is used to assess the severity of organ system damage. SOFA has a better predictive validity for sepsis than SIRS criteria with better prognostic accuracy and ability to predict in-hospital mortality.

Septic shock: Sepsis with hypotension (SBP <90 mm Hg or 40 mm Hg <patient's normal BP) for at least 1 hour after adequate fluid replacement or need for vasopressors to maintain SBP >90 mm Hg or MAP >70 mm Hg. To reduce the complexity of calculating the SOFA, qSOFA was introduced which includes:

- Abnormal mental status
- RR>22 and
- SBP <100

If qSOFA score >2, then SOFA score to be calculated.

Eclampsia

Eclampsia is a type of hypertensive disorder of pregnancy associated with convulsions, often followed by coma, and posing a threat to the life of mother and the baby. It is associated with sudden onset of seizures. Eclampsia is preceded by preeclampsia.[11]

Apart from resuscitative measures, the mainstay of treatment of eclampsia is delivery. Magnesium sulphate is administered as an anti-convulsant as per Pritchard's regimen, 4 g in a 20% solution given IV over 5 minutes and 10 g in a 50% solution intramuscular 5 g. In each buttock to a total of 14 g as a loading dose, followed by 5 g repeated every 4 hours in alternate buttocks, till 24 hours of delivery or till the signs of magnesium toxicity appear. IV labetalol, hydralazine or nifedipine can be used as anti-hypertensive.[11]

Amniotic Fluid Embolism

The incidence of AFE is 2-3/1,00,000 deliveries. Amniotic fluid embolism (AFE) is a rare and typically catastrophic condition that occurs when amniotic fluid enters maternal circulation. The pathogenesis of AFE is not clear. It is hypothesized that entry of amniotic fluid (which contains fetal cells and other antigenic material) into the maternal systemic circulation via a breach in maternal/fetal interface leads to abnormal activation of humoral and immunological processes and release of vasoactive, and procoagulant substances, similar to the systemic inflammatory response syndrome.[12]

Clinical features: Sudden collapse due to profound hypotension, hypoxemia, DIC.

Factors that may be associated with AFE: Advanced maternal age, multiparty, meconium-stained liquor, obstructed labor, intrauterine fetal death, polyhydramnios, uterine rupture, placenta accreta

Investigations: Coagulation profile, ECG, ABG (arterial blood gases), Chest X-ray

Treatment:

- Multidisciplinary, team-based approach involving maternal-fetal medicine, anesthesia, critical care, respiratory, and nursing is desirable to increase the chances of stabilization and avoid further deterioration[11]
- CPR is to be performed.
- Management is supportive and symptomatic.
- Maintain oxygen saturation
- Provide hemodynamic support
- Control hemorrhage
- Correction of coagulability
- Termination of pregnancy after the initial management.

RESUSCITATION IN POSTPARTUM COLLAPSE[1]

Multidisciplinary team, including senior obstetrician and senior obstetric anesthetist/intensivist, should manage women with postpartum collapse.

- *Airway:* The airway should be protected as soon as possible by intubation with a cuffed endotracheal tube.
- *Breathing:* Supplemental oxygen should be administered as soon as possible. High flow oxygenation should be given.
- *Circulation:* Chest compression should be started immediately. Compressions should be performed at a ratio of 30:2 ventilations unless the woman is intubated, in which case chest compressions and ventilations should be desynchronized, with compressions being performed at a rate of 100/minute and ventilations at a rate of 10/minute.
- Urgent abdominal ultrasonography is required to rule out concealed hemorrhage.
- *Defibrillator:* Same energy level is used as in non-pregnant women.
- No alteration in algorithm of drugs or their doses.
- Identify the cause and manage accordingly.

MEDICOLEGAL IMPLICATIONS

Obstetrics is a very litigious specialty. Patients and their families are frequently involved in legal processes related with professional and emotional stress, and because pregnancy is viewed as a natural event, any unexpected consequence is deemed to be the result of medical malpractice.[13] The majority of the time, it is connected with a breakdown in communication, both vertically (between patient and doctor) and horizontally (between various medical departments).

CASE STUDIES

(As per the Author's Personal Experience during Clinical Practice)

Case 1

The dangerous placenta: Placenta accreta percreta in a woman with history of previous cesarean sections has become a common presentation in today's practice and the outcome is varied. We had many such cases in recent past. A well-documented consent prior to the operative procedure is mandatory so as to avoid medicolegal implications.

An unbooked woman with previous three cesareans was admitted in the labor ward emergency at 35 weeks pregnancy with APH. After all the investigations and USG, she was diagnosed to be a case of placenta accreta spectrum (PAS). An elective cesarean was planned, and a classical cesarean was done so as to avoid torrential hemorrhage from the placental site and the placenta was left in situ to be removed at a later date after the vascularity decreases and blood loss minimized. At a later date, she was again taken up for surgery and total abdominal hysterectomy was done. The patient was fine and was discharged in due course of time in a healthy condition.

Case 2

Another such emergency arose when a similar patient was taken up because of almost the same episode. She was G7P4L1A2; POG 34 weeks 1 day with gestational hypertension and placenta previa along with placental accreta with history of previous 1 LSCS, with Hb 7 gm%.

She was referred from a district hospital. The patient underwent cesarean section. Intraoperatively, there was placenta percreta; as there was no active bleeding from placental site so placenta was left in situ. But the patient had sudden about of postpartum hemorrhage on third postoperative day and emergency exploratory laparotomy and interval hysterectomy was done. She had cardiac arrest on the operation table. All resuscitative measures were taken but the patient could not be revived and she succumbed to the loss.

These two women both had placenta accreta spectrum (PAS). The management was individualized. *Case 1* was multigravida with the previous three cesareans and she tolerated both the surgeries well and without any untoward incident. However, *Case 2* was anemic grand multipara with previous one cesarean but with comorbidities. She bled in the postoperative period and though immediately taken up for intervention, could not tolerate the loss and succumbed to the condition.

Case 3

An unbooked, 35-year-old women *G3P2L2*, 36 weeks of gestation, with previous two cesareans came with APH, and was diagnosed as a case of accidental hemorrhage. On the table, her ECG recording was showing marked tachycardia. Risk associated with surgery and her condition was documented and explained to the relatives in their own language and a written informed consent was taken. Without losing more time, she was immediately taken up for surgery under general anesthesia, in view of the concealed hemorrhage. The uterus was Couvelaire. A dead baby was extracted, and there were marked retroplacental clots which were removed. CG Balloon was kept as a preventive measure for postpartum hemorrhage and stepwise devascularization was also done by ligating both uterine and ovarian vessels. On reversal, she had ventricular fibrillation for which DC shock was given and thereafter she was shifted to ICU. Massive transfusion protocol (MTP) was also done. On third day, she had cardiac arrest but was revived. And the conservative management continued. But in spite of best measures next day again, she had cardiac arrest, and she died.

She was an unbooked case, belonged to lower middle socioeconomic group. She had reached hospital late, after being first managed at a private setup but left to take second opinion.

Case 4

A woman G3P2L2, later after her demise the true formula revealed was G9P7A1 was admitted in the labor ward with multiple pregnancy in advanced labor. Immediate relevant and very necessary investigations were done, as there was no record of any antenatal check-up with her. And she delivered two stillborn babies. She had a bout of bleeding PV and succumbed to the loss. Herein, the concern was, grand multi, multiple pregnancy with no antenatal check-ups succumbed because could not tolerate even a small amount of blood loss. The hiding of proper history was also a concern.

Case 5

A 22-year-old was referred from a Civil Hospital as primi gravida with 27 weeks 4 days period of gestation (POG) with pregnancy-induced hypertension (PIH) and anasarca ?allergic reaction. She was admitted and was diagnosed as severely anemic. Her USG showed F/S/O FGR with high-resistance flow in umbilical artery. The patient had sudden rise in BP with sudden fall in O_2 saturation associated with bilateral chest crepitations. She was shifted to ICU where she developed cardiac arrhythmias. All resuscitative measures were taken but the patient could not be revived and declared dead on the same day.

Case 6

A 36-year-old patient P6 L5 D1 was referred to our institute from district level Civil Hospital, where she had delivered a stillborn male baby. At the time of admission, the general condition of the patient was very sick, and she was already intubated. The patient was admitted in ICU. ECHO was done in view of persistent hypertension which revealed grade 3 diastolic dysfunction and ejection fraction 30% indicating peripartum cardiomyopathy. The patient also had AKI for which dialysis was scheduled but was not possible due to very sick general condition of the patient. The patient had sudden cardiac arrest and could not be revived.

As we see today, the scenario has changed dramatically over the decades. The litigations are increasing constantly and steadily and unluckily gynecologists are the ones to rank first in these. In spite of being very particular, the scenario can change anytime, and the labor which was going smoothly may end in a catastrophe. So reasonable care along with proper documentation is a must in every case.

Antenatal/labor ward protocols should be followed with adequate supervision and monitoring of each patient. Communication, counseling and consent is a must along with documentation and record keeping.

We must foresee and anticipate the worst, with prompt diagnosis and necessary investigations. Postoperative care by operating surgeon, especially when he has operated on someone else's set-up is a must. And must always engage a qualified anesthesiologist.

Every minute a woman is dying not because of some no preventable causes but of some preventable too. A regular monthly audit of cases should be done for a better future.

Early recognition, prompt investigation and treatment are the key to prevent many obstetrical catastrophes. Multifaceted team-based strategies such as use of checklists, bundles, early warning systems and simulation trainings need to be designed and followed to decrease medical errors and improve the maternal outcomes, not just by the providers but largely by everyone.

REFERENCES

1. Chu J, Johnston TA, Geoghegan J, on behalf of the Royal College of Obstetricians and Gynaecologists. Maternal Collapse in Pregnancy and the Puerperium. BJOG. 2020;127:e14-52.
2. Registrar General of India. Special Bulletin on Maternal Mortality in India 2016-2018.

[Internet]. New Delhi: Office of the Registrar General and Census Commissioner, India; 2020 [cited 2024 Jul 10].
3. Gopalan PD, Muckhart DJ. The critically ill obstetric patient what's the score? Int J Obstet Anaesth. 2004;13:144-5.
4. Khan KS, Wojdyla D, Say L, Gülmezoglu AM, Van Look PF. WHO analysis of causes of maternal death: a systematic review. Lancet. 2006;367(9516):1066-74.
5. American College of Obstetricians and Gynaecologist (ACOG). Thromboembolism in Pregnancy. ACOG Practice Bulletin No 196. Obstet Gynecol. 2018;132:e1-17.
6. Bowyer L. The Confidential Enquiry into Maternal and Child Health (CEMACH). Saving Mothers' Lives: reviewing maternal deaths to make motherhood safer 2003-2005. The Seventh Report of the Confidential Enquiries into Maternal Deaths in the UK. Obstet Med. 2008;1(1):54.
7. Sharma C, Mistry K. Postpartum collapse. In: Sharma A (Ed). A Practical Guide to Third Trimester of Pregnancy and Puerperium. New Delhi: Jaypee Brothers Medical Publishers; 2016. ISBN 9789385891294.
8. Varatharajan L, Chandraharan E, Sutton J, Lowe V, Arulkumaran S. Outcome of the management of massive postpartum hemorrhage using the algorithm "HEMOSTASIS". Int J Gynaecol Obstet. 2011; 113(2):152-4.
9. Chandraharan E, Rao S, Belli AM, Arulkumaran S. The Triple-P procedure as a conservative surgical alternative to peripartum hysterectomy for placenta percreta. Int J Gynaecol Obstet. 2012;117(2):191-4. doi: 10.1016/j.ijgo.2011.12.005.
10. Bamfo JE. Managing the risks of sepsis in pregnancy. Best Pract Res Clin Obstet Gynaecol. 2013;27(4):583-95.
11. Salha O, Walker JJ. Modern management of eclampsia. Postgraduate Medical Journal. 1999;75(880):78-82.
12. Kaur K, Bhardwaj M, Kumar P, Singhal S, Singh T, Hooda S. Amniotic fluid embolism. J Anaesthesiol Clin Pharmacol. 2016; 32(2):153.
13. Jha S, Ferriman E. Medicolegal Issues in Obstetrics and Gynaecology. Springer; 2018. ISBN 9783319786834.

CHAPTER 21

Sepsis and Critical Care in Pregnancy

Prashanth Prabhu J

SEPSIS

Puerperal sepsis is defined as an infection of the genital tract occurring at any time between rupture of membrane or labor and 42 days postpartum in which two or more of the following are present; pelvic pain, fever (temperature ≥38.5°C on any occasion), abnormal vaginal discharge, delay in the rate of uterine involution. It is a leading cause of pregnancy-related maternal morbidity and mortality in developing countries.[1] Medicolegal aspects related to puerperal sepsis involve legal liability towards prevention, diagnosis, and appropriate management of puerperal sepsis. It is extremely crucial for the healthcare providers to be aware of these medicolegal aspects to ensure patient safety and minimize the medicolegal risks. Common terminologies related to sepsis are provided in **Box 1**.

Signs and Symptoms

- *Fever and shivering:* Fever is induced by cytokine activation. Hyperthermia is an increase in body temperature due to thermoregulation failure. Sepsis causes peripheral vasodilation and loss of endothelial integrity, hampering the body ability to regulate its core temperature leading to shivering.
- *Altered mental status:* Sepsis causes activation of cerebral endothelial cells resulting in blood-brain barrier dysfunction and release of various mediators into the brain resulting in altered mental status.
- *Increased breathing (tachypnea):* Sepsis causes the release of endotoxins and other inflammatory mediators causing stimulation of medullary ventilator center causing tachypnea. In sepsis due to tissue hypoperfusion, it leads to metabolic acidosis which is compensated by tachypnea.
- *Increased heart rate:* In sepsis, blood flow decreases to vital organs. The heart tries to compensate for this by increasing heart rate leading to tachycardia.

BOX 1: Common terminologies related to sepsis.[2]

Sepsis	It is a life-threatening organ dysfunction caused by a dysregulated host response to infection. It is an infection with systemic manifestation of infection
Maternal Sepsis	Sepsis, that occurs during pregnancy
Puerperal Sepsis	An infection of the genital tract occurring at any time between rupture of membrane or labor and 42 days postpartum
Severe sepsis	Sepsis + organ dysfunction or tissue hypoperfusion induced by sepsis
Septic shock	Persistence of hypoperfusion despite adequate fluid replacement therapy

- *Weak pulse, Low blood pressure:*[3] Sepsis leads to cardiac dysfunction characterized by impaired contractility, diastolic dysfunction, reduced cardiac index and reduced ejection fraction. This leads to weak pulse and low blood pressure. It is due to either elevated inflammation or suppression of both fatty acid and glucose oxidation and eventual ATP depletion. The cardiac adrenergic signaling is also compromised in sepsis.
- *Low urine output:* Sepsis causes a decrease in glomerular filtration rate because of decrease in renal blood flow and renal perfusion pressure leading to decreased urine output.
- *Cyanotic or mottled skin:* Cyanosis is classified into three types:
  1. *Central cyanosis:* Generalized bluish discoloration of the body and mucous membrane
  2. *Peripheral cyanosis:* Bluish discoloration of distal extremities and also involve circumoral, periorbital areas
  3. *Differential cyanosis:* Bluish discoloration between upper and lower extremities. Bluish discoloration despite adequate oxygenation is called pseudo-cyanosis. Skin mottling is defined as a patchy skin discoloration. It is a sign of cutaneous hypoperfusion and usually manifests around knees.
- *Cold extremities:* When the heart is unable to pump enough blood to the extremities, it leads to cold extremities.
- *Extreme body pain or discomfort*: Group B *Streptococcus* and *Escherichia Coli* are the leading causes of maternal sepsis.[4]

Stages of Sepsis

Sepsis can progress through stages, each with increasing severity and there is a risk for organ dysfunction or failure. Early recognition and appropriate management are crucial to prevent progression through these stages. The progression of sepsis may be categorized as the following stages:

- *Systemic inflammatory response syndrome (SIRS):* It includes the following:
  1. Temperature greater than 100.4° F or lesser than 96.8° F
  2. Respiratory rate greater than 20/min
  3. Heart rate greater than 90/min
  4. White blood cells count greater than 12000 cells per microliter or less than 4000 cells per microliter or greater than 10% of band cells.
  5. Partial pressure of carbon dioxide (PCO_2) is less than 32 mm Hg.
- The second step involves sepsis. It includes the following:
  1. Any two components of SIRS
  2. Confirmed or suspected infection
- The third step is severe sepsis. It includes the following:
  1. Components of sepsis+
  2. Signs of end organ failure+
  3. Hypotension (systolic blood pressure <90 mm Hg)
  4. Serum lactate >4 mmol
- *Septic shock:* It includes the following:
  1. Severe sepsis with persistent signs of end organ failure
  2. Hypotension (Systolic blood pressure <90 mm Hg)
  3. Serum lactate >4 mmol

How to Prevent Sepsis?

1. Prevent microbial transmission and infection. The most important step to avoid sepsis is by prevention of microbial transmission.
   a. *Effective hygiene practices (hand washing, safe preparation of food):* Hand washing is an important preventive step to avoid sepsis.

The hand can have normal bacterial flora like *Staphylococcus Epidermidis, S. Hominis, Coryneform* bacteria which may cause infections in sterile body cavities, eyes, and non-intact skin. Hand care associated infection leads to increased resistance of microorganisms. There are five stages of hand transmission of infection:

i. Germs are present on patient skin and immediate environment surfaces.
ii. This germ transfer onto health-care worker's hands
iii. These germs are present on healthcare worker hands for some time.
iv. Suboptimal handwashing or no handwashing will keep the healthcare worker's hand contaminated.
v. This contaminated hand will transmit infection onto others.

Thus, hand washing is very important. The steps of hand washing are important, which covers palm to palm, back of hands, fingers interlaced, base of thumb, base of the fingers, fingernails, and wrist. The hand hygiene has to be maintained before touching a patient, before any aseptic procedure, after body fluid exposure, after touching a patient and patient surroundings in order to avoid transmission of infection.

b. *Improving sanitation and water quality: World Health Organization (WHO) with UNICEF has given practical steps to achieve universal access to quality care and to prevent infections. It has termed it as Water, Sanitation and Hygiene (WASH) in healthcare facilities.*[5] *There are eight practical steps to improve WASH in healthcare facilities:*
   i. Conduct situation analysis and assessment
   ii. Set targets and define roadmap
   iii. Establish national standards and accountability mechanisms
   iv. Improve and maintain infrastructure
   v. Monitor and review data
   vi. Develop health workforce
   vii. Engage communities
   viii. Conduct operational research and share learning
c. Providing access to vaccines. In which all individuals and community are free from vaccine preventable diseases.
d. *Appropriate nutrition:* It helps in building immunity which can help a person to fight infections.

2. Prevention of infection evolving to sepsis. Any infection contracted by a person should be avoided going into sepsis.
   a. *Appropriate antibiotic treatment of infection:* Different organisms lead to infection which in-turn leads to sepsis. These different organisms have to be treated by specific antibiotics. Using multiple antibiotics and higher antibiotics can lead to resistance. Therefore, appropriate antibiotic treatment is required to treat any infection. Hence, it is recommended to send for culture and sensitivity to start appropriate antibiotic.
   b. *Promptly seeking medical care:* Any person or patient with an infection should seek physician/hospital care to avoid its progression to sepsis. Some serious patients require early ICU care to avoid mortality and morbidity. Hence prompt seeking medical care is very important.

c. *Early detection of sepsis signs and symptoms:* Early detection of signs and symptoms reduces mortality of the patient. It can be done by formulating using protocols and educating the healthcare workers. The protocols can be developed depending on the facility, infrastructure and using scoring systems.

RAPID RESPONSE SYSTEM (RRS)[6]

It has four limbs:

1. *Afferent limb:* They monitor patients according to criteria and protocols and raise alarm when necessary.
2. *Efferent limb:* They are trained to handle sick patients. Efferent limb of Obstetric RRS contains: ICU Team, Anesthesiologist, Obstetrician, Neonatal Resuscitation Team, Interventional Radiologist, Surgeon, Blood Bank Officer.
3. *Quality improvement limb:* They record the whole scenario and provide necessary feedbacks.
4. *Administrator limb:* They provide human resources and equipment.

RISK FACTORS FOR MATERNAL SEPSIS IN PREGNANCY[7]

- *Obesity:* Body mass index (BMI) is calculated by weight (in kg)/height (in meter)^2. Obesity is subdivided into three categories:
  - i. *Class 1:* BMI of 30 to <35
  - ii. *Class 2:* BMI of 35 to <40
  - iii. *Class 3* (severe obesity): BMI >40
- *Impaired glucose tolerance/diabetes:* Impaired glucose tolerance is defined as two-hour glucose levels of 140–199 mg/dL on the 75 g oral glucose.[8]
- *Impaired immunity/immunosuppressant medication:* An impaired immune system cannot protect a person effectively against infection. The causes of the impaired immune system are any autoimmune disease (lupus, rheumatoid arthritis, Type 1 diabetes), infections (HIV, pneumonia), lymphoma, leukemia, sickle cell disease and immune cell deficiency. Immunosuppressant medication are drugs that suppress the immune system, e.g., Biologics (adalimumab, infliximab), Calcineurin inhibitors (tacrolimus, cyclosporine), Antiproliferative agents (mycophenolate mofetil, mycophenolate sodium, azathioprine), mTOR inhibitor (Sirolimus), Steroids (Prednisone).
- *Anemia:* There is a lack of enough red blood cells to carry adequate oxygen to body tissues. Anemia can be of different forms and due to different reasons, like iron deficiency anemia, vitamin deficiency anemia, sickle cell anemia, hemolytic anemia, aplastic anemia, anemia associated with bone marrow disease, anemia of inflammation.
- *Vaginal discharge:* Certain types of vaginal discharge can indicate an infection. It is categorized based on color and consistency. Examples are white discharge with cottage-cheese like consistency—yeast infection, yellow or green discharge with thick consistency and unpleasant smell—trichomoniasis.
- *History of pelvic infection:* Pelvic inflammatory disease is the infection of female reproductive organs.
- *History of Group B Streptococcal infection*
- *Amniocentesis and other invasive procedures:* Amniocentesis is a procedure where amniotic fluid is removed from uterus for testing or treatment.
- *Cervical cerclage:* It is a medical procedure where a stitch is placed around cervix to prevent late miscarriage or preterm delivery.

- *Prolonged spontaneous rupture of membranes:* Any tear or hole in amniotic sac is called as rupture of membranes.
- GAS (Group A *Streptococcus*) infection in close contacts or family members.

CHALLENGES IN DIAGNOSING SEPSIS IN PREGNANCY[9]

Diagnosing sepsis in pregnancy can be challenging due to various factors related to pregnancy. Pregnancy-related changes in vital signs, white blood cell count, and other laboratory values can mask or mimic sepsis. Symptoms due to sepsis can be like those of normal pregnancy or other pregnancy-related complications. Sometimes healthcare providers may attribute symptoms to pregnancy rather than sepsis, which may result in delayed diagnosis. The systemic inflammatory response syndrome (SIRS) criteria, commonly used to diagnose sepsis, have limited accuracy in pregnant women. Conditions like preeclampsia, HELLP syndrome, and placental abruption can present similarly to sepsis. Sepsis in pregnancy can present atypically, making diagnosis more challenging. Laboratory results, such as white blood cell count and C-reactive protein, can be affected by pregnancy. Comparison of physiological changes in pregnancy, changes during sepsis and cumulative effect are provided in **Table 1**.

Remedies to the Difficulties in Diagnosis

- Any abnormality or uneasiness by the pregnant woman has to be reported early.
- Early evaluation of these pregnant women is important.
- Monitoring of pregnant women has to be done with increased frequency if admitted in-hospital.
- Early transfer to ICU if any abnormality detected.
- Initiation of early treatment of sepsis
- Involvement of multispecialty of doctors is required to treat pregnant woman with sepsis.

SCORING SYSTEMS IN SEPSIS

Sequential Organ Failure Assessment (SOFA) Score

It is used to track a patient organ (respiratory system, nervous system, cardiovascular system, renal system, liver, and coagulation) status in ICU (Intensive Care Unit). Sequential organ failure assessment score has been provided in **Table 2**.

Interpreting the SOFA Score

Depiction of mortality according to the SOFA score has been provided in **Table 3**.

SOMANZ (Society of Obstetric Medicine Australia and New Zealand) recommends obstetrically modified SOFA (om SOFA) score to assess evidence of end organ dysfunction.[12] It is performed after screening for sepsis using omSOFA score. Parameters related to obstetrically modified SOFA score have been provided in **Table 4**.[12]

How qSOFA score is different from SOFA score?

- Score 2 shows end organ dysfunction. Scores of 3 and 4 are removed for making it easy.
- GCS is a little difficult to assess regularly in obstetrics wards.

Quick Sequential Organ Failure Assessment (qSOFA)

It helps to identify patients with suspected sepsis outside ICU with poor outcome. qSOFA scoring has been provided in **Table 5**.

TABLE 1: Comparison of physiological changes in pregnancy—changes during sepsis and cumulative effect.[2]

	Physiological changes in Pregnancy	*Changes during sepsis*	*Cumulative effect*
Cardiovascular system	• Decrease systemic vascular resistance (25–30%) • Decreased blood pressure • Increased blood volume (40–45%) • Increased heart rate (10–20 bpm) • Increased cardiac output (40%)	• Decreased systemic vascular resistance • Decreased blood pressure • Increased heart rate • Vasodilatation • Myocardial depression	Rapid hemodynamic collapse
Respiratory system	• Decreased pulmonary vascular resistance • Decreased plasma colloid pressure • Decreased residual volume • Decreased functional residual capacity • Increased tidal volume • Increased minute ventilation • Compensated respiratory alkalosis	• Increased pulmonary microvascular pressure and permeability • Acute lung injury	• Susceptible to pulmonary edema • Decrease in oxygenation • Adult respiratory distress syndrome • Decreased ability to compensate for metabolic acidosis
Renal system	• Increased renal plasma flow • Increased glomerular filtration rate • Renal collecting system dilatation	• Ischemia • Vasoconstriction • Cytokine- mediated renal cell injury	Acute kidney injury
Coagulation	• Increased factors I, II, VII, VIII, IX, XII • Increased plasminogen activator inhibitors (PAI) I and II • Decreased protein S • No change in anti-thrombin and Protein C	• Increased procoagulant effects • Increased thrombin production • Decreased activated protein C • Fibrinolysis • Increased PAI I	• Increased microvascular thrombus formation • Microcirculation dysregulation • Tissue hypoperfusion • End organ dysfunction

Obstetrically Modified qSOFA (omqSOFA) Score

- Systolic blood pressure of 90 mm Hg or less
- Respiratory rate of 25/min or greater
- Altered mentation

National Early Warning Score (NEWS)[14]

It is a tool developed by Royal College of Physicians which helps in detection and clinical deterioration of adult patients. National Early Warning Scoring system has been provided in **Table 6**.

TABLE 2: Sequential organ failure assessment (SOFA) score.[10]

SOFA score	*0*	*1*	*2*	*3*	*4*
Respiratory system PaO_2/FiO_2 (mm Hg) SaO_2/FiO_2	>400	<400 221–301	<300 142–220	<200 67–141	<100 <67
CNS GCS (Glasgow Coma Scale)	15	13–14	10–12	6–9	<6
CVS Hypotension	No hypotension	MAP <70	Dopamine ≤5 or dobutamine (any)	Dopamine >5 or norepinephrine ≤0.1	Dopamine >15 or norepinephrine >0.1
Renal Creatinine (mg/dL) or urine output (mL/day)	<1.2	1.2–1.9	2.0–3.4	3.5–4.9 or <500	>5.0 or <200
Liver Bilirubin (mg/dL)	<1.2	1.2–1.9	2.0–5.9	6.0–11.9	>12.0
Coagulation Platelets ($10^3/mm^3$)	>150	<150	<100	<50	<20

TABLE 3: Depicting mortality as per SOFA score.[11]

SOFA score	*Mortality*
0–6	<10%
7–9	15–20%
10–12	40–50%
13–14	50–60%
15	>80%
16–24	>90%

TABLE 4: Parameters related to obstetrically modified SOFA score.[12]

System parameter	*Score 0*	*Score 1*	*Score 2*
Respiration: PaO_2/FiO_2	>400	300–400	<300
Coagulation: Platelets $\times 10^6$/L	>150	100–150	<100
Liver: Bilirubin (μmol/L)	<20	20–32	>32
Cardiovascular: Mean arterial pressure (mm Hg)	MAP >70	MAP <70	Vasopressors required
Central nervous system	Alert	Rousable by voice	Rousable by pain
Renal: Creatinine (μmol/L)	<90	90–120	>120

FiO_2: fraction of inspired oxygen, PaO_2: partial pressure of oxygen.

- *If NEW score:* 0 (aggregate 1-4), clinical risk is low.
- *If NEW score:* 3 (any individual score) with aggregate 5–6, clinical risk is medium.
- *If NEW score with aggregate:* 7 or more, clinical risk is high.

Sepsis in Obstetrics Score (SOS)

It is a model to identify risk of morbidity from sepsis in pregnancy. SOS scoring has been provided in **Table 7.**[15]

Systemic Inflammatory Response Syndrome (SIRS) Criteria

SIRS response: 2 or more of the following:

- *Temperature:* >38.3°C or <36°C
- Heart rate >90 bpm
- Respiratory rate >20 breaths/min or $PaCO_2$ <32 mm Hg (<4.3 kPa)
- White cell count <4 or >12g/L or >10% immature (band) forms
- Blood glucose >140 mg/dL (7.8mmol/L) in non-diabetic
- New altered mental state

Usage of scoring:

- SOFA score shows a good predictive value for maternal death and is used for evaluation of the severity in complicated obstetric patients.[16]
- qSOFA requires only clinical data for assessment, hence can be done quickly.
- A woman's gravid state will impact some variables of qSOFA, hence omqSOFA is used.
- NEWS scoring is easier score for the healthcare workers to check the status of any pregnant woman in non-ICU wards.
- SOS identifies the risk of morbidity from sepsis in pregnancy.

How to proceed with Sepsis in Obstetric Patients?

- *Recognize sepsis:* If the woman has 2 or more in omqSOFA, it is a high-risk of poor outcome. It is advisable to consult

TABLE 5: Sequential organ failure assessment (Quick).[13]

Assessment	*qSOFA score*
Low blood pressure (SBP ≤100 mm Hg)	1
High respiratory rate (≥22 breaths/min)	1
Altered mentation (GCS ≤14)	1
0 or 1 points: Not high risk. Continue management as appropriate *2 or 3 points:* High risk of poor outcome Assess for evidence of organ dysfunction	

TABLE 6: National early warning score (NEWS).[14]

	Score						
Element	*3*	*2*	*1*	*0*	*1*	*2*	*3*
Respiratory rate (bpm)	≤8		9–11	12–20		21–24	≥25
O_2 saturation (%)	≤91	92–93	94–95	≥96			
Any supplemental oxygen		Yes		No			
Systolic BP (mm Hg)	90	91–100	101–110	111–219			≥220
Pulse (bpm)	≤40		41–50	51–90	91–110	111–130	≥131
AVPU score				Alert			VPU
Temperature (°C)	≤35.0		35.1–36.0	36.1– 38.0	38.1– 39.0	≥39.1	

TABLE 7: Sepsis in obstetrics score.[15]

	Score Value								
Variable	***+4***	***+3***	***+2***	***+1***	***0 (Normal)***	***+1***	***+2***	***+3***	***+4***
Temperature (OC)	>40.9	39–40.9		38.5–38.9	36–38.4	34–35.9	32–33.9	30–31.9	<30
SBP (mm Hg)					>90		70–90		<70
HR (bpm)	>179	150–179	130–149	120–129	≤119				
RR (breaths/minute)	>49	35–49		25–34	12–24	10–11	6–9		≤5
SpO_2 (%)					≥92	90-91		85–89	<85
Leukocytes (number/microliter)	>39.9		25–39.9	17–24.9	5.7–16.9	3–5.6	1–2.9		<1
Immature neutrophils (%)			≥10%		<10%				
Lactic acid (mmol/L)			≥4		<4				

a physician and senior obstetrician for appropriate management of the patient.

- Maintain patent airway and oxygenate.
- *Intravenous access:* Establish 2 large bore IV cannula
- *Obtain blood culture prior to antibiotic administration.*
- *Send for Blood tests:* Complete blood count, electrolytes, urea, creatinine, C-reactive protein, liver function tests, coagulation studies, blood culture and lactate.
- *Fluid administration:* IV crystalloid given to maintain SBP >90 mm Hg, Even after 2 Liter fluid, SBP is inadequate call ICU Team.
- Administer broad spectrum antibiotics within 60 minutes. A combination of either piperacillin/tazobactum or a carbapenem plus clindamycin provides one of the broadest ranges of treatment for severe sepsis.[7]
- Assess fetus (ultrasound and electronic fetal monitoring) and reassess pregnant woman.
- Look for signs of sepsis deterioration using omqSOFA score.
- Continue targeted assessment and monitoring.

INDICATIONS FOR TRANSFER OF OBSTETRIC PATIENTS TO THE INTENSIVE CARE UNIT[17]

- *Cardiovascular system:* Hypotension or raised serum lactate persisting despite fluid resuscitation, suggesting need for inotrope support. If the blood pressure is not within the normal limits in spite of fluid resuscitation, the woman has to be shifted to ICU as the patient will require inotropes. Any patient requiring inotropes need constant cardiac monitoring and ICU admission.
- *Respiratory system:* Pulmonary edema, mechanical ventilation, airway protection. Pulmonary edema might require mechanical ventilation due to respiratory distress. Any patient requiring mechanical

ventilation will need cardiac monitors and ICU care.
- *Renal system:* Renal dialysis. Renal dialysis leads to lot of fluid shifts and electrolyte abnormalities requiring constant cardiac monitoring in ICU.
- *Neurological system:* Significantly decreased conscious level.
- Decreased conscious level can lead to aspiration, hence airway protection is important in these patients. ICU care is required for constant monitoring and management of these patients.
- *Others:* Multi-organ failure, uncorrected acidosis, hypothermia. The trauma triad of death is combination of hypothermia, acidosis and coagulopathy requiring ICU care.

Concept of Maternal Delays

In 1994, Thaddeus and Maine proposed Three Delays Model (3DM) that contribute to maternal mortality.[18]
- *First delay:* Delay in pregnant woman to seek help
- *Second delay:* Delay in woman reaching health care
- *Third delay:* Delay in appropriate treatment in healthcare facility

What to do, once a Woman is Admitted with Sepsis?

Hour-1 Bundle[19] *(Initial Resuscitation for Sepsis and Septic Shock):*
1. Measure lactate level. Remeasure lactate if initial lactate elevated (>2 mmol/L)
2. Obtain blood cultures before administering antibiotics
3. Administer broad-spectrum antibiotics
4. Begin rapid administration of 30 mL/kg crystalloid for hypotension or lactate ≥4 mmol/L
5. Apply vasopressors if hypotensive during or after fluid resuscitation to maintain a mean arterial pressure ≥65 mm Hg.

The above five steps are to be tried preferably within the first hour of recognition of sepsis.

Blood culture, full blood count and blood lactate, hourly urine output, oxygen, intravenous fluid challenge and IV antibiotics are the components of '*sepsis six*'.

IMPORTANT UPDATES

(2021 Surviving Sepsis Campaign Guidelines)[20]
- To maintain performance improvement program for sepsis in the hospitals.
- Do not use qSOFA as a single screening tool for sepsis and sepsis shock.
- Measuring blood lactate is important in suspected sepsis patients.
- Treatment and resuscitation should begin simultaneously in sepsis patients.
- Atleast 30 mL/kg of IV crystalloid to be given in septic shock within first 3 hours of resuscitation.
- Use dynamic measures to guide fluid resuscitation.
- Resuscitation done to decrease serum lactate levels in patients.
- Capillary refill time used as one of the methods to guide resuscitation of perfusion.
- Adults with septic shock on vasopressors, maintain mean arterial pressure (MAP) of 65 mm Hg.
- Patients with sepsis require ICU admission within 6 hours.
- Adults with suspected sepsis but unconfirmed infection, if any alternate cause of illness is strongly suspected, discontinue empirical antimicrobials.
- If there is highly likelihood of sepsis, antimicrobials to be given within 1 hour.

- Rapid assessment of infectious versus noninfectious causes of acute illness is important.
- For adults with high risk of MRSA, use antimicrobials with MRSA coverage.
- Any old intravascular access devices, possible source of sepsis should be removed once other vascular access has been established.
- Daily assessment for de-escalation of antimicrobials is recommended.
- Adults with adequate source control of sepsis, shorter duration of antimicrobial is suggested.
- Crystalloids are first-line fluid for resuscitation.
- Balanced crystalloids are better than normal saline for resuscitation.
- Albumin is suggested after large volumes of crystalloids.
- Starches not to be used for resuscitation.
- Gelatin too not suggested for resuscitation.
- Norepinephrine is always the vasopressor of choice.
- If adequate MAP is not achieved, the next vasopressor of choice is vasopressin.
- After vasopressin it is epinephrine.
- Terlipressin is not recommended.
- Septic shock and cardiac dysfunction with persistent hypoperfusion despite adequate volume status and arterial blood pressure, add dobutamine to norepinephrine or use epinephrine alone. Levosimendan is not recommended.
- Once it is practically possible and resources available, use invasive monitoring of arterial blood pressure.
- Start vasopressors peripherally to restore MAP rather than delaying for central venous access.
- No evidence available regarding which is better for the first 24 hour resuscitation, restrictive or liberal fluid strategies.
- For sepsis-induced hypoxemic respiratory failure, high flow nasal oxygen is better than noninvasive ventilation.
- For sepsis-induced ARDS (Acute Respiratory Distress Syndrome), low tidal volume ventilation (6 mL/kg) is recommended over high tidal volume strategy (>10 mL/kg) and to use an upper limit goal for plateau pressures of 30 cm H_2O.
- Use higher PEEP and low tidal volume for sepsis-induced ARDS.
- Recruitment maneuvers suggested as traditional recruitment maneuvers. Incremental PEEP titration/strategy is not recommended.
- In sepsis induced ARDS, prone ventilation >12 hour/day is recommended.
- Intermittent NMBA (Neuro Muscular Blocking Agent) is recommended rather than continuous infusions.
- Venovenous ECMO (Extra Corporeal Membrane Oxygenation) is suggested when conventional mechanical ventilation fails.
- Septic shock with vasopressors, IV corticosteroids is suggested, polymyxin B is not recommended.
- Restrictive transfusion strategy is recommended with septic shock.
- IV immunoglobulins is not recommended.
- In those with risk of gastrointestinal (GI) bleeding, stress ulcer prophylaxis is recommended.
- For adults with sepsis, pharmacological venous thromboembolism (VTE) prophylaxis is to be given, unless a contraindication exists. Mechanical VTE prophylaxis is not recommended.
- Adult with sepsis and AKI, either continuous or intermittent renal replacement therapy is advised.
- If glucose level ≥180 mg/dL (10 mmol/L), insulin therapy is recommended.

- IV Vitamin C is not advised.
- Adult with septic shock and hypoperfusion-induced lactic academia, using sodium bicarbonate therapy to improve hemodynamics is not recommended.
- If there is severe metabolic academia (pH ≤7.2) and acute kidney injury (AKIN score 2 or 3), sodium bicarbonate therapy is recommended.
- Early initiation of enteral nutrition (within 72 hours) is recommended.
- Discussing goals of care and prognosis with patient and patient attenders is suggested best practice.
- Adult survivors of sepsis with mechanical ventilation >48 hour or an ICU stay >72 hour, post-hospital rehabilitation program is suggested.

MEDICOLEGAL ASPECTS

Tubectomy failure, maternal deaths, issues related to medical termination of pregnancy, postpartum complications and procedure done without valid consent are cases passed against medical profession.[21]

The standard of care which has to be maintained by medical professional is outlined in Medical Council of India Act 2021. In maternofetal supremacy, maternal autonomy takes precedence.

In ICU pregnant patients, "acting in good faith" always upholds provided with the principle of not harming is followed.

The consent in ICU is to establish the fact that the patient has willingly consented for treatment. Hence consent in ICU is very important. Day-to-day proceedings of the patient improvement and status needs to be updated to patient and patient attenders to have a good doctor–patient relationship.

Documentation is also very important in ICU. Any procedure/treatment/ intervention/ investigation done on the patient needs to be documented as early as possible and updated with patient and patient attenders.

CONCLUSION

Sepsis in pregnancy has high mortality and morbidity. It is always better to avoid sepsis by preventing microbial transmission and prevent infection evolving. There are risk factors for sepsis during pregnancy. Pregnant woman in these criteria should be cautious. There is difficulty in diagnosing sepsis in pregnancy due to physiological changes in pregnancy. Hence multiple scoring systems are used depending on the situation, time, healthcare worker to triage the pregnant woman requirement to ICU. Sometimes RRS is initiated for early care of septic pregnant woman. There are specific management of sepsis patients in ICU. The surviving sepsis campign international guideline provide protocols in management of sepsis patients. Early admission, initiation of resuscitation and treatment within the golden first hour to pregnant woman are the factors which reduce the mortality and morbidity.

Critical care is highly voluminous and a constant-evolving subject. Important topics are discussed here pertaining to obstetrics. All attempts are made to provide up-to-date information.

REFERENCES

1. Olutoye AS, Agboola AD, Bello OO. Puerperal Sepsis at University College Hospital, Ibadan: a 10-year review. Ann Ib Postgrad Med. 2022;20(1):32-9.
2. Bridwell RE, Carius BM, Long B, Oliver JJ, Schmitz G. Sepsis in Pregnancy: Recognition and Resuscitation. Western Journal of Emergency Medicine. 2019;20(5):822-32. DOI: 10.5811/westjem.2019.6.43369.
3. Drosatos K, Lymperopoulos A, Kennel PJ, Pollak N, Schulze PC, Goldberg IJ. Pathophysiology of Sepsis-related cardiac

dysfunction: driven by inflammation, energy mismanagement, or both? Current Heart Failure Reports. 2015;12(2):130-40. Doi: 10.1007/s11897-014-0247-z. PMID: 25475180.
4. Royal College of Obstetricians and Gynaecologists. Bacterial Sepsis in Pregnancy. Green-top Guideline No. 64a. London: RCOG; 2012 [https://www.rcog.org.uk/en/guidelines-research-services/guidelines/gtg64a/].
5. https://www.unicef.org/documents/eight-practical-steps.
6. S Anushapreethi, Pandey A, Ahmed A. Obstetric Rapid Response Teams (Chapter 78). Critical Care Update 2021. Jaypee Brothers Medical Publishers. 2022. Pp. 391-5.
7. Royal College of Obstetricians and Gynaecologists. Bacterial Sepsis following Pregnancy. Green-top Guideline No.64b. London: RCOG; 2012 [https://www.rcog.org.uk/en/guidelines-research-services/guidelines/gtg64b/].
8. Rao SS, Disraeli P, Mcgregor T. Impaired glucose tolerance and impaired fasting glucose. Am Fam Physician. 2004;69(8):1961-8.
9. Greer O, Shah NM, Johnson MR. Maternal sepsis update: current management and controversies. The Obstetrician & Gynaecologist. 2019;22(1):45-55. https://doi.org/10.1111/tog.12623.
10. Vincent JL, Moreno R, Takala J, et al. The SOFA (Sepsis-related Organ Failure Assessment) score to describe organ dysfunction/failure. On behalf of the Working Group of Sepsis-Related Problems of the European Society of Intensive Care Medicine. Intensive Care Med. 1996;22(7):707-10. DOI: 10.1007/BF01709751.
11. Tekade T, Manohar T. Utility of SOFA (Sequential Organ Function Assessment) score to predict outcome in critically ill patients at a tertiary care hospital, Nagpur. Panacea Journal of Medical Sciences, 30th December 2017. Corpus ID: 80590239.
12. Bowyer L, Robinson HL, Barrett H, et al. SOMANZ Guidelines for the Investigation and management sepsis in pregnancy. Australian and New Zealand Journal of Obstetrics and Gynecology. 2017;57(5):540-51. https://doi.org/10.1111/ajo.12646.
13. Seymour CW, Liu VX, Iwashyna TJ, et al. Assessment of clinical criteria for sepsis. JAMA. 2016;315(8):762. Doi: 10.1001/jama.2016.0288.
14. Kolic I, Crane S, McCartney S, Perkins Z, Taylor A. Factors affecting response to National Early Warning Score (NEWS). Rapid Response Systems. 2015;90:85-90.
15. Agarwal R, Yadav RK, Mohta M, Sikka M, Radhakrishnan G. Sepsis in Obstetrics Score (SOS) utility and validation for triaging patients with obstetric sepsis in the emergency department: evidence from a low income health care setting. Obstet Med. 2019;12(2):90-6. Doi: 10.1177/1753495X18761522. PMID:31217814.
16. Esquivel LAB, Urbina JM, Zeron HM. Approach to an obstetric prognosis scale: The modified SOFA scale. Ghana Med J. 2016;50(3):129-35. PMID: PMC5044792.
17. Danna VA, Bedwell C, Wakasiaka S, Lavender T. Utility of the three-delays model and its potential for supporting a solution-based approach to accessing intrapartum care in low- and middle-income countries: a qualitative evidence synthesis. Glob Health Action. 2020;13(1):1819052. DOI: 10.1080/16549716.2020.1819052. PMID: 33040697.
18. Thaddeus S, Maine D. Too far to walk: maternal mortality in context. Soc Sci Med. 1994;38(8):1091-110. DOI: 10.1016/0277-9536(94)90226-7.
19. https://www.sccm.org/getattachment/SurvivingSepsisCampaign/Guidelines/Adult-Patients/Surviving-Sepsis-Campaign-Hour-1-Bundle.pdf?lang=en-US.
20. Evans L, Rhodes A, Alhazzani W, et al. Surviving Sepsis Campaign: International Guidelines for Management of Sepsis and Septic Shock. Critical Care Medicine. 2021;49(11):e1063-143.
21. Samavedam S. Medicolegal aspects of obstetric critical care. Indian J Crit Care Med. 2021;25(Suppl 3):S279-82.

SECTION 7

Medicolegal Issues in Gynecology

CHAPTER 22

Polycystic Ovary Syndrome

Deepti Gupta, Jyoti Sharma

INTRODUCTION

Polycystic ovarian syndrome (PCOS) is a complex, multifactorial, hyperandrogenic, and hyperinsulinemic condition which presents with myriad of symptoms form being completely asymptomatic to menstrual irregularity, hirsutism, acne, obesity, infertility, etc. Normal ovulation is a well-coordinated and complex interaction of neuroendocrine, intraovarian and endometrial mechanisms acting at various levels of hypothalamo-pituitary-ovarian axis. Polycystic ovary syndrome is an aberration in this fine-tuned orchestrated hormonal symphony. PCOS remains the most common condition associated with chronic anovulation. Even though it was officially first described by Stein and Leventhal in 1935,[1] literature finds its mention dating as back as 1721.[2]

DEFINITION

Exact incidence of PCOS is not known because of the differences in diagnostic criteria, evaluation strategies, and ethnic variations, but it has been estimated to affect 4–20% women in reproductive age group.[3] Indian studies have reported incidence varying from 3–22.5%.[4] After years of research, it is agreed that it is an ill-defined, heterogeneous, multifactorial condition with complex pathophysiology. Multiple classification systems have evolved over the past few years, most common used being *Rotterdam criteria*[5] which requires presence of 2 out of 3 for diagnosis of PCOS. Comparison of different diagnostic criteria is provided in **Table 1**.

TABLE 1: Comparison of different diagnostic criteria.[6]

National Institute of Health (NIH) Consensus 1990 (all required)	*Rotterdam consensus 2003 (two out of three required)*	*Androgen Excess PCOS Society (AEPCOS) definition 2006 (Androgen excess and one another criterion)*
1. Clinical and/or biochemical hyperandrogenism 2. Oligo/amenorrhea, anovulation	1. Clinical and/or biochemical hyperandrogenism 2. Oligo/amenorrhea, anovulation 3. Polycystic ovaries appearance on ultrasound	1. Clinical and/or biochemical hyperandrogenism 2. Oligo/amenorrhea, anovulation 3. Polycystic ovaries appearance on ultrasound
Exclusion of other androgen excess disorders NC-CAH (non-classical congenital adrenal hyperplasia), Cushing's syndrome, Androgen secreting tumors, Hyperprolactinemia and Thyroid disease, Drug-induced androgen excess. Other causes for anovulation should also been excluded.		

BOX 1: Phenotypes of polycystic ovary syndrome (Rotterdam criteria).[7]

Classic polycystic	All three chronic anovulation PCOM and hyperandrogenism present
Classic noncystic	Anovulation and hyperandrogenism present ovaries have normal morphology
Nonclassic ovulatory	PCOM and hyperandrogenism present regular menses
Non-classic mild or normo-androgenic	Anovulation, PCOM, and normoandrogenism present

1. Oligo- and/or anovulation
2. Clinical and/or biochemical hyperandrogenism with exclusion of other causes of androgen excess
3. Polycystic ovaries

PCOS PHENOTYPES[7]

Based on presence or absence of two or more features out of 3, various phenotypes have been established. Phenotypes of polycystic ovary syndrome (Rotterdam criteria) are provided in **Box 1**.

ETIOPATHOGENESIS

PCOS is considered to occur due to a combination of genetic factors and lifestyle/environmental factors. It is well-recognized that there is definite genetic predisposition for developing PCOS with risk in first degree relative being around 24% of mothers and 32% of sisters.[8] On the basis of small twin pair-based studies, it is suggested to be X-linked polygenic disorder, rather than autosomal dominant or monogenic.[9] Expectedly major susceptibility locus are genes involved in biosynthesis and metabolism of androgens with likely autosomal dominant mode of inheritance. P450 CYP-11a and gene for follistatin are ones most often implicated **(Fig. 1)**.

Role of lifestyle and environmental factors has gained more and more importance with deeper understanding of disease. BMI is a key risk factor associated with the incidence of PCOS (mean BMI: 29.3 ± 7.5 vs. 25.6 ± 5.8 kg/m^2, $p < 0.001$ in women with and without PCOS).[10] Especially BMI changes during adolescence are associated with likelihood of developing PCOS.

Commonly encountered abnormality in PCOS is abnormality in GnRH pulsatility as a result of abnormality in steroid hormone feedback or increased circulating androgen levels. There is robust evidence to suggest that in utero exposure to increased androgen levels (due to genetic and/or environmental factors) also predisposes the female fetus to increased pituitary LH secretion and ovarian hyperandrogenism.[11,12]

Mechanism of Anovulation

PCOS is a multisystem endocrine/metabolic disorder exhibiting dysfunction of both gonadotropic and somatotropic axis. The common endpoint is hyper-insulinemic insulin resistance and hyperandrogenism.

Hyperandrogenism: Approximately 70% of women with PCOS have elevated androgen levels with major androgens being androstenedione, DHEA-S and testosterone.[12] In normal course, it is converted to estradiol by FSH-dependent aromatase. But with excess levels, excess is converted to estrone which exerts tonic effect on LH production and partial suppressive effect on FSH. This in turn leads to further increased production of androstenedione and decreased conversion to estradiol setting a vicious cycle.

Gonadotropic axis dysfunction leads to excessive androgen, elevated LH, excessive stromal/thecal hyperplasia. Chronic elevation

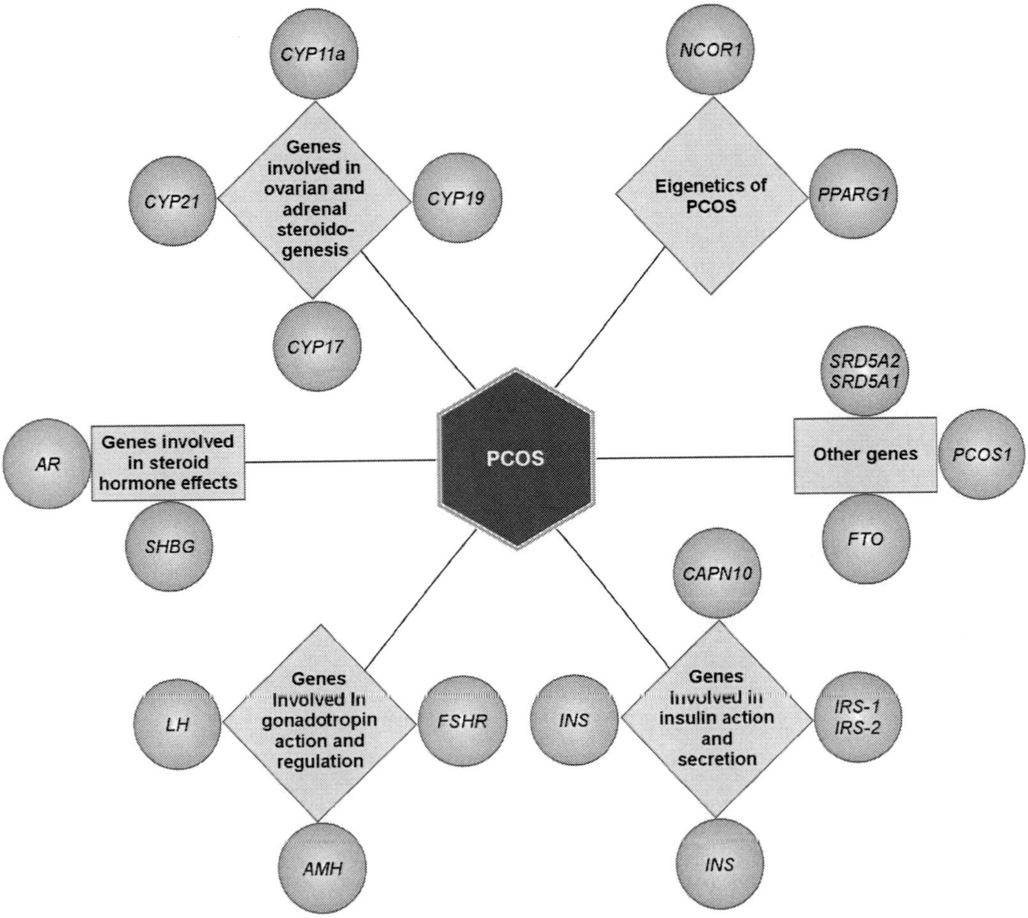

Fig. 1: Summary of genes involved in pathogenesis of PCOS.[9]

in estrogen levels exerts negative feedback on FSH preventing stimulation or sustenance of progressive follicular growth. In non-PCO ovulatory women, sequential rise and fall of estrogen allows for intercycle rise in FSH which allows for recruitment of next cohort of follicles. But in PCOS women, sustained high levels of estrogen lead to chronic anovulatory state. Likewise poor follicular growth does not generate and sustain enough estrogen to stimulate ovulatory LH surge.

Two-cell-two gonadotrophin theory also emphasizes the importance of local androgen concentrations in ovarian steroidogenesis and ovulation. Ovarian androgens act as substrate for FSH induced aromatization and estrogen production at low levels, however, at high levels, ovarian androgens:

1. Converted to more potent 5α-reduced androgens
2. These cannot be converted to estrogens
3. They further inhibit aromatase activity and FSH induced LH receptors.

All these lead to hamper follicular maturation, promote follicular atresia and a chronic anovulatory state ensues:

- Hyperinsulinemia leading to hyperandrogenism
- Elevated insulin

- LH mediated thecal androgen production through IGF 1 receptors, suppresses hepatic SHBG (Sex hormone-binding globulin) synthesis

DIAGNOSIS

Before forming diagnosis of PCOS, ethnic variation in the presentation and manifestations of PCOS should be kept in mind including: a relatively mild phenotype in Caucasians, higher body mass index (BMI) in Caucasian women, especially in North America and Australia, more severe hirsutism in Middle Eastern, Hispanic, and Mediterranean women, increased central adiposity, insulin resistance, diabetes, metabolic risks, and acanthosis nigricans in South East Asians and Indigenous Australians, Lower BMI and milder hirsutism in East Asians, higher BMI and metabolic features in African.

Clinical Features

a. *Amenorrhea/Oligomenorrhea:* 28% of all women report irregular menses throughout their reproductive years. 20% reported to have regular menses for a few years post-menarche which became irregular later on.[7] Ovulatory dysfunction refers to oligomenorrhea (cycles more than 35 days apart but less than six months apart) or amenorrhea (absence of menstruation for 6–12 months after a cyclic pattern has been established).

   Irregular menstrual cycles are defined as: Normal in the first year post-menarche as part of the pubertal transition, >1 to <3 years post-menarche <21 or >45 days, >3 years post-menarche to perimenopause: <21 or >35 days or <8 cycles per year, >1 year post-menarche >90 days for any one cycle, Primary amenorrhea by age 15 or >3 years post-thelarche (breast development). When irregular menstrual cycles are present a diagnosis of PCOS should be considered and assessed according to the guidelines. For adolescents who have features of PCOS but do not meet diagnostic criteria, an "increased risk" could be considered, and reassessment advised at or before full reproductive maturity, 8 years post-menarche.
b. *Hirsutism/Acanthosis Nigricans/Acne:* 90–100% women with severe resistant acne will have PCOS.[13] Hirsutism is defined as terminal hair growth in male pattern. It must be differentiated from hypertrichoism. Standardized visual scales should be preferred when assessing hirsutism, such as the modified Ferriman-Gallwey score (mFG) with a level ≥4–6 indicating hirsutism. Acanthosis nigricans is a sign of insulin resistance and seen in 5% women with PCOS. HAIR-AN syndrome stands for Hyperandrogenism, Insulin Resistance and Acanthosis nigricans.
c. *Obesity:* Obese PCOS women have higher plasma androgen, higher incidence of insulin resistance, hypersecretion of LH and lower sex-hormone binding globulin (SHBG) levels. BMI >30 or waist-hip ratio >0.82 considered as obese.
d. Diabetes/hypertension/endometrial hyperplasia in perimenopausal women.

Biochemical Abnormalities

e. *Abnormal androgen levels:* Elevated-free androgen/DHEA/androgen index. Although free and total testosterone is used in the diagnosis of PCOS, the recommended baseline biochemical test for hyperandrogenism is free androgen index (total testosterone divided by sex-hormone binding globulin [SHBG] × 100).[14] If there are signs of virilization (e.g., deep voice, reduced breast size, increased muscle bulk, clitoral hypertrophy), rapidly progressing hirsutism (less than 1 year between hirsutism being noticed and seeking medical advice) or high total testosterone levels (greater than 5 nmol/L or more than twice the upper limit of normal reference range), androgen-secreting tumors and late-onset/nonclassical congenital adrenal hyperplasia (CAH) should be excluded. Calculated-free testosterone, free-androgen index or calculated bioavailable testosterone should be used to assess biochemical hyperandrogenism in the diagnosis of PCOS. High-quality assays such as liquid chromatography–mass spectrometry (LCMS)/mass spectrometry and extraction/chromatography immunoassays, should be used for the most accurate assessment of total or free testosterone in PCOS.

f. LH:FSH ratio >3
g. Fasting glucose: insulin ratio <4.5

Ultrasound Assessment

h. Polycystic ovarian morphology of >12 FNPO (*follicle number per ovary*) in at least one or both ovaries
i. Ovarian volume >10 mL
j. Ultrasound should not be used for the diagnosis of PCOS in those with a gynecological age of <8 years (<8 years after menarche), due to the high incidence of multifollicular ovaries in this life stage.
k. The transvaginal ultrasound approach is preferred in the diagnosis of PCOS, if sexually active and if acceptable to the individual being assessed. Using endovaginal ultrasound transducers with a frequency bandwidth that includes 8 MHz, the threshold for PCOM on either ovary, a follicle number per ovary of R20 and/or an ovarian volume 10 mL on either ovary, ensuring no corpora lutea, cysts or dominant follicles are present.
l. In patients with irregular menstrual cycles and hyperandrogenism, an ovarian ultrasound is not necessary for PCOS diagnosis; however, ultrasound will identify the complete PCOS phenotype.
m. Clear protocols are recommended for reporting follicle number per ovary and ovarian volume on ultrasound. Recommended minimum reporting standards include:
   - Last menstrual period
   - Transducer bandwidth frequency
   - Approach/route assessed
   - Total follicle number per ovary measuring 2–9 mm
   - Three dimensions and volume of each ovary
   - Reporting of endometrial thickness and appearance is preferred; 3-layer endometrial assessment may be useful to screen for endometrial pathology.
   - Other ovarian and uterine pathology, as well as ovarian cysts, corpus luteum, dominant follicles
n. Ovaries with higher resistance (PI and RI) in intraovarian vessels tend to be resistant to medical management.

These should be differentiated from multifollicular ovaries or MFO which are often physiological, found in delayed normal puberty, hypothalamic anovulation, hyperprolactinemia and usually have larger follicles, lesser stromal echodensity, normal ovarian volume and usually associated growing dominant follicle.

Histological changes of PCOS include the following:

- Whole ovarian hypertrophy
- Thickened capsule

- Increased subcapsular follicle cysts
- Scarcity of corpus lutea/albicartia
- Hyperplasia and fibrosis of ovarian stroma
- Decreased thickness of granulosa layer
- Atretic pattern of granulosa layer
- Increase thickness of theca interna
- Premature luteinization of theca cells

NEOHORMONES IN PCOS

Leptin is an important hormone linked with PCOS. Bound form of leptin was found to be lower in lean PCOS women. Adiponectin is almost exclusively produced in adipose tissues and has insulin sensitizing action. This hormone is decreased in obese women. Adiponectin was also found to be lower in PCOS women. Resistin hormone impairs insulin action on hepatic glucose production and inhibits glucose uptake. It may be a link between obesity and metabolic disorders seen in PCOS. Ghrelin appears to be involved in food intake and energy balance. This might act as a signal between peripheral mechanisms sensing caloric intake with brain centers controlling energy homeostasis.

Insulin Resistance in PCOS

Even though it is not an essential criterion in diagnosis of PCOS but its association in both lean and obese PCOS is well established now. It is also associated with increased risk of various disorders like Type II DM, hypertension, dyslipidemia, etc. Insulin resistance in PCOS is due to postbinding defect in signaling and associated with constitutive serine phosphorylation of the insulin receptor. Ovarian cytochrome P450, 17α activity in women with PCOS is due to stimulation by insulin and can be recovered by decreasing the secretion of insulin.

Metabolic Syndrome and PCOS

There is an increased incidence of type 2 DM, cardiac disease, dyslipidemia, sleep apnea and non-alcoholic fatty liver (NAF-LD) even after adjusting for BMI. Metabolic syndrome in PCOS is defined by presence of 3 or more of following criteria:

a. Insulin resistance leading to hyperinsulinemia
b. Obesity, high BMI
c. Hypertension
d. Triglycerides >150 mg/dL
e. HDL-cholesterol <50 mg/dL
f. Fasting glucose >110 mg

Considering the above associations, ACOG have recommended that patients' blood pressure should be evaluated at every visit and lipid levels at the time of diagnosis, and screen for type 2 diabetes with a two-hour oral glucose tolerance test regardless of a patient's body mass index. Patients should have repeat diabetes screening every three to five years, or more often if other indications for screening are present. The Endocrine Society further recommends depression screening, as well as screening for symptoms of obstructive sleep apnea in overweight and obese patients with PCOS.[15] However, routine screening for non-alcoholic fatty liver disease or endometrial cancer (using ultrasonography) is not recommended as per RCOG recommendations.[17]

Psychological issues should be considered in all women with PCOS. Depression and/or anxiety should be routinely screened for and, if present, assessed. If a woman with PCOS is positive on screening, further assessment and appropriate counseling and intervention should be offered by a qualified professional.[6] The lifetime risk for CVD is higher in women with PCOS and mostly preventable, all women with PCOS should be assessed for CVD risk by assessing individual CVD risk factors (obesity, lack of physical activity, cigarette smoking, family history of type II diabetes, dyslipidemia, hypertension, impaired glucose tolerance, type II diabetes) at baseline and treated accordingly.

MANAGEMENT OF PCOS

Because PCOS is not a single pathological disease, it does not have a single treatment option. Also because of its long-term nature, lifestyle and weight management remains the crux with symptom-specific drug treatment at different stages of life. Downregulation of somatotropic axis is the primary modality in all patients.

Lifestyle Modification[18]

- *Exercise*: In adults from 18–64 years, a minimum of 150 min/week of moderate intensity physical activity or 75 min/week of vigorous intensities or an equivalent combination of both, including muscle strengthening activities on 2 non-consecutive days/week is recommended. In adolescents, at least 60 minutes of moderate-to-vigorous intensity physical activity/day, including those that strengthen muscle and bone at least 3 times weekly should be advised. Activity is performed in at least 10-minute bouts or around 1000 steps, aiming to achieve at least 30 minutes daily on most days. Health professionals should encourage and advise the following for modest weight loss, prevention of weight-regain and greater health benefits: A minimum of 250 min/week of moderate intensity activities or 150 min/week of vigorous intensity or an equivalent combination of both, and muscle strengthening activities involving major muscle groups on two non-consecutive days/week. There should be stress on minimized sedentary, screen, or sitting time. Physical activity includes leisure time physical activity, transportation such as walking or cycling, occupational work, household chores, games, sports or planned exercise, in the context of daily, family and community activities. Daily, 10000 steps are ideal, including activities of daily living and 30 minutes of structured physical activity or around 3000 steps. Structuring of recommended activities needs to consider women's and family routines as well as cultural preferences.
- *Dietary changes*: It is recommended to follow calorie-restricted diet (low carbohydrate and fat, high protein) in consultation with dietician and lifestyle modification as first-line therapy for at least 6 months, then add metformin as second-line therapy. To achieve weight loss in those with excess weight, an energy deficit of 30% or 500–750 kcal/day (1200–1500 kcal/day) could be prescribed for women, also considering individual energy requirements, body weight and physical activity levels. In women with PCOS, there is no or limited evidence that any specific energy equivalent diet type is better than another, or that there is any differential response to weight management intervention, compared to women without PCOS. Tailoring of dietary changes to food preferences, allowing for a flexible and individual approach to reducing energy intake and avoiding unduly restrictive and nutritionally unbalanced diets, are important, as per general population recommendations.
- *Weight reduction*: Achievable goals such as 5–10% weight loss in those with excess weight yields significant

clinical improvements and is considered successful weight reduction within six months. Ongoing assessment and monitoring are important during weight loss and maintenance in all women with PCOS. SMART (Specific Measurable, Achievable, Realistic and Timely) goal setting and self-monitoring can enable achievement of realistic lifestyle goals. Weight reduction leads to decrease in androgen and increase in SHBG, decreases LH pulse amplitude reducing ovarian androgen production.

- *Supportive drugs*: Low-dose OCP remains the choice of treatment. Non-androgenic progestin like norgestimate or desogesterel-containing OCP or spironolactone analog drosperinone OCP are preferred. In women with PCOS, metformin is not recommended as first-line therapy for the management of menstrual irregularity. In women with PCOS, spironolactone is not recommended for menstrual irregularity. *Menstrual regularity:* 4 cycles/year in adolescents of 12–16 years.
- The ideal time to stop hormonal therapy for hyperandrogenism cannot be established with existing evidence, however minimum 6 month–1 year therapy is needed for symptom relief. Risk of thromboembolism with use of COCs can be managed by identifying susceptible patients and/or pausing treatment for 3 months after one year of treatment. In adolescents with hyperandrogenism, if glucose intolerance is not established by OGTT, metformin should not be started. Due to insufficient evidence, alternative (acupuncture) and complementary therapeutic options (e.g., myoinositol, omega-3 fatty acids) are not recommended for the management of hyperandrogenism.
- *Insulin sensitizers: Metformin*—it is a biguanide which suppresses endogenous glucose production and improves peripheral tissue sensitivity to insulin. Currently, it is considered first-line drug in hyperinsulinemic PCOS at 1500–1700 mg per day in divided doses. Studies have also shown improvement in spontaneous, and clomiphene-induced ovulation. Where metformin is prescribed the following need to be considered: Adverse effects, including gastrointestinal side effects that are generally dose dependent and self-limiting, need to be the subject of individualized discussion, starting at a low dose, with 500 mg increments 1–2 weekly and extended release preparations may minimize side effects, metformin use appears safe long-term, based on use in other populations, however, ongoing requirement needs to be considered and use may be associated with low vitamin B_{12} levels, use is generally off-label and health professionals need to inform women and discuss the evidence, possible concerns and side effects. Pioglitazone-thioglitazones are not recommended as additional therapy for any of PCOS conditions. D Chiro Inositol–Inositol (in any form) should currently be considered an experimental therapy in PCOS, with emerging evidence on efficacy highlighting the need for further research.
- Ovarian electrocautery/drilling should be reserved for selected anovulatory women. Similarly, bariatric surgery may be considered in morbid obese women unresponsive to routine weight loss measures.

Symptom-specific management options in women with PCOS is provided in **Table 2** and treatments for polycystic ovary syndrome is provided in **Table 3**.

TABLE 2: Symptom-specific management options in women with PCOS.[18]

PCOS with main symptom	*Preferred management*
Adults with PCOS showing menstrual irregularity	Progesterone withdrawal bleed
Adults with PCOS who do not intend to conceive	COCs (drospirenone and desogestrel as progestin component)
Adults and adolescents with PCOS, if there is no improvement of menstrual irregularity with COCs or COCs are not tolerated	Insulin sensitizers such as metformin (with or without progestins) but not thiazolidinediones
Adolescents with PCOS	Low-dose COCs (with or without anti-androgenic progestins drospirenone and desogestrel) for the management of MI. Between 12–16 years of age, low-dose COCs only to be used, for short period (up to 7 days)
Management of Hirsutism	
First line	Cyproterone acetate alone or in combination with EE
Adult women with PCOS who do not intend to conceive	Low-dose COCs with anti-androgen progestin (cyproterone acetate, drospirenone, or desogestrel)
Second line if no improvement with COCs or COCs are not tolerated	Spironolactone or finasteride but recommended to stop 6 months before planned pregnancy
If menstrual irregularity and hirsutism are diagnosed	Low-dose COCs with anti-androgenic activity (CPA, drospirenone, desogestrel)
Adolescents/children with hyperandrogenism, obesity and signs of insulin resistance	Lifestyle modification is first-line therapy; metformin is second-line therapy with a wait period of 2 years post-menarche in children
Management of Acne	
Adults and adolescents	Topical medication along with pharmacological interventions based on the clinical presentation of acne as early as possible, in consultation with dermatologist
Adults with PCOS	Oral contraceptives (cyproterone acetate, drospirenone, or desogestrel as progestin component) as first-line therapy for management of all types of acne lesions
Adolescents with PCOS and acne	Oral contraceptives (cyproterone acetate, drospirenone, or desogestrel as progestin component) based on the clinical presentation of acne, in consultation with dermatologist

TABLE 3: Treatment for PCOS.[16,19]

Medication or device	*Description*	*Manifestation treated*	*FDA Pregnancy Category*
Clomiphenet	Ovulation induction agent, selective estrogen receptor modulator	Infertility (First-line therapy)	X
Eflornithine (Vaniqa)	Inhibits hair growth	Mild hirsutism (Second-line therapy)	C
Finasteride (Proscar)	alpha-reductase inhibitor	Hirsutism (weak recommendation because of inconsistent study result)	X
Flutamide	• Nonsteroidal antiandrogen used • Mostly for prostate cancer	Hirsutism (safe and effective according to low- to very low-quality evidence)	D
Hormonal contraceptives (pill, patch, vaginal ring)	See article for details	Menstrual irregularities, hirsutism, acne (first-line therapy)	X
Letrozole (Femara)	Nonsteroidal competitive inhibitor of aromatase; inhibits conversion of adrenal androgens	Infertility (First-line therapy)	C
Levonorgestrel-releasing intrauterine system (Mirena)	Intrauterine device	• Endometrial hyperplasia • Abnormal uterine bleeding (FDA approved)	X
Metformin	Insulin-sensitizing agent	• Insulin resistance (First-line therapy) • Menstrual irregularities (Second-line therapy added to hormonal contraceptives) • Hirsutism (Third-line therapy added to hormonal contraceptives and spironolactone)	B
Spironolactone	• Antiandrogenic • Antimineralocorticoid	• Hirsutism (Second-line therapy added after 6 months of oral contraceptive therapy if not improved) • Acne (Second-line therapy)	C

FDA: US Food and Drug Administration; MI: myocardial infarction; PCOS: polycystic ovary syndrome

PCOS AND PREGNANCY

High LH in these women has been shown to be associated with miscarriage rate of 65% compared to 12% in normal women. In women with PCOS planning to have children, it is recommended to screen for markers of obesity, hypertension and IR to reduce the risk of pregnancy-related complications. These women should also be evaluated for homocysteine levels to rule out hyperhomocysteinemia-mediated repeated pregnancy loss.

Long-term Sequel of PCOS[21]

Women with PCOS are at higher risk of developing type II diabetes mellitus, dyslipidemia, cardiovascular disease and cancer. As many as 30–40% women have IGT and 10% have type II DM by 4th decade.[20] Dyslipidemia is characterized by reduced HDL and elevated triglycerides. They are likely to develop hypertension during pregnancy with persistent HTN later. Prolonged unopposed estrogen is probably associated with higher risk of endometrial cancer in women with PCOS, hence withdrawal bleed every 3–4 months is recommended. In PCOS, endometrium of <7 mm unlikely to be hyperplasia.

Diagnostic Dilemmas in Adolescents

In normal adolescents, also there is transient physiological hyperinsulinemia which usually reverts spontaneously in the majority. However, if it persists, it can lead to the development of PCOS. In addition, hyperactivity of gonadotropic and adrenocorticotropic axis also causes hyperandrogenicity. At this juncture, genetic predisposition, coupled with unhealthy lifestyle, sedentary habits, and lack of physical exercise can all lead to full blown PCOS.

Prevention/Prediction

Recommendations on risk factors for assessment of PCOS. It is recommended that Indian women showing at least one biochemical characteristic in conjunction with one clinical symptom should be considered for further evaluation for the likelihood of PCOS.

1. *Biochemical characteristics:* High BMI for overweight/obesity >23 kg/m^2 for adults and >97.5th percentile for age in adolescents), insulin resistance (acanthosis nigricans as clinical marker of insulin resistance), family history of diabetes or PCOS, obesity and inadequate lifestyle, any marker of lipid metabolic dysregulation (elevated serum total cholesterol, triglyceride and LDL-C levels).
2. *Clinical symptoms:* Pubertal deviations (early or late), disturbances in periodicity/timing of menstrual cycle, presence of PCOS and clinical signs of hyperandrogenism such as early acne or hirsutism, persistent severe acne, frequent relapse in acne, acne in facial 'V' area, persistent acne and hirsutism for more than two years. In women suspected to have PCOS, it is recommended to screen and appropriately document all clinical and biochemical risk factors in the case history. It is recommended that patients who currently show either a clinical symptom, or fit into a biochemical characteristic may be referred for further diagnosis when feasible or should be regularly monitored for appearance of other presentations of PCOS. It is recommended that individual patients with two or more clinical risk factors be subjectively assessed by the gynecologist and referred to an appropriate healthcare provider for further diagnosis of PCOS.

SECONDARY PCOS

This is an emerging concept which means that a woman presents with typical PCOS phenotype but due to an underlying primary well-defined cause of hyperandrogenism. When the primary cause is treated the woman undergoes remission of PCOS which does not happen in true PCOS. New nomenclature has been proposed HA-PODS (hyperandrogenism and persistent ovarian dysfunction syndrome) which is further classified as primary or secondary.

MEDICOLEGAL ASPECTS

PCOS is a complex multifactorial pathology with varying symptomatology. It is extremely important to give time and attention to all details, use appropriate tools/questionnaires for identifying associated complications. Elaborate counseling about long-term nature of disease with influence on all phases of reproductive life-including pregnancy and menopause should be done. Radical interventions like ovarian electrocautery which are likely to affect fertility potential adversely should be used only when absolutely indicated after thorough evaluation and counseling.

Key Points

- Patient presentation is variable ranging from asymptomatic to having multiple gynecologic, dermatologic, or metabolic manifestations.
- Adolescent evaluation should be deferred until 2 years post-menarche and thereafter all three criteria should be fulfilled in adolescents for diagnosis of PCOS.
- Twice as likely to develop metabolic syndrome.
- Four times more likely than the general population to develop type 2 diabetes mellitus.
- Clomiphene and letrozole are first-line medications for infertility. Metformin is the first-line medication for metabolic manifestations, such as hyperglycemia.
- Hormonal contraceptives are first-line therapy for irregular menses and dermatologic manifestations.

CONCLUSION

PCOS continues to remain an enigma. Newer concepts are emerging. The long-term nature of disease and multifactorial nature makes it a challenge. There is an urgent need for community-based cross-sectional studies and awareness programs. There should be interdisciplinary meetings to exercise uniform diagnostic criterion and therapeutic measures.

REFERENCES

1. Stein IF, Leventhal ML. Amenorrhea associated with bilateral polycystic ovaries. Am J Obstet Gynecol. 1935;29(2):181-91.
2. Stein IF, Leventhal ML. History of discovery of polycystic ovary syndrome. Adv Clin Exp Med. 2017;26(3):555-8.
3. Deswal R, Narwal V, Dang A, Pundir CS. The prevalence of polycystic ovary syndrome: a brief systematic review. J Hum Reprod Sci. 2020;13(4):261-71.
4. Ganie MA, Vasudevan V, Wani IA, Baba MS, Arif T, Rashid A. Epidemiology, pathogenesis, genetics and management of polycystic ovary syndrome in India. Indian J Med Res. 2019;150(4):333-44.
5. Rotterdam ESHRE/ASRM-Sponsored PCOS consensus workshop group. Revised 2003 consensus on diagnostic criteria and long-term health risks related to polycystic ovary syndrome (PCOS). Hum Reprod. 2004; 19(1):41-7.
6. Williams T, Mortada R, Porter S. Diagnosis and treatment of polycystic ovary syndrome. Am Fam Physician. 2016;94(2):106-13.
7. Dahlgren E, Johansson S, Lindstedt G, Knutsson F, Odén A, Janson PO, Mattson LA, Crona N, Lundberg PA. Women with polycystic ovary syndrome wedge resected in 1956–1965: a long-term follow-up focusing on natural history and circulating hormones. Fertil Steril. 1992;57(3):505-13.
8. Kahsar-Miller MD, Nixon C, Boots LR, Go RC, Azziz R. Prevalence of polycystic ovary syndrome (PCOS) in first-degree relatives of patients with PCOS. Fertil Steril. 2001;75(1):53-8.
9. Khan MJ, Ullah A, Basit S. Genetic basis of polycystic ovary syndrome (PCOS): current perspectives. Appl Clin Genet. 2019;12:249-60.

10. Moran LJ, Ranasinha S, Zoungas S, McNaughton SA, Brown WJ, Teede HJ. The contribution of diet, physical activity and sedentary behaviour to body mass index in women with and without polycystic ovary syndrome. Hum Reprod. 2013;28(8):2276-83.
11. Abbott DH, Kraynak M, Dumesic DA, Levine JE. In utero androgen excess: a developmental commonality preceding polycystic ovary syndrome? Front Horm Res. 2019;53:1-17.
12. Ashraf S, Nabi M, Rasool SuA, et al. Hyperandrogenism in polycystic ovarian syndrome and role of *CYP* gene variants: a review. Egypt J Med Hum Genet. 2019;20:25.
13. Amuzescu A, Tampa M, Matei C, Georgescu SR. Adult female acne: recent advances in pathophysiology and therapeutic approaches. Cosmetics. 2024;11:74.
14. Abdalla MA, Deshmukh H, Mohammed I, Atkin S, Reid M, Sathyapalan T. The effect of free androgen index on the quality of life of women with polycystic ovary syndrome: a cross-sectional study. Front Physiol. 2021;12:652559.
15. Legro RS, Arslanian SA, Ehrmann DA, et al.; Endocrine Society. Diagnosis and treatment of polycystic ovary syndrome: an Endocrine Society clinical practice guideline. J Clin Endocrinol Metab. 2013;98(12):4565-92.
16. Williams T, Mortada R, Porter S. Diagnosis and treatment of polycystic ovary syndrome. Am Fam Physician. 2016;94(2):106-13. PMID: 27419327.
17. Royal College of Obstetricians and Gynaecologists. Long-term Consequences of Polycystic Ovary Syndrome (Green-top Guideline No. 33). London: RCOG; 2014. Available from: https://www.rcog.org.uk/media/qmtlp2b0/gtg_33.pdf
18. Teede HJ, Tay CT, Laven JJE, Dokras A, Moran LJ, Piltonen TT, et al; International PCOS Network. Recommendations from the 2023 international evidence-based guideline for the assessment and management of polycystic ovary syndrome. Eur J Endocrinol. 2023;189(2):G43-64.
19. Malik S. Indian Fertility Society good clinical practice PCOS guidelines. Womens Health (Lond). 2016;12(1):91-3.
20. Teede HJ, Misso ML, Costello MF, et al. Recommendations from the international evidence-based guideline for the assessment and management of polycystic ovary syndrome. Hum Reprod. 2018;33(9):1602-18. [Published correction appears in Hum Reprod 2019;34(2):388]
21. Legro RS. Polycystic ovary syndrome. Long-term sequelae and management. Minerva Ginecol. 2002;54(2):97-114.

CHAPTER 23

Endometriosis

Anjali Suneel Mundkur

INTRODUCTION

Endometriosis is an enigmatic disease with the presence of ectopic endometrium (tissue similar to the endometrium that grows outside the uterus) in the ovary, peritoneum, bladder, bowel, and ureter. This results in pelvic pain and infertility. It commonly affects age group of 25–29 years. The overall incidence of endometriosis is 10%, with a 50% prevalence amongst infertile women.[1] Endometriosis is a hormone-responsive inflammatory disease, which continues to be a diagnostic and therapeutic challenge to the gynecologist worldwide. There are currently no clear guidelines that allow clinical diagnosis. Yet, physicians frequently do make a clinical diagnosis of endometriosis and treat it with first-line therapies. Pain is subjective, and it is challenging to discern normal from abnormal, except in the extremes. It is a chronic disease that is associated with severe physical and psychological morbidity. Common symptoms are pain during periods, sexual intercourse, bowel movements and/or urination, chronic pelvic pain, abdominal bloating, nausea, fatigue, and sometimes depression, anxiety, and infertility. It is very important to understand and appreciate that, the disease has associated medicolegal implications which must be considered while taking clinical decisions including patient counseling, consent and documentation.

ETIOLOGY[2]

There are speculative theories concerning to etiology of the endometriosis.

Retrograde menstruation theory: Menstrual blood containing endometrial cells flows back through the fallopian tubes and into the pelvic cavity, at the time when the blood is flowing out of the body through cervix and vagina during periods. Retrograde menstruation can result in endometrial-like cells deposited outside the uterus, where they can implant and grow.

Cellular metaplasia theory: Cells change from one form to another. Cells outside the uterus change into endometrial-like cells, which start to grow.

Stem cells theory: Stem cells give rise to disease, spreading through the body via blood and lymphatic vessels.

Other factors contributing to the growth of the endometrial tissue are hormone-sensitive tissues responding to estrogen and progesterone, which facilitates the inflammation, progression of the disease, and pain associated with the disease. Altered or impaired immunity, localized complex hormonal influences, genetics, and potential environmental contaminants may also promote the growth of the ectopic endometrium.[3]

Endometriosis is a severe threat to a woman's reproductive potential. These lesions respond less often to medical treatment. They can potentially destroy and damage healthy ovarian tissue, reducing the ovarian reserve leading to premature ovarian failure.

Endometriomas can lead to destructive and potentially damaging pelvic surgeries leading to complete/partial loss of ovarian function and other neighboring structures like the colon, small bowel, or bladder. These cysts are known to represent a medical dilemma for women receiving fertility treatments. Thus, endometriosis has associated medicolegal implications which must be considered diligently while taking clinical decisions.

DIAGNOSIS

Endometriosis can be diagnosed with the help of its associated symptoms and signs. Pain associated with menstruation is a common symptom suggestive of endometriosis. Symptoms can be described with the *pneumonic 6 Ds* as provided hereunder (*Source:* Dr Pratap Kumar, Professor and Head, Department of Reproductive Medicine and Surgery, Kasturba Medical College, Manipal, Karnataka, India):

6 Ds—associated with the Diagnosis of Endometriosis

1. **D**ysmenorrhea (painful periods)
2. **D**yspareunia (painful sexual activity)
3. **D**yschezia (painful defecation)
4. **D**isorders of menstruation—abnormal menstrual pattern ranging from frequent cycle to heavy menstruation
5. **D**eep pelvic pain—chronic pelvic pain disturbing the daily activity
6. **D**ifficulty in conception—infertility is a common symptom

High index of suspicion is required, very often missed in adolescents presenting with dysmenorrhea. Unusual symptoms are catamenial diarrhea, rectal bleeding, constipation, small bowel obstruction, urgency, frequency, hematuria. It is important to be aware of the fact that the Stage of disease does not necessarily correlate with the severity of the symptoms.

In some cases, the endometriosis may remain asymptomatic, especially if the disease is isolated to the peritoneum. There may not be any systemic sign, unless the endometriosis is infected.

On per-abdomen examination—a cystic mass may be palpable, which may be of any size. Borders may be felt but of restricted mobility. The fixity of the mass is due to adhesions.

On per-speculum examination—bluish nodules in posterior fornix may be present, cervix may appear deviated to either side depending on the presence of the ovarian endometrioma.

Bimanual examination—may suggest the fixed uterus, the adnexal mass of varying size.

Per rectal examination—may suggest nodules in Pouch of Douglas.

However, a regular and thorough pelvic examination may not be able to rule out endometriosis. It is advisable that women in the reproductive age group with any of the symptoms described above should undergo pelvic ultrasonography. Transabdominal sonography for women who are not sexually active and transvaginal sonography for sexually active women is advised.

Endometriosis presents in classic implants on the surface of one or both ovaries. It can be deep within the ovaries. These are commonly called *chocolate cysts.* The diagnosis of endometriosis can be made by ultrasound imaging, but the final confirmation of diagnosis, microscopic examination of the cyst is recommended.

Common Locations of the Endometriosis

Ovaries 75%, anterior/posterior cul-de-sac 70%, posterior broad ligament 50%, uterosacral ligament 35%, uterus 10%, colon 5%.[5]

Consensus Opinion by the International Deep Endometriosis Analysis (IDEA)[6]

Diagnosis of endometriosis particularly deep endometriosis is difficult. Transvaginal sonography and magnetic resonance imaging are used for the diagnosis. A careful TVS by experienced sonographer picking up the subtle findings of endometriosis is important. The following are various findings which help in diagnosis of endometriosis:

- *Transvaginal ultrasonography:* An anteverted, retroflexed uterus (*question mark sign*) is often seen with severe posterior compartment, deep infiltrating endometriosis. Ovarian endometriomas, typically unilocular cystic lesions containing uniform low-level echoes (ground-glass appearance) and no blood flow on color Doppler (color score 1). It may be single or multiple, can have an atypical appearance including multiple locations and papillary projection. Decidualization of endometriosis can occur in pregnancy often confused with malignancy of the ovary. Ovaries are adherent to each other and to the posterior wall of the uterus called *Kissing ovaries sign.*
- *Ovarian sliding sign:* On gentle pressing of the ovaries with the transvaginal probe, the ovaries slide on the lateral pelvic wall, however, in the presence of endometriosis, the ovaries are adherent and do not move. Even in the absence of an obvious ovarian cyst, the absence of the sliding ovary may help in suspecting occult endometriosis.
- *Fallopian tubes:* Often, hydrosalpinx is observed during the transvaginal sonography.
- *Urinary bladder nodules* are commonly found on bladder base and bladder dome. Hypoechoic linear or spherical lesions, with or without regular contours involving the muscularis (most common) or (sub) mucosa of the bladder may be present.
- *Ureters* may appear dilated with deep infiltrating endometriosis either due to extrinsic compression or intrinsic infiltration.
- *Uterovesical regional adhesions* are less common than the Pouch of Douglas. These can be assessed by moving the transvaginal probe back and forth. Up to 1/3rd of women with a previous cesarean section will have adhesions in this region.
- *Rectovaginal septum:* Deep infiltrating endometriosis (DIE) nodule on transvaginal ultrasound in rectovaginal space below the line passing along the lower border of the posterior lip of the cervix. DIE on the rectovaginal septum is very rare.
- *Posterior vaginal wall/posterior vaginal fornix:* Vaginal wall thickening with discrete hypoechoic nodules with regular or irregular margins may be seen within the peritoneal fat surrounding the uterosacral ligament. There may also be thickening of the white line of the uterosacral ligaments (>5.8 mm) have shown to have a strong association with endometriosis on or near the uterosacral ligaments.[7]
- *Rectosigmoid colon:*[8] The nodules on the bowel are hypoechoic, or a 'tail' is noted at one end, resembling a comet (*Comet sign*). Retraction and adhesion possible, resulting in the so-called *Indian Headdress or Moose Antler sign.*
- *Pouch of Douglas:* The pouch of Douglas is considered obliterated if the *sliding sign* is negative (i.e., if the rectum and uterus do not slide apart).
- Repeated bleeding into the endometrioma is common; however, findings of acute

hemorrhage such as reticular pattern or retractile thrombus is seen in <10%.[5] MRI is a valuable adjunct when suspecting deep-infiltrating endometriosis before the surgery for the same. Histopathology showing endometrial glands and stroma with varying degrees of inflammation and fibrosis is a definitive diagnosis of endometriosis which can be made only after surgical excision.

CA-125 levels can be elevated in endometriosis but have limited value in making a diagnosis as it is also elevated in many peritoneal conditions.

TREATMENT OF ENDOMETRIOSIS

Treatment of endometriosis can be expectant, medical, or surgical. The choice of treatment depends on the age, presenting complaints, findings of the patient.

Medical Treatment

Medical treatment is the option for women not contemplating pregnancy and also it is a preferred choice in the extremes of the age group. The hormonal and non-hormonal medical options are available. The goals of treatment are to control pain and to stop the growth of endometriotic tissue. NSAIDs, oral contraceptive pills, GnRH agonists, aromatase inhibitors are some of the commonly used medications.

Selective progesterone receptor modulators, anti-angiogenic factors, and immunomodulators are newer therapy for endometriosis. In women who do not respond to medical therapy or have severe symptoms, or suffering from subfertility, surgical excision of the endometrial lesions and adhesions is often helpful and offers confirmatory diagnosis by histopathology.

Hormonal Therapy

- Combined oral contraceptives—suppresses ovulation and reduces the pain of endometriosis.
- *Progesterone-containing contraceptives:* Oral or injectable, implant, levonorgestrel-containing intrauterine system (LNG-IUS)
- *Selective progesterone receptor modulators:* Mifepristone, ulipristal acetate, onapristone
- *Gonadotropin-releasing hormone agonists:* Leuprolide acetate, nafarelin, goserelin
- *Gonadotrophin releasing hormone antagonists:* Cetrorelix

Nonhormonal Therapy

- NSAIDs
- Aromatase inhibitors
- Danazol

Endometriosis is hormone-sensitive; combined pills can be used to inhibit ovulation and suppress endometriotic tissue. It can be prescribed in a sequential or continuous manner. Reduction in number of bleeding episodes can reduce the size of endometriotic tissue.

Surgery in Endometriosis

Surgery is the choice of treatment in patients with infertility. All patients undergoing conservative surgical treatment need to be explained regarding the recurrence of endometriosis. Complete excision may not be possible. In the presence of bowel adhesions, injury to the bowel may need to be tackled intraoperatively. For Patients with suspected deep infiltrating endometriosis, surgical management of pain should be balanced with risks associated with surgery. Adequate surgical expertise is required in managing patients with DIE. Colostomy consent needs to be taken when operating such patients.[4,8] Laparoscopic surgery is the preferred mode (conservative surgery).

Laparoscopic Cystectomy

- Peeling of the cyst wall with the drainage of fluid
- Adhesion lysis can be combined with cystectomy.
- Excision of the peritoneal endometriosis
- Most of them see and treat patients with chronic pelvic pain undergoing diagnostic laparoscopy.

Laparotomy

- Patients with completed family symptomatic
- Hysterectomy and oophorectomy followed by hormone replacement therapy.

COMPLICATIONS

- Torsion of the endometriotic cyst is unlikely, as most often, adhesions are present.
- Rupture of the cyst with peritonitis can occur presenting with acute abdomen can be managed with conservative management but may require surgical management. Multiple hemorrhages into the cyst are often occurring with or without pain.
- Infection of the cyst with intraovarian abscess is not uncommon, presenting with pain, fever with chills, and rigor. Pelvic infection associated with endometriosis is treated with antibiotics and drainage of abscess most often with laparotomy as severe adhesions with bowel may be present.
- Malignant transformation of endometriosis is very rare <1%. It may be in the form of endometrioid carcinoma or, less commonly, clear cell carcinoma. Annual transvaginal sonography is advocated by some, which may help in making the diagnosis of malignant transformation.[7]

DIFFERENTIAL DIAGNOSIS

The differential diagnosis of endometriosis includes tubo-ovarian abscess, dermoid cyst, corpus luteal hemorrhagic cyst, malignant ovarian tumors. All necessary investigations must be done so as to rule out/diagnose the diseases considered in the differential diagnosis.

PREVENTION OF ENDOMETRIOSIS

Primary prevention of endometriosis may not be possible; however, early diagnosis and intervention may prevent the progression of the disease.

In adolescents with pelvic pain or dysmenorrhea not responding to the simple analgesics, the possibility of endometriosis be considered and treated with combined oral contraceptive pills.

Early diagnosis may help women of childbearing age not to postpone the conception. Pregnancy and the progesterone of pregnancy may help in the suppression of the disease.

During the surgical excision or cystectomy, free endometriotic cells may be released into the peritoneal cavity, which re-adhere, grow, and invade, leading to recurrent endometriosis.[8,9]

Barrier agents are frequently used to prevent postoperative adhesion. A combined medical and surgical approach could reduce the recurrence.

RECENT UPDATES

Gel sonovaginography in diagnosing deep infiltrating endometriosis: About 20 mL of ultrasonography gel is inserted into the vagina, and a transvaginal probe is slowly inserted into the vagina, looking into the rectovaginal septum, nodules in the pouch of Douglas.[10]

Precise delineating of pelvic endometriosis by ultrasonography by trained sonographers is achievable. The International Society of Gynaecologic Endoscopy (ISGE) recommends the acquisition of the lexicon and methodology proposed by the International Deep Endometriosis Analysis (IDEA) group and the #Enzian classification system for US assessment of patients with suspected or known endometriosis. The ISGE good practice recommendations for the structured reporting of the findings of the endometriosis during the surgery. The structured reporting and documenting will help the sonographers/radiologists and clinicians counseling and treating women with adenomyosis, adhesions, endometriomas and/or DIE.[11]

MEDICOLEGAL ASPECTS

- Thorough counseling and explanation during informed written consent before the surgery has a vital in avoiding medicolegal issues that may emerge later on due to unexpected outcomes. The risk of recurrence and other complications should be explained to the patient and attendants. Informed consent should be signed by the patient, treating doctor, and the witness. Endometriosis is not a malignant condition however, it may present with all the features of malignancy except the mitotic activity. Hence, it may not be potentially life-threatening but causes severe morbidity. This is a crucial aspect to be explained to the patient. Endometriosis due to inflammatory reaction causes many adhesions among the bowel, bladder, uterus, and ovary. This needs adequate consent before the surgery.
- Adequate facility for managing the potential complication in OT, instruments, anesthesia, surgical help, and ICU facility. The benefits of removal of deep-infiltrating endometriosis should balance against the risks associated with it. Patients need to understand that removing deep endometriosis may compromise the organ function and may require colostomy, etc.
- Early diagnosis is critical in preventing medicolegal implications related to allegation of delay in diagnosis resulting in harm to the patient, medical negligence or deficiency in services on the part of treating doctor. All these aspects have potential medicolegal implications, and the treating doctor may be held responsible and may have to face the brunt of the aggression at times.

CONCLUSION

Endometriosis is a severely debilitating disease to some and asymptomatic in many. Accurate clinical and serological diagnosis is vital for management. A medical or surgical line of management can be chosen. The patient needs to understand that there is no permanent cure for endometriosis till menopause. It may not be life-threatening but debilitating, causing physical absence for work and economic burdens to the patient and healthcare system. A high index of suspicion early diagnosis and management reduces morbidity associated with it. Appropriate referral, adequate counseling, and detailed documentation may help in litigation and avoidance of compensation.

Key Points

- Adolescents and young women presenting with dysmenorrhea need to be adequately evaluated.
- Symptoms of endometriosis do not directly correlate with severity of the disease.
- Transvaginal sonography in addition to transabdominal sonography with various signs during the ultrasound in the grey scale makes the diagnosis clear.
- MRI may be of additional benefit in deep-infiltrating endometriosis.
- Medical management of pain in patients not for fertility treatment.
- Progesterone and estrogen may help in decreasing the size of endometriosis.
- Laparoscopy is the treatment option when fertility is the issue.
- Careful dissection during the laparoscopy helps in retaining the ovarian reserve and less damage to the normal ovarian tissue.
- Prevention of endometriosis is the current challenge in the medical field.
- Early diagnosis is critical in managing endometriosis and prevention of progression of the disease.

REFERENCES

1. Cranney R, Condous G, Reid S. An update on the diagnosis, surgical management, and fertility outcomes for women with endometrioma. Acta Obstet Gynecol Scand. 2017;96:633-43.
2. Zondervan KT, Becker CM, Missmer SA. Endometriosis. N Engl J Med. 2020; 382:1244-56.
3. Wen X, Xiong Y, Qu X, et al. The risk of endometriosis after exposure to endocrine-disrupting chemicals: a meta-analysis of 30 epidemiology studies. Gynecol Endocrinol. 2019;35:645-50.
4. Dmowski WP, Lesniewicz R, Rana N, et al. The changing trends in the diagnosis of endometriosis: a comparative study of women with pelvic endometriosis presenting with chronic pelvic pain or infertility. Fertil. Steril. 1997;67(2):238-43. doi:10.1016/S0015-0282(97)81904-8.
5. Jones, J., Knipe, H. Endometrioma. Reference article, Radiopaedia.org. (accessed on 17 Oct 2021) https://doi.org/10.53347/rID-9042.
6. Aas-Eng MK, Montanari E, Lieng M, Keckstein J, Hudelist G. Transvaginal sonographic imaging and associated techniques for diagnosis of ovarian, deep endometriosis, and adenomyosis: a comprehensive review. Semin Reprod Med. 2020;38(2-03):216-6.
7. Krawczyk N, Banys-Paluchowski M, Schmidt D, Ulrich U, Fehm T. Endometriosis-associated malignancy. Geburtshilfe Frauenheilkd. 2016;76(02):176-81.
8. Guerriero S, Condous G, Van den Bosch T, Valentin L, Leone FP, Van Schoubroeck D, et al. Systematic approach to the sonographic evaluation of the pelvis in women with suspected endometriosis, including terms, definitions and measurements: a consensus opinion from the International Deep Endometriosis Analysis (IDEA) group. Ultrasound Obstet Gynecol. 2016;48(3): 318-32.
9. Renner SP, Strissel PL, Beckmann MW, Lehmann J, Burghaus S, Hackl J, et al. Inhibition of adhesion, proliferation, and invasion of primary endometriosis and endometrial stromal and ovarian carcinoma cells by a nonhyaluronan adhesion barrier gel. Biomed Res Int. 2015:2015:450468.
10. Venkatesh S, Anjali M, Vasudeva A, Kumar P. Sliding sign and gel sonovaginography: a sneak peek prior to laparoscopy in patients with endometriosis. J Hum Reprod Sci. 2020;13(1):26-30.
11. Djokovic D, Pinto P, van Herendael BJ, Laganà AS, Thomas V, Keckstein J. Structured report for dynamic ultrasonography in patients with suspected or known endometriosis: Recommendations of the International Society for Gynecologic Endoscopy (ISGE). Eur J Obstet Gynecol Reprod Biol. 2021:263: 252-60.

CHAPTER

24

Urological Injuries in Obstetric and Gynecological Practice

T Srikala Prasad

INTRODUCTION

Urological injuries are not uncommon in Obstetrics and Gynecology practice,[1-3] because of the anatomic proximity of the reproductive tract and the lower urinary tract. The altered anatomy arising out of common clinical conditions like endometriosis, pelvic inflammatory diseases (PID), malignancy and previous lower segment cesarean section (LSCS), etc. lead to a situation of vulnerability causing inadvertent urological injury. It is imperative to identify patients with potential risk factors, take all measures to prevent any inadvertent injuries and at the same time be vigilant enough to recognize any possible injury and provide appropriate remedial measures.

BLADDER INJURIES

Bladder injuries are three times more likely than ureteric injuries.[4] The incidence of bladder injury during cesarean section ranges from 0.08 to 0.94%.[5] Obstructed labor, overdistended bladder, previous LSCS, and placenta previa/placenta accreta spectrum (PAS) are common obstetric causes of bladder injuries. Endometriosis, malignancy, adhesions as a result of previous surgeries, especially previous LSCS are common causes of bladder injuries in gynecological practice. The incidence of bladder injuries in gynecologic procedures is around 0.049%.[1] Laparoscopic hysterectomy and laparoscopic associated procedures are now the leading cause of such iatrogenic injuries.[4]

Prevention of Bladder Injuries

The first and the most important step is to keep the bladder empty in all obstetrics and gynecology surgeries. The distended bladder is prone to inadvertent iatrogenic injury as the bladder wall becomes thin. While planning surgeries on patients with history of previous surgeries including LSCS, it is advisable to counsel the patient and her attendants about the possible difficulties in entry; chances of adhesions with the bowel and omentum; possible difficulty in mobilizing the bladder in case of morbid adhesion of the bladder. Patients and their attendants need to be informed (*verbally as well as in writing*) that, in spite of following all safety precautions, the bladder and or the bowel can inadvertently get injured and need to be duly repaired.

The rate of iatrogenic bladder injury during abdominal hysterectomy is between 0.5% and 1.0%.[1] Care must be exerted right from opening the abdomen, especially when we are operating on a patient who has already been operated on or on whom adhesions may be expected because of endometriosis, PID, malignancy, etc. It is possible that the bladder is drawn up and be present at the incision site itself.

Simple measures like confirming that there is no underlying bladder prior to making an opening in the peritoneum will be helpful. The underlying bladder will make the tissue between the two hemostats feel thicker. A more cranial approach will help in opening the peritoneum safely.

If we get clear fluid, we must ensure that we have not opened the bladder. The Foley's catheter will guide us whether it is the bladder or not. It is the dome of the bladder which is usually injured during entry into the abdomen. Instilling a sterile solution of methylene blue through the Foley's catheter will identify any bladder injuries.

The next important place to safeguard the bladder is during mobilization of bladder. In normal conditions, the UV (uterovesical) fold of the peritoneum is easily opened and there is no difficulty in pushing the bladder down. But we can face difficulties in mobilizing the bladder which shows morbid adhesion to the lower uterine segment especially in patients who have undergone one or multiple LSCS. With counter traction on the bladder, we can safely mobilize the posterior wall of the bladder using sharp dissection.

Partially distending the bladder with a sterile and dilute solution of methylene blue will help identify the posterior wall of the bladder and allow prompt diagnosis of bladder injury if any, facilitating repair immediately. The bladder must be sufficiently pushed down especially while performing a total hysterectomy so that there is enough place to do a colpotomy and do vault closure comfortably without any compromise on the bladder, thereby preventing a fistula formation.

Dense adhesions formed between the bladder and the lower abdomen as well as the lower uterine segment are responsible for causing inadvertent injury. The most common time for bladder injury in repeat LSCS was during the creation of the bladder flap (43–60%) followed by, during entry into the peritoneal cavity (30–33%), and finally during the uterine incision or delivery (10–24%).[6]

The urgent, abrupt, stressful nature of the surgery may be more responsible rather than the scar tissue from the surgery.[6] This is also proven by the fact that the number of bladder injuries is more in emergency LSCS as compared to elective LSCS where the added anxiety of delivering the baby soon is present.[5] Distorted anatomy as a result of the head being deep in labor and bladder being drawn up also can be causative. When we need to deliver a very big baby which is deep down in the pelvis, an inverted T-shaped incision or delivering the baby as breech may be helpful in preventing extension of the uterine incision.[7]

Accessing the Sheth's space in relation to the lateral one-fifth of the bladder on both sides in women with a previous history of LSCS would help us to prevent bladder injuries.[8]

Patients with PAS need to be counseled not only of the possibility of postpartum hemorrhage (PPH) and need for obstetric hysterectomy, but also the possibility of inadvertent bladder and ureteric injury (Overall injuries was 21.7%, with bladder 11.7%, ureter 4.7%, and bladder with ureter 5.3%).[9]

Detection of Bladder Injury

Bladder injury is usually detected intra-operatively and repaired immediately. The following are pointers to bladder injury:

- Blood-stained urine
- Intraoperative detection of rent in the bladder with Foley's catheter seen inside.
- Metal catheter introduced into the bladder during a vaginal hysterectomy can pass through the rent in the bladder.
- In laparoscopic surgeries, distension of the Urobag with gas occurs as a result of bladder injury.

- In suspicious cases, retrograde filling of the bladder with saline can decipher its boundaries. We can instill a dilute and sterile solution of methylene blue into the bladder and watch for leaks.
- Cystoscopy can also be used to diagnose bladder injury. This not only diagnoses bladder injury but also evaluates the ureters by assessing the efflux of urine from both orifices and also the distance of the rent from both the ureteric orifices. Cystoscopy can also identify any suture material inside the bladder which can be removed so as to prevent any nidus for stone formation or vesicovaginal fistula (VVF) occurrence.

Preventing Bladder Injury in Vaginal Hysterectomy

The incidence of bladder injuries in vaginal hysterectomy is around 1.7%.[1] Opening the anterior pouch is the first step in vaginal hysterectomy. The metal catheter is used not only to empty the bladder but also to assess the extent of the bladder.

The circular incision is made at the level of the bladder crease. The anterior lip of the cervix is held with a volsellum at 12 O'clock position and traction are given. Counter traction is given by holding the anterior vaginal wall and cystocele and the bladder is safely mobilized from the uterus. In case the bladder is densely adherent, sharp dissection can be used to safely mobilize the bladder. The UV fold of the peritoneum is safely opened, and a bladder retractor keeps the bladder and ureters away.

BLADDER INJURY IN INCONTINENCE PROCEDURES

The incidence of bladder injury is very less in mid-urethral sling surgeries using the transobturator approach compared to the retropubic approach.[10] Keeping the bladder empty is a good preventive step. Intraoperative check cystoscopy with the trocar or the needle carrier inside will facilitate diagnosis of inadvertent bladder entry. Blood-stained urine, presence of the trocar or the needle carrier inside the bladder are diagnostic. The sling can be removed, and another attempt can be made. This must be followed by a check cystoscopy to ensure that there is no inadvertent bladder entry. Catheter drainage for a week helps to heal the bladder.

Repair of Bladder Injuries

It is imperative to assess the bladder injury, the site, the relation to the ureteric orifices, whether there is any other site of injury, and also whether the bladder needs to be mobilized to facilitate a good repair. Most of the bladder injuries are fortunately detected on the table. The rich vascularity of the bladder is an important factor that helps the bladder to heal well when repaired. Most of the bladder injuries can be repaired by the gynecologists themselves. They can also utilize the services of the urologists in the following scenario:

- Large defect which extends into the posterior bladder wall extending into the trigone.
- Irregular tears
- Tears which are closer to the ureteric orifice.
- When the bladder wall is stuck to the lower uterine segment and needs to be mobilized prior to repair.
- Any situation in which the gynecologist does not have the necessary experience or feels the need for expertise.

Technique of Bladder Repair

The rent in the bladder is usually repaired on two layers. The first layer involves suturing the mucosa and the muscle with 3-0 delayed absorbable sutures. The second layer involves suturing the muscle and serosa with 2-0 delayed absorbable sutures. The bladder heals well when it is in a decompressed state with continuous bladder drainage. It is sufficient to achieve that with urethral catheter drainage alone, without suprapubic cystostomy (SPC) (AUA Urotrauma Guideline Statement 18).[12] Urethral catheters are good enough to adequately drain the bladder. Good nursing care also ensures that there is continuous drainage. They help to shorten the hospital stay and decrease morbidity. However, clinicians may choose to perform SPC in certain cases like complex bladder repairs, where the repair had been difficult and tenuous and there is blood-stained urine (for fear of clot retention disturbing a good repair). Postoperative care involves ensuring that the catheter is draining well, in addition to the usual fluids, antibiotics, and anticholinergics (which helps to keep the bladder quiescent). Catheter removal can be done around 7–14 days. Cystogram can be taken prior to catheter removal to ensure complete healing and that there is no leak.[11] Usually bladder heals well because of its excellent vascularity. The incidence of fistula after hysterectomy is estimated to be roughly 0.1–0.2%.[1]

URETERIC INJURY

Adequate knowledge of anatomy and points of possible risks must be known. The ureter is commonly at risk in one of the following areas, at the pelvic brim where it crosses over the common iliac vessels, in the mid-pelvis where it is crossed over by the uterine artery, and near the cervix at the level of the internal os.

Good history-taking will give us good clues regarding possible risks. A thorough physical examination will give us a lot of information including the scars, the nature of the fibroid or the mass, possible endometriosis, mobility of the mass, the possibility of adhesions, and any pelvic organ prolapse (POP). Preoperative investigations should include a whole abdomen USG (ultrasonogram) which will not only evaluate the pelvic pathology in detail but also assess the kidney, look for hydroureteronephrosis, and any anomalies. There is no proof that preoperative IVU (intravenous urogram) or computed tomography (CT) urography reduces the risk of ureteric injury and is used in only select conditions. Similarly, conditions like endometriosis, pelvic inflammatory disease (PID), and previous intra-abdominal surgeries which are associated with an increased risk of ureteric injury, are not associated with an increased prevalence of abnormal IVU findings.

Types and Causes of Ureteric Injury

Only around 30% of ureteral injuries are picked up intraoperatively and we need to have a high index of suspicion to pick-up them. The rate of ureteral injury in a large Finnish study was 0.3% for abdominal, 0.04% for vaginal, and 0.3% for laparoscopic hysterectomy.[13] Intraoperative ureteric injury may result from ligation with suture, crushing with misapplication of a clamp, or transection which may be partial or complete, avulsion, devascularization. Ureteric injuries can also be caused by energy sources. The ureter may be damaged by the lateral thermal spread of heat from the various sources of energy used. It may not be possible to identify these injuries immediately and these patients have a delayed presentation.

Preventive Strategies

One needs to choose the appropriate operative procedure for the patient, based on the combined clinical assessment and investigations and expertise available.

Prevention in Abdominal Hysterectomy

Adequate exposure, good lighting, good assistance, necessary equipment is very essential for meticulous surgery.

We need to exercise care and caution in all surgeries and more so when there is an 'altered anatomy' as a result of factors like procidentia, large ovarian masses, fibroids (especially broad ligament fibroids, cervical fibroids), endometriosis and PID, malignancies, previous pelvic surgeries and prior pelvic irradiation for cancers. These patients need to be counseled that in spite of taking all safety precautions, there is a possibility of inadvertent injury to the ureters which needs to be tackled in addition. They also need to be told that there is a possibility that there may be a delayed presentation in some cases.

Efforts must be taken to apply clamps as close as possible to the uterus. This ensures that the clamps are at a safer distance from the ureter. We need to be sure what we are clamping and cutting is not the ureter. In cervical fibroid, preliminary myomectomy or enucleation of the fibroid can be done after mobilizing the bladder. A midline vertical incision can be made on the fibroid till the level of the pseudo-capsule (which is the compressed tissue). We would now be able to see a relatively bloodless plane through which we can enucleate the myoma in toto. The ureter is not in danger as we have removed the fibroid by working within the capsule of the fibroid. The uterus now looks normal in shape. It would now be possible to apply clamps as close to the uterus as possible.

Similarly, in cases of broad-ligament fibroid, enucleation of the fibroid can be done by opening the leaves of the broad ligament. We will be able to visualize the ureter and safeguard it. The hysterectomy can now proceed in the usual way.

Normally, it is not necessary to open the retroperitoneum. In case of extension of bleeding into the broad ligament or while operating on a broad-ligament fibroid or whenever we are in doubt, we can enter the retroperitoneum by opening the leaves of the broad ligament by entering the peritoneal reflection between the round ligament (lateral) and infundibulopelvic ligament (medial). We need to exercise great care and caution as the ureter can cling on to the medial leaf of the broad ligament. A small nick is made after catching the leaves of the broad ligament and ensuring that it is thin and there is nothing underneath. It can be extended under vision. The loose areolar tissue will help in blunt dissection. The iliac vessels and the ureter crossing over are well visualized and can be safeguarded. Hemostasis can be safely achieved without any blind clamping.

The next step is to be careful and safely mobilize the bladder and push it down. With this step, the ureter also moves out of danger. It is imperative to check for bleeding from the pedicles before the closure of the vault. It is better to take superficial bites at the angles of the vault so as to avoid the inadvertent inclusion of the ureters.

Adnexal Surgery

Great care has to be exercised while performing adnexectomy in ovarian tumors and post-hysterectomy ovarian cyst, where they may be adherent to the lateral pelvic wall. In such cases, it is safer to open the retroperitoneum and safeguard the ureter. The ureter may often be found stuck to the medial leaf of the broad ligament.

Laparoscopic Hysterectomy

Laparoscopic hysterectomy is now becoming increasingly the cause of ureteric injuries. Knowledge of ureteric anatomy is essential. The location of the ureter can be visualized through the peritoneum. In case of doubt, the retroperitoneum can be opened, and the course of the ureter be visualized. Extreme care must be exercised while using the energy sources near the ureter. Lateral spread of the thermal damage may occur which may have a delayed presentation.

Role of Preoperative Stenting

Preoperative stenting may not prevent ureteric injury. It will help in the intraoperative diagnosis of ureteric injury and facilitate repair. It can be difficult to feel the stent inside the ureter in cases of severe fibrosis especially in cases of endometriosis, PID, malignancy. It may predispose the ureter to damage as a result of the immobility it imparts to the ureter. Stenting-related complications like ureteral perforation, edema, hematuria, stent malposition, and stricture can also occur. It may be technically difficult to stent where there is a lot of distortion as in huge cervical fibroid. Tackling the fibroid by enucleation may be much simpler.

OBSTETRIC URETERIC INJURIES

Obstetric ureteric injuries are uncommon. These can happen in cases of extension of the uterine angle during cesarean section, leading to broad-ligament hematoma, especially in obstructed labor where there had been difficulty in delivery of the head particularly a deflexed head. Blind clamping into the broad ligament in a desperate attempt to obtain hemostasis can jeopardize the ureter. It is better to open the retroperitoneum, safeguard the ureter and then obtain accurate hemostasis. Ureters are not generally involved while doing a subtotal hysterectomy. Cesarean hysterectomy for placenta accreta spectrum is a condition where total hysterectomy is done and here the ureters need to be safeguarded.

Safeguarding the ureter in vaginal hysterectomy and urogynecology procedures. Opening the anterior pouch and safely mobilizing the bladder is the first step. A bladder retractor can now be placed to safeguard the bladder. With the bladder pushed above, the ureter also goes away. By applying traction on the anterior lip of the cervix, the ureter moves away from the uterus. Following the standard guidelines of applying the clamps close to the uterus, also will protect the ureters.

While dealing with long-standing, irreducible procidentia with gross hydroureteronephrosis, the ureters are dragged down resembling the knee of the ureter. A period of pessary insertion will help reduce the chances of ureteric injury. Single clamp application on the uterosacral ligament also is useful in safeguarding the ureter.

High uterosacral ligament (HUSL) suspension procedures are associated with a higher incidence of intraoperative ureteric injuries (between 1 to 11%) and therefore it is better to do a check cystoscopy at the end of the procedure as it is easy to manage any inadvertent ureteric inclusion immediately. Low rates of ureteral obstruction were seen in sacrospinous ligament fixation and McCall culdoplasty.[14]

What to do in Case of Suspicious Ureteric Injury?

The presence of ureteric peristalsis does not rule out ureteric injury. It is better to directly inspect the ureters during laparotomy in patients with a suspected ureteral injury

(AUA Urotrauma Guidelines 9b).[12] Injectable dyes like methylene blue or indigo carmine, if available can be given to help identify ureteral injuries but is not readily available in many places. The retroperitoneum can be opened, and the ureter can be visualized in its entirety. Cystoscopy can be done and the urinary efflux visualized on both sides. Preoperative administration of a single tablet of Pyridium 200 mg. One hour prior to the surgery will impart a yellowish-orange color to the urine and will facilitate easy visualization of the efflux from the ureters. Using 50% dextrose as the cystoscopic distension medium will offer a contrast in viscosity between the urine and the cystoscopy fluid and will enable better detection of the ureteric efflux.[15]

Endoscopic stent placement, preferably with a long duration stent should be tried as an initial step in the management of patients diagnosed postoperatively with incomplete ureteral injuries or even when presented in a delayed fashion. Guidance with retrograde ureteral imaging would be an added advantage. This will safeguard the kidney from possible damage because of the distal obstruction and will facilitate healing of the fistula. These patients, however, need to be monitored for the development of ureteric stricture. In case, it is not possible to stent the ureter from below, an attempt at stenting the ureter by an antegrade approach can be done. If it is not possible through one or both approaches, they require a definitive repair (urotrauma Guideline Statement 11a).[12] If an immediate repair is not feasible, the renal system can be protected by percutaneous nephrostomy (PCN) and a corrective surgery done later (AUA Urotrauma Guideline Statement 11b).[12] Thermal injury will manifest only days after the injury.

Management of Injury to the Ureter

The incidence of the ureterovaginal fistula is around 0.5–2.0% following a simple hysterectomy.[16] The incidence is increased to 10–20% following radical hysterectomy.[16] It is not always possible to prevent intraoperative injuries to the ureter in spite of the best possible care. Only one-third of ureteric injuries are detected during the surgery. A high index of suspicion and constant vigilance is extremely crucial. A watery leak or excessive fluid collection may raise doubts. Flank pain and tenderness in the costovertebral angle, low-grade fever, and ileus in the postoperative period should alert the possibility of ureteric injury. A bedside USG showing hydroureteronephrosis further points towards ureteric injury. Good urine output does not rule out unilateral injury. Elevated levels of creatinine in the drain fluid are a marker of ureteric injury. CT urogram is the gold standard investigation which will not only tell us whether there is any injury to the ureter or the bladder but also the level of obstruction. It is imperative that we manage the ureteric injury as early as possible in order to prevent compromise to the renal unit. In case, the patient is found to be unfit for the procedure, a PCN will help us tide over the crisis.

The retroperitoneum is explored, and the ureter is mobilized with its adventitia down to the level of the obstruction, clamped and disconnected. The distal end is ligated. The cut end of the ureter is assessed for its vascularity and if found not satisfactory, the ureter can be cut till the level of the viable ureter. We now need to assess the length needed to bridge. The length of the ureter lost, the level at which the ureter is looking healthy, and the degree of bladder mobility will decide the type of surgery.

The distal ureter is the site of most of the gynecologic-related ureteric injuries. Ureteroureterostomy as a modality of managing them is not a feasible one as the lower portion of the ureter is amalgamated in the obstruction, included in the ligature and therefore a viable portion of the ureter is not available for anastomosis.

Ureteroneocystotomy

Ureteroneocystotomy without a psoas hitch is a preferred procedure that can be done in most patients, if the length lost is around 4–5 cm. If psoas hitch is performed in addition, we can easily tackle 6–10 cm length of ureteral loss. There is no need to dissect further in the area and mobilize the ureter as it will not be viable. We will be bypassing the injured portion of the ureter. If the length of the ureter lost is more than this, a ureteroneocystostomy using a Boari flap repair can be done which can bridge around 12–15 cm loss of the ureter. It is very important not to have tension on the anastomosis. It is not necessary to have anti-refluxing anastomosis in adults. A simple refluxing anastomosis will not only reduce the chances of ureteric obstruction but also make subsequent ureteroscopy if needed easier.

The Boari flap repair will be sufficient to tackle almost all gynecological ureteric injuries and therefore it will usually not be necessary to do other surgeries like transureteroureterostomy, renal descensus, or ileal interposition.

Boari Flap

The bladder is mobilized all around. Additional mobility is obtained by ligating the opposite superior vesical pedicle. The desired length of the pedicle is marked on the bladder. An oblique flap with a width of 4 cm at the base and 3 cm at the tip is planned in which the ratio of the flap length to width should not be greater than 3:1. This helps to minimize flap ischemia. A tongue-shaped flap of the bladder is swung cephalad and tubularized and anastomosed to the injured ureter. A double J-stent safeguards the anastomosis.

Injuries of the Urethra

Injuries can occur following urethral diverticulectomy, urethropexy, sub-urethral sling procedures, and in cases of urethral diverticulum which was mistakenly thought of as anterior vaginal wall cyst. They can be repaired immediately with 3-0 delayed absorbable sutures with an indwelling catheter left in situ for 10–14 days.

RELEVANT JUDGMENTS

Smt. B Jyothi vs. Geetha Maternity Nursing Home (5th July 2010)

State Consumer Disputes Redressal Commission

- The patient underwent a hysterectomy for the fibroid uterus. In the immediate postoperative period, the patient had hematuria for which she got evaluated by a urologist. The urologist did a diagnostic cystoscopy and found bladder injury.
- Laparotomy was done and found to have bladder injury with left ureteric injury. Bladder repair and left ureteric reimplantation with DJ stenting were done.
- The patient later developed VVF which was operated on at another hospital.
- Experts examined the records and all of them in one voice confirmed that there was *no negligence on the part of the doctor.* These injuries are inevitable, being close proximity to the organs attached to the part where the operation was conducted

Mrs Anuja Shah vs. Dr NV Pai (3rd Sep 2020)

State Consumer Disputes Redressal Commission

- The patient underwent cesarean section and was discharged. She developed abdominal pain and fever for which she consulted the operating surgeon. She was started on medications. Since symptoms persisted and developed urine leak through the vagina (UVF).
- The patient consulted an apology. As per his advice, she underwent an ultrasound which showed the right hydroureteronephrosis with a mid-ureteric stricture.
- The patient underwent the right percutaneous nephrostomy initially and later underwent right Boari flap ureteric implantation.
- *Judgment:* The operating surgeon was held negligent for not having documented the circumstances that led to the intraoperative injury, not informing the patient attendants about the same and no steps were taken in anticipation of the postoperative complication. The Court ordered to pay for the medical expenses and pay ₹6,00,000 as compensation within one month failing which will carry interest @12% p.a.

Bharti Yadav & Ors vs. Bansal Nursing Home (19th May 2017) (First Appeal No 1372 of 2013)

State Consumer Disputes Redressal Commission

- The patient underwent a hysterectomy and in the postoperative period, the patient had abdominal pain. On evaluation, she was found to have grossly right hydroureteronephrosis with DTPA showing only 7% function. Eventually, the patient underwent a right nephrectomy.
- *Judgment:* The operating Surgeon (General Surgeon) was held negligent because he had not taken the opinion of gynecologist or urologist. The name of anesthetist was not documented in the records which inferred that anesthesia was administered by the surgeon himself. The Court ordered the doctor to pay ₹5,00,000 with interest @7% p.a.

Smt. Chandrawati Rai vs. Santokba Durlabhji Merorial (19th May 2017)

State Consumer Disputes Redressal Commission

- Patients underwent abdominal hysterectomy. Postoperatively, she developed urinary leak through vagina. She consulted the operating surgeon. She was initially advised to do pelvic floor exercises and usage of diapers, later referred to urologist.
- The urologist evaluated and found that the patient had UVF and VVF, which was eventually repaired.
- *Judgment:* The operating surgeon was held negligent for not evaluating the patient symptoms (postoperative urinary leak) and delaying the urologist opinion. The Court ordered the doctor to pay ₹20,00,000.

MEDICOLEGAL ASPECTS

- A dedicated history taking, complete examination, necessary investigations are the first steps in the prevention of urologic injuries in Obs/Gyne practice.
- It is important to counsel all patients regarding your planned procedure, discuss specifically the possible problems which can be encountered and the additional management which may be necessary.

- Patients with risk factors should be identified and necessary preoperative investigations have taken. A detailed informed consent should be obtained.
- All possible care should be taken to ensure meticulous and careful surgical techniques. This has to be followed by good postoperative care.
- Never hesitate to call for the help of other experts if needed.
- The patient and the attenders need to be clearly informed of any technical difficulties encountered during surgery and the follow-up needed for such problems. It is also better to document all these in the case sheet and get their signature.
- Following standard protocols in all aspects of patient care will go a long way in safeguarding the interests of both the patients and the treating doctors. We definitely need to be conscious of bladder and ureter, but stress or anxiety will have a negative impact and compromise our work efficiency.
- Intraoperative cystoscopy to assess the integrity of the urinary tract in doubtful cases and stenting may be helpful in obviating the need for ureteric reimplantation or other definite procedures as may be needed. This may be supplemented with appropriate imaging studies as the need may be. It is extremely important to be vigilant even during the postoperative period and not to ignore any complaints like watery discharge or loin pain. CT urogram will help identify fistula and ureteric injury.
- Unrecognized ureteric obstruction can lead to the kidney becoming a non-functioning one and ultimately requiring nephrectomy. In fact, patients presenting with urinary leaks as a result of ureteric injury are fortunate that we are able to do a corrective procedure and stop the urinary leaks and at the same time safeguard their kidney. Patients who are present with urinary leak due to vesicovaginal fistula (VVF), usually need to undergo a delayed corrective procedure. The exact timing is tailored according to the condition.
- Prevention is always the best. This includes both prevention of injuries and prevention of possible litigation. An unrecognized bladder or ureteric injury or urologic injury in the absence of any abnormal anatomy or risk factor may be a difficult issue to handle. Prevention of urological injuries is the desire of every obstetrician or gynecologist. If not, prompt recognition and repair of injuries should be the next attainable goal.

REFERENCES

1. Partin A, Campbell M, Walsh P, Wein Alan J. Campbell-Walsh-Wein Urology. Amsterdam: Elsevier; 2021.
2. Neuman M, Eidelman A, Langer R, Golan A, Bukovsky I, Caspi E. Iatrogenic injuries to the ureter during gynecologic and obstetric operations. Surg Gynecol Obstet. 1991; 173(4):268-72.
3. Pal D, Wats V, Ghosh B. Urologic complications following obstetrics and gynecologicai surgery: Our experience in a tertiary care hospital. Urology Annals. 2016;8(1):26.
4. Wong J, Bortoletto P, Tolentino J, Jung M, Milad M. Urinary tract injury in gynecologic laparoscopy for benign indication. Obstetrics & Gynecology. 2018;131(1):100-8.
5. Awonuga A, Fletcher N, Saed G, Diamond M. Postoperative adhesion development following cesarean and open intra-abdominal gynecological operations. Reproductive Sciences. 2011;18(12):1166-85.
6. Tarney C. Bladder injury during cesarean delivery. Current Women's Health Reviews. 2014;9(2):70-6.

7. Jeve Y, Navti O, Konje J. Comparison of techniques used to deliver a deeply impacted fetal head at full dilation: a systematic review and meta-analysis. BJOG: An International Journal of Obstetrics & Gynaecology. 2015;123(3):337-45.
8. Sheth S. Vaginal hysterectomy, 2nd edn. New Delhi: Jaypee Brothers Medical Publishers; 2014.
9. Alanwar A, Al-Sayed H, Ibrahim A, Elkotb A, Abdelshafy A, Abdelhadi R, et al. Urinary tract injuries during cesarean section in patients with morbid placental adherence: retrospective cohort study. The Journal of Maternal-Fetal & Neonatal Medicine. 2017;32(9):1461-7.
10. Barisiene M, Cerniauskiene A, Matulevicius A. Complications and their treatment after midurethral tape implantation using retropubic and transobturator approaches for treatment of female stress urinary incontinence. Videosurgery and Other Miniinvasive Techniques. 2018;13(4):501-6.
11. Baggish MS, Karram MM. Atlas of Pelvic Anatomy and Gynecologic Surgery, 5th edn. Elsevier; 2020.
12. Morey A, Broghammer J, Hollowell C, McKibben M, Souter L. Urotrauma Guideline 2020: AUA Guideline. Journal of Urology. 2021;205(1):30-5.
13. Brummer TH, Jalkanen J, Fraser J, Heikkinen AM, Kauko M, Mäkinen J, et al. FINHYST, a prospective study of 5279 hysterectomies: complications and their risk factors. Hum Reprod. 2011;26(7):1741-51.
14. Berek J, Berek D, Novak E. Berek and Novak's gynecology/Novak's gynecology, 16th edn. Philadelphia, Pa: Wolters Kluwer; 2020.
15. Narasimhulu D, Prabakar C, Tang N, Bral P. Use of 50% Dextrose as the distension medium during cystoscopy for visualization of ureteric jets. Obstetrics & Gynecology. 2016;127(1):78-80.
16. Gordon D, Katlic M. Pelvic floor dysfunction and pelvic surgery in the elderly, 1st edn. Springer; 2017.

SECTION

8

Miscellaneous Topics

CHAPTER 25

Communication Skills in Obstetrics and Gynecology

Ritu Sharma, Monika Singh

INTRODUCTION

Doctor-patient relationship is based on trust, and good communication remains the cornerstone for building the same. Good communication skills are an asset not only for the physician but also for the patient resulting in improved satisfaction in both and overall good outcome of the disease. Though Western world has acknowledged the importance of communication skills long before, the same is lacking in Indian medical education. An enormous increase in the number of lawsuits filed against Obstetricians and Gynecologists has been reported predicting more severe menace in future and poor communication is a crucial factor in this regard. Patient autonomy and introduction of Consumer Protection Act have further emphasized its importance.[1]

After recognizing its importance, communication skill has been introduced as the core competency in the new medical curriculum along with emphasis on the regular conduction of workshops focusing on this pivotal issue. According to the five roles expected from the Indian Medical Graduate (IMG), one of them is a good communicator who can communicate with patients, attendant and their families effectively and respectfully.[2]

COMMUNICATION

The word communication is derived from Latin word *"communis"* which means common/sharing. Communication means "to share information via different ways like verbal, written and body language. The key purposes served by communication in medicine include: (i) Exchange of information, (ii) therapeutic decisions, and (iii) creating interpersonal rapport.

Components of Communication

Effective communication has three important components:[3,4]

1. *Verbal component* includes verbal content of the message consisting of an appropriate choice of words with detailed explanation by the doctor to the patient and his/her family regarding the disease, its outcome, investigations required and various management options along with their pros and cons. It is also equally important to discuss with them the financial implications. The active participation of patient party should be encouraged by the obstetricians and gynecologists through empathetic, supportive and non-judgmental attitude. Though it is considered to be a major part of communication, it delivers only 10% of the message to be conveyed.
2. *Non-verbal component* includes body language which depends on facial expression, eye contact, posture, gesture and interpersonal distance. This component decides the compliance and satisfaction of the patient.

3. *Paraverbal component* is related to the qualities of the voice like loudness, pitch, intonation, rhythm and speed.

Non-verbal and paraverbal components deliver 90% of the intended information. Doctor–patient communication includes two types of behaviors:[5,6]

1. *Instrumental behavior/technical behavior:* This is based on cognitive domain, i.e., problem-solving skills of the expert and are cure oriented. It mainly includes the verbal component associated with information sharing and management of medical condition.
2. *Affective behavior/socioemotional behavior:* This is based on empathy and is care oriented. It mainly includes the choice of words, active listening (verbal), voice quality (paraverbal) and body language (non-verbal) associated with building interpersonal relationships.

It is interesting to note that affective behavior is often difficult to be perceived verbally, which contributes only 7% of this while 22% is transmitted by paraverbal component and a majority of 55% is conveyed via nonverbal component.

EFFECTIVE COMMUNICATION IN OBSTETRICS AND GYNECOLOGY

Effective communication is considered as a need of the hour in Obstetrics and Gynecology. Doctors should be open in discussion regarding the disease and help the patient and attendants to reach a shared decision. Effective communication should be patient centered and needs skill training.

Communication with Attendants[7]

This is of immense importance especially in the case of critically-ill patients/when medical error occurs/while breaking bad news. Preferably, the senior most members of the team should address the attendants and patients. Inform the progress of patients at each step with proper documentation (by treating the doctor himself and not by other members of the team as interpretation may differ), sort out their queries and do not hesitate in taking second opinion as it will help in confidence building and satisfying the attendants. Difficult encounters occur when there is imbalance between the expectations, perceptions and behavior; but irrespective of the scenario Obstetrician–Gynecologist is ethically and professionally bound to continue managing the patient.

Communication with the Team

Patient care is teamwork. Talking ill of team members or scolding juniors in front of patients or attendants is not advocated. Be a leader, be courteous and give meaningful feedback as and when required.[8,9]

Communication with the Victims of Sexual Abuse

A victim-centered approach giving priority to compassionate care and respecting privacy after informed consent is advocated[10] to win the confidence and facilitate information gathering. Communication with children requires more experience and should take place in the presence of parents or guardians. Consent from appropriate authority needs to be documented.

Several models are available to help Obstetrician–Gynecologist for clinical interview and dealing with challenging situations **(Table 1)**.[11-17] In *partnership model,* there is equal participation of doctor and patient leading to a consensus-building on the treatment plan, thereby increasing the prospects of appropriate diagnosis, long-term compliance and reduced litigations.[18]

TABLE 1: Different protocols for communication in various clinical scenarios.[11-17]

Clinical scenario	*Protocol*	*Description*
Clinical interviews	AIDET[11]	• Acknowledge (greet, pay attention) • Introduce (yourself) • Duration (adequate time) • Explanation (explain, get it confirmed) • Thank you (for being cooperative)
	Kalamazoo Consensus Statement[12]	• Build the doctor–patient relationship • Open the discussion • Gather information • Understand patient's perspective • Share information • Reach agreement on problems and plans • Provide closure
Breaking bad news	SPIKES[13]	• Setting up the conversation • Perception • Invitation • Knowledge • Emotions (EVE protocol) • Strategy and summary
Medical error (or sudden deterioration or sudden death)	CONES[14]	• Context (senior most members should update, anticipate reaction, be calm) • Opening shot (alert them for some important news) • Narrative (sequence of events, avoid blame instead offer clear apology) • Emotions (EVE protocol) • Strategy and summary (investigate cause of error, strategize further plan)
Cultural competence (cross-cultural medical encounters)	RESPECT[15]	• Rapport (be courteous, be non-judgmental) • Empathy (understand patient's perspective and feelings) • Support (reassure, involve family) • Partnership (encourage equal participation) • Explanations (answer queries, confirm understanding) • Cultural competence (be sensitive to cultural, religious and regional beliefs) • Trust (build a trustworthy relationship)
	BALANCE[16]	• Belief and values (influencing perception) • Ambience (society and family) • Language and health literacy (require interpreter) • Affiliations (with respect to religion, community) • Network (social support) • Challenges (related to disease, personal) • Economics (socioeconomic status)
Challenging conversations	BUSTER[17]	• Be prepared (anticipate emotions from both ends, plan to deal them) • Use non-judgmental listening • Six second rule (wait for six seconds to calm down your emotions) • "Tell me more" statements (try to explore) • Empathize and validate emotions (EVE protocol) • Respond with a wish statement

BOX 1: Kalamazoo Consensus Statement for Clinical Interviews.[12]

Build the doctor-patient relationship	Make patient comfortable by greeting; address the patient by name; use appropriate verbal, nonverbal and paraverbal communication giving due consideration to gender, religion and cultural issues; maintain privacy; and show interest in patient
Open the discussion	Encourage the patient to come up with his/her complaints; do not interrupt the patient before completion of her/his statement
Gather information	Collect information using both open-ended as well as closed-ended questions; summarize the information at the end-giving chance to the patient to add more information and correct wrongly interpreted information, if any. Active listening is advocated to gather adequate information
Understand patient's perspective	Understanding the complaints with respect to patient's sociocultural concerns; addressing their needs, concerns and beliefs; and positively responding to their queries help to gain their confidence
Share information	Explain the patient clearly, using understandable words, about the problem, its outcome, the management options with pros and cons; answer their queries and check for their understanding
Reach agreement on problems and plans	Try to reach a shared decision with active participation of patients and attendants, without forcing our own decision, taking into account their individual needs, affordability and compliance; respect their decision
Provide closure	Summarize the opted management plan; clarify any concern, schedule follow-up, document the informed consent and the shared decision and close the interview

Several guidelines now emphasize shared decision making, e.g., the decision for mode of delivery after cesarean (VBAC or repeat cesarean) should be a shared decision.[19] The important steps in clinical interview as per Kalamazoo consensus statement have been outlined in **Box 1**.[12]

Breaking bad news is complex skill with a major role of empathy to tackle the impact on the recipient.[20] One has to ascertain the concerns, understanding and the coping ability of the patient and attendants. The steps involved in SPIKES model for breaking bad news have been described in **Box 2**.[13]

TYPES OF COMMUNICATION AND THE IMPORTANCE IN OBSTETRICS AND GYNECOLOGY

Good Communication and its Impact[21]

Good and open communication benefits both Obstetrician-Gynecologist and the patient via information sharing. The former gets benefitted by reaching to the accurate diagnosis, deciding the most appropriate management plan considering patient's needs, getting job satisfaction and reduced work-related stress. The latter gets benefitted by being more satisfied, more compliant, and good health outcome. Effective communication leads to shared decision making with equal and active participation from patients and family, thereby reducing future unhealthy encounters.

Bad Communication and its Impact[1,22]

Bad/ineffective communication has a negative impact on both clinical and medicolegal fronts.

Clinical Aspects

The passive role of the patient will be a hurdle in reaching the accurate diagnosis due to incomplete medical history; unsatisfied

BOX 2: SPIKES Model for Breaking Bad News.[13]

S	*Setting up the conversation*	Conversation should take place in front of key people, maintaining privacy and making patients comfortable in an undisturbed area
P	*Perception*	Try to understand the take of patients/attendants on the condition and any discrepancy in relation to actual condition
I	*Invitation*	Transfer the information to the patients only if they want, and only that much knowledge which they want to know; try to sort out their queries, if any
K	*Knowledge*	Explain the condition in clear, simple and understandable language; try to confirm their understanding and clear any gap
E	*Emotions*	EVE protocol (Explore and validate the emotion, deal with patient's emotions in *empathic* manner and avoid giving false reassurances, while controlling your own emotions)
S	*Strategy and Summary*	Reach to a plan of management by shared decision, schedule follow-up and document the same. Summarize the whole discussion and be patient to answer the queries till end

patient will be less compliant with the treatment advised leading to poor outcome of the disease. The Obstetrician-Gynecologist will have increased job-related stress and reduced job satisfaction.

Medicolegal Aspects

Inactive and unequal participation of patients in clinical interviews causes stress, frustration and resentment among them adversely affecting the doctor–patient relationship. Inefficient documentation of informed consent and the management plan; lack of shared decision coupled with outbursts of anger and misunderstanding lead to spurt in medicolegal encounters.

Barriers to Good Communication

As per various studies, only 50–61% of patients were satisfied after the medical consultation.[23,24] Differences in gender, religion, culture and race can lead to biased communication which can affect the health outcome. There are various barriers to good communication between Obstetrician-Gynecologist and patient which include:[25-27]

1. Inadequate knowledge and training in communication skills
2. Inadequate knowledge about the disease or treatment options available
3. Inadequate information communicated to patients or their attendants
4. Inadequate time for consultation
5. Neglecting nonverbal skills like lack of eye contact, negative facial expression
6. Lack in active listening to patients and attendants
7. Lack of empathy and respect for patients
8. Language barrier arising due to several local languages in Indian scenario.
9. *Adverse working circumstances of doctors:* Overburden, tiredness, stress at workplace
10. Sociocultural diversity

Clinical encounters eliciting good and bad communication have been tabulated in **Table 2**.

IMPROVING THE COMMUNICATION SKILLS WITH PATIENT AND ATTENDANTS

Obstetrician-Gynecologist should be sensitized to various dos and don'ts with respect to various clinical encounters and tailor the management accordingly.

TABLE 2: Case scenarios with different types of communication.

Case scenario	*Bad communication*	*Good communication*
Mrs X *(Para 2)* visits postnatal OPD of government hospital, two weeks postpartum with complaints of pain abdomen	• When she entered the inside room, there were already two patients for whom the doctor was giving instructions to the junior resident to write the prescription • Doctor, without looking up, in a flat voice asks her complaints • The patient wants to add something, but doctor interrupted saying that there is nothing to worry • Doctor checked the vitals and without going for local examination writes the prescription and hand it over to junior resident to explain to her	• Doctor calls the patient when no other patient is inside *(maintains privacy)*, greets, offers chair and introduce himself/herself *(building rapport)* • Doctor politely asks the patient what brings her to the hospital? *(opens discussion, paraverbal component)* • Doctor then attentively listens to all her problem without interruption, maintaining eye contact and came to know of the continuous character of pain *(active listening, non-verbal component, empathy, adequate time)* • To gather more information, relevant history was asked, and history of foul-smelling vaginal discharge could be extracted *(gather information)* • She was afebrile, local examination after verbal consent revealed forgotten swab in vagina which was removed • Patient was explained her condition, her queries were clarified and the management plan including follow-up was decided with equal participation of patient *(understand patient's perspective, share information, shared decision making)* • Further counseling regarding family planning and newborn immunization was done • She was appreciated for co-operation. The opted plan was summarized and documented *(appreciation, provide closure)*
Mrs Y, 65 years, (Para 4), a known case of cervical cancer visits gynecology OPD for follow-up and was looking low	The doctor asks her to sit. Ask staff to take out her records and write down the further plan without interacting much with her	Doctor greets her with name, makes her sit comfortably *(acknowledge, compassionate care)* and asks about the reason of her looking low *(open discussion)*. She breaks down. The doctor holds her hand and tried to calm her *(empathy, non-verbal component)*. She came out with apprehension related to radiotherapy sessions due to which she had not slept for two days *(gather information)*. She was counseled and referred for psychological counseling where she was diagnosed with depression. Her further plan was charted out with participation of family, documented and she was encouraged to participate in group counseling *(shared decision, provide closure)*

Effective Communication in Obstetrics and Gynecology—Recommendations by ACOG (American College of Obstetricians and Gynecologists)[28]

- Training of the doctors and staff though workshops
- Patient-centered interviewing and caring communication skills
- Use sustainable practice models with adequate duration to address multiple concerns
- Encourage patients to list down their queries prior to the interview
- Appoint trained and experienced staff (nurses and physician assistants) for assistance

Other key points worth mentioning include developing good rapport; providing sufficient information at each step to the patient: the risks and benefits of investigations and procedures; acknowledging their concerns; using understandable language avoiding medical jargons; patient listening; tailoring the management as per individual needs; addressing vast cultural diversities in India; balancing the emotions while breaking bad news and in challenging encounters; documenting informed consent and shared decision; and respecting their decision without being judgmental.

The need for regular dedicated workshops and effective communication skills training program for medical professionals in India has been recognized so as to ensure the best standards of care.

Further the communication skill training should be continuous and longitudinal with the aim to incorporate these skills in the routine behavior of the practitioner. The module for Attitude, Ethics and Communication (AET-COM) skills training introduced by MCI in new CBME curriculum is a step towards this direction.[29] Role plays, video recordings, doctor-patient interaction in skill labs with a simulated patient and with a real patient at workplace, supplemented with feedback are considered to be the best educational tools for teaching communication skills—both verbal and non-verbal. The level of competence achieved can be assessed by different assessment tools like OSCE, mini-CEX, multi-source feedback and other workplace-based assessments. After acquiring basic communication skills, the next level will be to overcome the challenging situations, and training should continue at regular intervals as a part of lifelong learning.[30]

ROLE OF COUNSELING IN OBSTETRICS AND GYNECOLOGY[31]

Communication skills form the basis for counseling. It is not a simple suggestion, but a support given by the medical practitioner in an understandable language and comfortable environment so as to unveil the root cause of the problem or reach the diagnosis of the disease and encouraging the patient to reach a shared voluntary decision giving due importance to the patient's perspective, without being emotionally involved or being judgmental.

Counseling provides psychological support enabling patients to take their own decisions. Counseling should always be followed by documentation. Counseling may be done in person, on telephone or online. One can opt for group counseling where other group members are having similar problems, e.g., issues related to breastfeeding. Counseling is not always related to the cure but helps the patient to deal with the situation with a positive approach, e.g., counseling a patient with stage IV ovarian cancer helps to overcome the stress and improves the quality-of-life.

In obstetrics and gynecology, the importance of counseling is immense- starting from pre-pregnancy counseling which relates to the effects of any pre-existing medical or genetic disorders on pregnancy; counseling in infertile couples related to the outcome of various procedures (intrauterine insemination, in-vitro fertilization); counseling in antenatal period focuses on routine antenatal care as well as managing high-risk pregnancies (pre-eclampsia, gestational diabetes, intrauterine growth retardation, vaginal birth after cesarean, cesarean delivery); postnatal counseling focuses on breastfeeding, family planning methods; and gynecological counseling related to the medical or surgical options available and the benefits and risks associated with various investigations and procedures (fibroids, endometriosis, ovarian tumors, cervical cancer).

Counseling involves two steps: First step of active listening and learning where Obstetrician–Gynecologist plays a passive role; and second step of confidence building and providing support where his/ her role is active. Each step involves different components of communication skills **(Flowchart 1)**.

Medicolegal Aspects/Minimizing Medicolegal Litigations[32-34]

The obstetrics and gynecology branch is a major contributor to the medical litigations as per Medscape Malpractice Report 2015.[1] The involvement of reproductive health, two lives (mother and fetus) and being an emergency surgical branch are the main factors behind this. The obstetrical litigations arise mostly due to inadequate counseling and documentation related to prenatal, antenatal and postnatal issues as discussed above; the common areas being antenatal complications, perinatal deaths (intrauterine deaths, stillbirth, early neonatal death), birth asphyxia and operative complications (third/ fourth degree tear, hematoma, retained swabs or instruments, anesthetic complications). Gynecological litigations are again the result of grey areas in counseling and documentation; the common areas responsible include failure of sterilization/contraception, injury to uterus, emergency hysterectomy, injury to ureter, missed pregnancy of undiagnosed location and complications associated with laparoscopic procedures.

To prevent these litigations comes the role of effective communication skills, adequate counseling and proper documentation. Compliance with the policies and procedures

Flowchart 1: Steps of counseling.

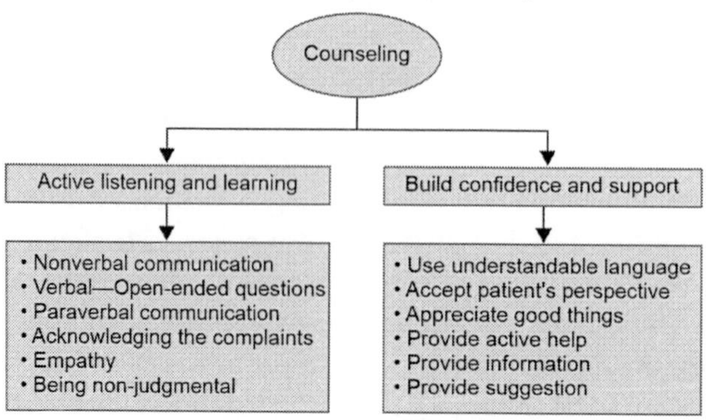

is the best defense against malpractice judgments. Detailed history, thorough physical examination, plan of management, operative and investigation details, record of discussions with patients and relatives, non-compliance of the patients, etc. should be properly documented. Various practice points, concluded from the feedback of bitter experiences, to be followed to reduce litigations in future include:

1. Be aware of medicolegal problems and medicolegal laws
2. Always take valid consent
3. Keep patient satisfied
4. Stay up-to-date on the standard of care required
5. Due care during treatment
6. Adequate pre- and postoperative care
7. Legally creditable documentation
8. Expert opinion/second opinion/timely referral
9. Adequate follow-up
10. Employing qualified staff
11. Morbidity and mortality audits
12. Continuing education (CME and workshops)
13. Avoiding cross pathy

LEGAL PROVISIONS[34]

As per Section 93 of the IPC (communication made in good faith), no communication made in good faith is an offense by reason of any harm to the person to whom it is made if it is made for the benefit of that person; provided the doctor can prove that the communication is based on scientific evidence, in a good faith for the benefit of the person, conveyed appropriately in the presence of spouse/guardian.

CONCLUSION

Effective communication in a challenging environment of Obstetrics and Gynecology requires a lot of commitment. Consider every patient to be a potential litigant. Apart from reducing future medicolegal litigations, good communication leads to improved satisfaction, compliance and hence better health outcomes. Shared decision making helps to mitigate future litigations. Longitudinal and continuous skill training is warranted to deal with difficult clinical encounters in emergency.

Key Points

- Good communication skills are the key component for developing trustworthy relations.
- Initial time investment in communication avoids later conflicts.
- Poor communication is a crucial factor responsible for the increase in lawsuits against obstetricians and gynecologists.
- The obstetrical and gynecological litigations arise mostly due to inadequate counseling and legally creditable documentation.
- Shared decision making helps to mitigate future litigations.
- Compliance with the clinical guidelines is the best defense against malpractice judgments.
- Do not neglect nonverbal and paraverbal components of communication skills as their contribution is immense.
- Effective communication should be patient centered.
- The four qualities considered indispensable for effective communication skills include making patient comfortable, accepting patient's attitude and perspective, positive response and empathetic attitude.
- For doctors to be effective communicator formal training is the need of the hour.
- Use sustainable practice models with adequate duration to address multiple concerns.
- Communication skill training should be continuous and longitudinal- AET-COM is a step towards achieving the same.

REFERENCES

1. Peckham C. Medscape Malpractice Report 2015: Why Most Doctors Get Sued? http://www.medscape.com/features/slideshow/malpractice-report2015/obgyn#page=2.
2. Regulations on Graduate Medical Education, 1997-Addition as part II for MBBS course starting from academic year 2019–2020 onwards, 6th Nov 2019. MCI Regulations. Gazette of India, Amendment notification. No-MCI-34 (41)/ 2019-Med./161726.
3. Robertson K. Active listening: more than just paying attention. Aust Fam Physician. 2005;34:1053-5.
4. Roter DL, Frankel RM, Hall JA, Sluyter D. The expression of emotion through nonverbal behavior in medical visits: mechanisms and outcomes. J Gen Intern Med. 2006;21: S28-34.
5. Ong LML, de Haes JCJM, Hoos AM, Lammes FB. Doctor-patient communication: a review of literature. Soc Sci Med. 1995;40(7): 903-18. doi: 10.1016/0277-9536(94)00155-m. PMID: 7792630.
6. Bensing JM. Doctor-patient communication and the quality of care: an observation study into affective and instrumental behavior in general practice. Dissertation. NIVEL, Utrecht, 1991.
7. Teutsch C. Patient-doctor communication. Med Clin North Am. 2003;87:1115-45.
8. Lerner S, Magrane D, Friedman E. Teaching teamwork in medical education. Mt Sinai J Med. 2009;76:318-29.
9. Ivers N, Jamtvedt G, Flottorp S, et al. Audit and feedback: effects on professional practice and healthcare outcomes. Cochrane Database Syst Rev. 2012;6:CD000259.
10. Guidelines and protocol: Medicolegal care for survivors/ victims of sexual violence. Ministry of Health and Family Welfare, Government of India 2014.
11. Studer Group. AIDET*: five fundamentals of patient communication. AIDET implementation guide. Gulf Breeze (FL): Studer Group; 2005.
12. Makoul G. Essential elements of communication in medical encounters: the Kalamazoo consensus statement. AcadMed. 2001; 76: 390-3.
13. Bailea WF, Buckmanb R, Lenzia R, et al. SPIKES: a six-step protocol for delivering bad news: application to the patient with cancer. The Oncologist August. 2000;5(4):302-11.
14. Margaret Llyod, Robert Bor, Lorraine Nobel. Clinical communication skills for medicine, 4th edition. Elsevier; 2018.
15. Mutha S, Allen C, Welch M. Toward culturally competent care: a toolbox for teaching communication strategies. San Francisco (CA): Center for the Health Professions, University of California, San Francisco; 2002.
16. Singer MK, Dadia AV, Yu MC, Surbone A, CA. Cancer, culture, and health disparities: time to chart a new course? CA Cancer J Clin. 2010;60:12-39.
17. Goleman D. The six-second rule. In: Emotional Intelligence. New York: Bantam Books; 1995.
18. Partnering with patients to improve safety. Committee Opinion No. 490. American College of Obstetricians and Gynecologists. Obstet Gynecol. 2011;117:1247-9.
19. National Institutes of Health Consensus Development Conference Statement: vaginal birth after cesarean: new insights March 8–10, 2010. National Institutes of Health Consensus Development Conference Panel. Obstet Gynecol. 2010;115: 1279-95.
20. Adebayo PB, Abayomi O, Johnson PO, et al. Breaking bad news in clinical setting—health professionals' experience and perceived competence in Southwestern Nigeria: a cross-sectional study. Ann Afr Med. 2013;12:205-11.
21. Zolnierek KBH, DiMatteo MR. Physician communication and patient adherence to treatment: a meta-analysis. Med Care. 2009;47:826-34.
22. Richard D. Communicate to win: Learn the secrets of successful communication and presentation, 2nd edn. Kogan Page; 2009. ISBN: 0749444355p 6-7
23. Steine S, Finset A, Laerum E. A new, brief questionnaire (PEQ) developed in primary

health care for measuring patients' experience of interaction, emotion and consultation outcome. Family Practice. 2001;18(4): 410-8. doi 10.1093/FAMPRA/18.4.410.

24. Sebastian NM, Jesha MM, et al. Gaps in doctor patient communication: a community based study. Int J Community Med Public Health. 2016;3(1):264-9.
25. Cultural sensitivity and awareness in the delivery of health care. Committee Opinion No 493. American College of Obstetricians and Gynecologists. Obstet Gynecol. 2011;117:1258-61.
26. Shendurnikar N, Thakkar PA. Communication skills to ensure patient satisfaction. Indian J Pediatr. 2013;80:938-43.
27. Silverman J, Kinnersley P. Doctors' non-verbal behavior in consultations: look at the patient before you look at the computer. Br J Gen Pract. 2010;60:76-8.
28. Effective patient-physician communication. Committee Opinion No 587. February 2014 (Reaffirmed 2016. Replaces Committee Opinion Number 492, May 2011). American College of Obstetricians and Gynecologists. Obstet Gynecol. 2014;123(2 Pt 1):389-93. doi: 10.1097/01.AOG.0000443279.14017.12.
29. Medical Council of India. Attitude, ethics and communication (AET-COM) competencies for the Indian medical graduate. New Delhi: Medical Council of India; 2018.
30. Chatterjee S, Choudhury N. Medical communication skills training in the Indian setting: Need of the hour. Asian J Transfus Sci. 2011;5:8-10.
31. Alka V Kuthe. Counseling—how and when? In: Malhotra Jaideep, Patel MC, Goel RN, Malhotra Narendra (Eds). FOGSI Focus Medicolegal Issues in Obstetrics and Gynecology Practice. 1st edn. New Delhi: Jaypee Brothers Medical Publisher; 2018. pp. 14-18 ISBN: 978-93-5270-397-5.
32. Buttigieg G. Minimizing obstetric medico-legal litigation. International Journal of Gynecological and Obstetrical Research. 2016;4:22-30.
33. Sharma RK. How to Face Medical Negligence in Clinical Practice? 1st edition. Noida: Institute of Medico-legal Publications; 2019. pp. 59-61. ISBN: 978-81-929895-1-8
34. Raveesh BN, Nayak RB, Kumbar SF. Preventing medico-legal issues in clinical practice. Annals of Indian Academy of Neurology. 2016;19(1):S15-20. doi:10.4103/0972-2327.192886.

CHAPTER 26

Breaking the Bad News

Shashwat K Jani

INTRODUCTION

Obstetrics is a branch where the clinician deals with two lives. There are physiological changes which occur during pregnancy, which increase the chances of aggravation of already present medical comorbidities, or even precipitate medical conditions in borderline patients. Even in normal pregnancy, even without any apparent complication, the maternal and/or fetal outcomes may not be optimal for various reasons. In such scenario, where patient/couple is not getting expected optimal results, it gets difficult for the clinician to manage. This chapter focuses on various factors causing problems, the barriers to breaking bad news and the solution/ways to deal with such a scenario with best possible outcome.

Bad news is defined as any information which adversely and seriously affects an individual's view of his/her future.[1]

It is a complex communication which has the following components:

- Responding to patients' emotional reactions
- Involvement of patients in decision making
- Managing stress on both sides
- Involving significant family members
- Giving hope and empathy to the patient/relative

CONSULTANT'S VIEWPOINT

Today's consultant faces work pressures and stress, along with emotional burnout and guilt at many points in their medical practice. An obstetrician who scans mother, is also in the process of acknowledging her anxiety when an anomaly is diagnosed. As per Brauer, it is necessary for the clinician to become supportive and professional friend foremost, rather than an expert complying with professional ethics codes.[2]

For most, pregnancy is a time of excitement, expectation, and joy. However, around 1 in 200 women will experience stillbirth, usually diagnosed in utero. Breaking the news of an intrauterine fetal death is one of the saddest, most challenging parts of the job. It can affect not only the patient but also the doctor.

Like anything breaking bad news becomes better with experience, but it is never easy.

The emotional burnout is real in case of obstetrician identifying fetal anomalies, informing about intrauterine fetal death and maternal morbidity or mortality increasing anxiety, mainly on how to break the news to the couple.[3]

Anxiety and apprehension on the part of doctors increase, as the patient faces unexpected outcomes. If the situation is not managed properly, it might land the doctor and/or staff in possibility of getting sued.

Because of the following points, consultants are worried about breaking bad news:

- Damage to reputation
- Facing questions of relatives
- Facing mob violence
- Handling police enquiry
- Medicolegal issues—arrest, court case, judgment
- Compensation amount
- Loss of confidence
- Stress in future cases

PATIENT'S PERSPECTIVE

Knowledge of patient/couple has increased over last few decades, majorly due to the advent of Internet. In such a scenario, apprehension from their side gets reflected in the form of their lack of patience and their urge of knowing the results instantly.

The loss of fetus/perinatal loss can be perceived as not only loss of a life, but also loss of expected outcome, loss of future dreams, loss of the loved one whom they were expecting with his/her probable name. Whenever fetal anomaly is diagnosed, impairing essential functions, the couple fears the negative approach of the society, and thus, puts more pressure on clinician's shoulders for the big "Why".

As there is advancement in technology, diagnosis of many of the fetal anomalies has become possible, and thus, it puts pressure on couple to decide the further course of action.

From the patient's perspective, there will be surge of emotions, like 'Is doctor correct on his/her diagnosis? Does this machine diagnose things correctly? Is there any scope of reversing what's been diagnosed?' etc. The couple would feel more confused, fearful, frustrated and at times, not able to decide anything in the moment.

In ever increasing legal cases against medical fraternity, there might be various purposes from the opposite side; either they would ask for financial compensation, or there might be reflection of their frustration/anger, which usually happens with improper communication.

Barriers to Effective Communication

- The receiving side of the bad news has anxiety, fear, and responsibility, making them strong emotions.
- Lack of training of the treating doctor and lack of guidelines in managing such situations.
- Already distressed relatives going into the zone of silence, known as 'MUM effect'.

Role of Strategies to Manage Such Situations of Breaking Bad News

- To increase confidence of the treating doctor
- To encourage and engage the patient/relative in the optimal management of further proceedings
- To have less stress and emotional turmoil on both sides

STEPS TO OPTIMALLY MANAGE THE SCENARIO

Doctors should be gradual in the process of breaking the bad news. For example, if there is some fetal scan is being performed, and some anomaly/absent fetal heart sound is diagnosed, clinician can continue conversation in a gradual manner, while taking patient in confidence. And then declare in soft spoken, yet clear words, his/her diagnosis, without using any medical jargon, and using much simpler and local words.

Counseling on fronts of both: explaining doctor's optimal efforts and removal of guilt on part of patient/relative, is of utmost importance.

There have been various strategies to manage 'Breaking Bad News'.

1. James Woods and Fay Rosovsky have suggested **"FEARED"** acronym for structured approach for the care provider dealing with such a situation as provided in **Box 1**.[4]

   Patient/relative should be interviewed for the following reasons:
   - Gathering patient's knowledge and expectations and their probable reactions on hearing bad news.
   - Provision of clear information as per the need of patient
   - An opportunity of supporting patients by reducing emotional impact
   - Making a plan for further management with full understanding and cooperation of patient.
2. *SPIKES strategy:* A six-step protocol for delivering bad news has been provided in **Box 2**.[5]
3. *ABCDE plan:*
   A: Advance preparation
   B: Build environment/relationship
   C: Communication
   D: Deal with reaction
   E: Encourage and Validate emotions

BOX 1: FEARED acronym for structured approach towards *Breaking Bad News*.[4]	
F	Get all the **Facts**
E	Express **Empathy** and **Educate**
A	Search for sources of **Anger**
R	Have the patient **Recite** back to you her understanding for your explanation
E	Evaluate the **Extended** family response
D	**Document** the conversation

4. *BLAT plan:*
   B: Build Trust
   L: Listen
   A: Apologize
   T: Thanks
5. *BREAKS approach:*
   B: Background: Knowledge of patient's perception, and background
   R: Rapport: Establish a good rapport with patient.
   E: Explore: Take patients from known segment of information to the bad news gradually.
   A: Announce: Announce in simple, short, easily comprehensible words.
   K: Kindling: Ask patient to come up with what they are perceiving.
   S: Summarize: Summarize the interview and try instilling courage in further course of action.

COMMUNICATE WELL

- Speak frankly but compassionately
- Avoid medical jargon
- Allow silence and tears; proceed at patient's pace
- Have the patient describe her understanding of the information given
- Encourage questions
- Write things down and provide written information
- Conclude each visit with a summary and follow-up plan

Deal with Patient and Family Reactions

- Assess and respond to emotional reactions
- Be aware of cognitive coping (denial, blame, guilt, disbelief, acceptance, intellectualization)
- Allow for "shut down", when patient turns off and stops listening.

BOX 2: SPIKES strategy for structured approach towards *Breaking Bad News.*[5]

S	*Setting up the interview:* Some privacy needs to be arranged. Significant decision makers should be involved. Comfortable space should be provided. Good rapport is recommended. Avoid any interruptions
P	*Patient's perception:* Open-ended questions are discussed, to know how things are perceived by the patient. Any misinformation must be corrected
I	*Invitation:* Questions should be asked to invite patients into communication. If the patient wants to know all, it opens the gate of revealing bad news. If the patient does not want to discuss in detail, offer to answer any specific questions they may have
K	*Knowledge:* Conversation can be started like, 'I am sorry to tell you…' Use simple plain words. Avoid using medical jargon. Look for body language. Avoid using statements such as 'There's nothing more we can do…'
E	*Empathy:* An empathic response to alleviate shock/grief/isolation would be of great help. It consists of 4 steps: i. Observe the emotions. ii. Identify emotion experienced by patient. Identify the reason for the emotion. iii. Give patient a brief period of time to express his/her feelings iv. Try to combine empathic, exploratory, and validating statements as a tool to provide support *Empathic statements:* • I know this is bad news for you • This is difficult for us also *Exploratory statements:* • Can you please elaborate what you mean? • Please tell me more details about it *Validating responses:* • You are correct in thinking that way • I can get it why you felt that way
S	*Strategy/Summary:* Patient's readiness is assessed. Answer any further questions. Summarize plan. Present them treatment options, and that would make them realize that their opinion matters

- Be empathetic; it is appropriate to say "I am sorry or I do not know." Crying may be appropriate.
- Do not argue or criticize colleagues.

What not to Do While Breaking Bad News?

- Do not start giving information until it is required.
- Do not hit and run.
- Do not leave the dirty job for someone else (your patient, your responsibility), unless necessary.
- Do not share information (e.g., to relatives), unless appropriate and after consent.

Response to Reactions

1. If the patient begins to cry:
   - Allow sometime to cry.
   - Could say, "I can see you are very upset."
   - Could touch the patient appropriately.
   - After a few moments you should continue talking even if the patient continues to cry.

2. If the patient becomes angry:
    - Defensive or irritation with patients is unhelpful.
    - Acknowledge patient's position and avoid talking about it.
3. If the patient refuses to accept the diagnosis:
    - Explore reasons for patient's denial.
    - Do not be combative.
    - Appreciate that there is an information gap and try to educate the patient.
    - Check that patient has a clear understanding of the problem.
    - Empathize with patient.
    - Get family members involved if appropriate.
    - Give time to adjust to new information.

BASIC COMMUNICATION SKILLS

Setting

- Schedule a meeting time:
    - This ensures we allocate time, says to the patient "big news" is coming, and allows family to be present.
    - Have face-to-face communication.
    - >50% of communication is nonverbal.
- Sit at eye level and within reach of the patient.
- *Minimize distractions:* Pager and phone off or on vibrate, door closed, ask colleagues not to disturb you, etc.

Information Exchange

- *Outline an agenda:* Why are we meeting and what should be accomplished by the meeting.
- *Ask open-ended questions:* See what they understand. This helps to define a starting point for the conversation. "What do you understand about your condition/diagnosis?" or "What have you been told about your condition?"
- Determine how much information or how many details the patient wants to know.
- Recognize that the patient and family may be different in their desire of information.
- Focus should be on the patients' concerns!

Listen

- *Responding:*
    - Address the patients' concerns.
    - Use nonverbal cues to demonstrate attentiveness.
    - Demonstrate empathy by acknowledging the patients' feelings as acceptable.
- Ask about perceived emotions: "You seem angry?" or "I feel you are scared. Do you want to tell me about how you are feeling?"
- Encourage and justify their emotions.
- Attend to all issues and needs, including physical, psychosocial, and spiritual.
- Review objectives
- *Summarize:*
    - Information, discussions, and decisions.
    - Ask open-ended questions.
    - Use nonverbal cues (nods, "uh-huh")
    - Provide empathic responses.
    - *Use repetition:* Repeat back to the patient what they said. Used to prove listening.
- Paraphrase your summary of what the patient said. Used to ensure understanding.
    - Confront emotions... yes, even difficult ones (anger).
    - Summarize.

Breaking bad news is a difficult but fundamentally important task for all healthcare professionals. Focused training in communication skills is essential and techniques to improve performance are required. It is an essential skill of good medical practice in modern obstetrics. The utmost caution should be practiced while breaking a bad news as it can significantly reduce the risk of grievances and litigations against treating doctors.

REFERENCES

1. Buckman R. Breaking bad news: why is it still so difficult? Br Med J. 1984;288(6430): 1597-9.
2. Brauer S. Moral implications of obstetric technologies for pregnancy and motherhood. Med Health Care Philos. 2016;19(1):45-54.
3. Singh N, et al. Occupational burnout among radiographers, sonographers and radiologists in Australia and New Zealand: Findings from a national survey. Journal of Medical Imaging and Radiation Oncology. 2017;61(3):304-10.
4. Woods Jr JR, Rozovsky FA. What do I say?: Communicating intended or unanticipated outcomes in obstetrics. ISBN: 978-0-787-96654-6, April 2003.
5. Baile WF, Buckman R, Lenzi R. SPIKES-A six-step protocol for delivering bad news: application to the patient with cancer. Oncologist. 2000;5(4):302-11.

Index

Page numbers followed by *b* refer to box, *f* refer to figure, *fc* refer to flowchart, and *t* refer to table.

D

E

F

J

K

L

W

Z